SCIENTIFIC AMERICAN

Molecular Cardiovascular Medicine

SCIENTIFIC AMERICAN Introduction to Molecular Medicine
Edward D. Rubenstein, M.D., Series Editor

SCIENTIFIC AMERICAN Molecular Cardiovascular Medicine
Edited by Edgar Haber, M.D.

Previously Published

SCIENTIFIC AMERICAN Introduction to Molecular Medicine
Edited by Philip Leder, M.D., David A. Clayton, Ph.D., and Edward Rubenstein, M.D.

Forthcoming

SCIENTIFIC AMERICAN Molecular Oncology
Edited by J. Michael Bishop, M.D., and Robert A. Weinberg, Ph.D.

SCIENTIFIC AMERICAN

MOLECULAR CARDIOVASCULAR MEDICINE

Edited by

Edgar Haber, M.D.

Elkan R. Blout Professor of Biological Sciences and Director, Center for the Prevention of Cardiovascular Disease, Harvard School of Public Health, Boston
Professor of Medicine, Harvard Medical School, Boston

Scientific American, Inc., New York

Cover Illustration by Tom Moore
Longitudinal Section of a Sarcomere with Bound Myosin Heads, *from Chapter 13.*

Library of Congress Cataloging-in-Publication Data
Scientific American molecular cardiovascular medicine/edited by Edgar Haber.
p. cm.
Includes bibliographical references and index.
ISBN 0-89454-021-1
1. Cardiology. 2. Molecular biology. I. Haber, Edgar, 1932 -
II Title: Molecular cardiovascular medicine.
[DNLM: 1. Cardiovascular Diseases--metabolism. 2. Molecular Biology. WG 120 S416 1995]
RC669.S343 1995
616.1'2—dc20
DNLM/DLC
For Library of Congress 95-15502
CIP

Vice President, Associate Publisher, Editorial Director: Hilary Evans
Executive Editor Aileen M. McHugh
Project Editor Ozzievelt Owens
Development Editor Thomas J. McVarish
Director of Art and Design Elizabeth Klarfeld
Art Assistant Talar Agasyan
Vice President, Associate Publisher/Production: Richard Sasso
Production Manager Christina Hippeli
Electronic Composition Jennifer Smith, Rolf Ebeling, Carol Hansen

ISBN: 0-89454-021-1

Scientific American, Inc., 415 Madison Avenue, New York, NY 10017

Contributors

William C. Aird, M.D. Instructor, Harvard Medical School; Attending Physician, Brigham and Women's Hospital, Boston

Anne Charru, M.D. College de France, INSERM U 36, Paris, France

Désiré Collen, M.D., Ph.D. Professor of Medicine, Center for Molecular and Vascular Biology, University of Leuven, Leuven, Belgium

Pierre Corvol, M.D. College de France, INSERM U 36, Paris, France

Victor J. Dzau, M.D. William G. Irwin Professor of Medicine, Stanford University School of Medicine; Chief, Division of Cardiovascular Medicine, Falk Cardiovascular Research Center, Stanford

Harry A. Fozzard, M.D. Otho S.A. Sprague Distinguished Service Professor, Department of Pharmacological and Physiological Sciences and Department of Medicine, The University of Chicago

Detlev Ganten, M.D., Ph.D. Max-Delbrück Center for Molecular Medicine, Berlin-Buch, Germany

Michael A. Gimbrone, Jr., M.D. Director, Vascular Research Division, Department of Pathology, Brigham and Women's Hospital; Elsie T. Friedman Professor of Pathology, Harvard Medical School, Boston

Edgar Haber, M.D. Elkan R. Blout Professor of Biological Sciences and Director, Center for the Prevention of Cardiovascular Disease, Harvard School of Public Health; Professor of Medicine, Harvard Medical School, Boston

Jacek Hawiger, M.D., Ph.D. Oswald T. Avery Professor and Chairman, Department of Microbiology and Immunology, Vanderbilt University School of Medicine, Nashville

Howard Hutchinson, M.D. Postdoctoral Research Fellow, Division of Cardiovascular Medicine, Falk Cardiovascular Research Center, Stanford University School of Medicine

Xavier Jeunemaitre, M.D. College de France, INSERM U 36, Paris, France

Michael Klagsbrun, Ph.D. Professor, Department of Surgery, Children's Hospital; Harvard Medical School, Boston

Reinhold Kreutz, M.D. Cardiovascular Division, Department of Medicine, Brigham and Women's Hospital; Department of Cardiology, Children's Hospital; Harvard Medical School, Boston

Jose E. Krieger, M.D., Ph.D. Assistant Professor of Medicine, Heart Institute, São Paulo, Brazil

Monty Krieger, Ph.D. Professor of Biology, Massachusetts Institute of Technology, Cambridge

Hiroki Kurihara, M.D., Ph.D. Assistant, The Third Department of Internal Medicine, University of Tokyo, Tokyo, Japan

Peter Libby, M.D. Director, Vascular Medicine and Atherosclerosis Unit, Brigham and Women's Hospital; Associate Professor of Medicine, Harvard Medical School, Boston

H. Roger Lijnen, Ph.D. Associate Professor, Center for Molecular and Vascular Biology, University of Leuven, Leuven, Belgium

Klaus Lindpaintner, M.D. Cardiovascular Division, Department of Medicine, Brigham and Women's Hospital; Department of Cardiology, Children's Hospital; Harvard Medical School, Boston

Elizabeth G. Nabel, M.D. Professor of Internal Medicine and Director, Cardiovascular Research Center, University of Michigan Medical Center, Ann Arbor

Gary J. Nabel, M.D., Ph.D. Professor of Internal Medicine and Biological Chemistry; Investigator, Howard Hughes Medical Institute, University of Michigan Medical Center, Ann Arbor

Peter Parham, Ph.D. Professor, Department of Cell Biology and Department of Microbiology and Immunology, Stanford University

Jordan S. Pober, M.D., Ph.D. Professor, Department of Pathology, Immunology and Biology, Yale University School of Medicine, New Haven

Daniel J. Rader, M.D. Director, Lipid Referral Center; Associate Professor, Department of Medicine, Division of Medical Genetics, University of Pennsylvania Medical Center, Philadelphia

Robert D. Rosenberg, M.D., Ph.D. Professor of Biology, Massachusetts Institute of Technology; William Bosworth Castle Professor of Medicine, Harvard Medical School, Boston

Russell Ross, Ph.D. Professor, Department of Pathology, University of Washington School of Medicine, Seattle

Frederick J. Schoen, M.D., Ph.D. Associate Professor and Vice Chairman, Department of Pathology, Brigham and Women's Hospital, Boston

Christine E. Seidman, M.D. Associate Professor of Medicine, Brigham and Women's Hospital and Harvard Medical School; Associate Investigator, Howard Hughes Medical Institute, Boston

Jonathan G. Seidman, Ph.D. Professor of Genetics, Harvard Medical School; Investigator, Howard Hughes Medical Institute, Boston

Florent Soubrier, M.D. College de France, INSERM U 36, Paris, France

James M. Wilson, M.D., Ph.D. Director, Institute for Human Gene Therapy; Professor and Chair, Department of Molecular and Cellular Engineering, University of Pennsylvania Medical Center, Philadelphia

Yoshio Yazaki, M.D., Ph.D. Professor and Chairman, Faculty of Medicine, University of Tokyo, Tokyo, Japan

Radovan Zak, Ph.D. Professor of Medicine, Department of Medicine, The University of Chicago

Contents

CHAPTER 1

The Impact of Molecular Biology on Cardiovascular Medicine

Edgar Haber, M.D.

Since the days of Willem Einthoven (1860–1927) and Sir Thomas Lewis (1881–1945), cardiologists have defined pathophysiology in terms of the electrical and mechanical properties of the heart, with scant attention to what cellular and molecular abnormalities might underlie gross changes in cardiac function. In the past decade, however, remarkable progress has been made in our understanding of the cellular and molecular mechanisms of cardiovascular disorders. Cardiologists are beginning to appreciate how to intervene in these disorders by controlling gene expression or modulating the function of essential receptors, ion channels, signaling molecules, and metabolic pathways.

Specific diagnosis and treatment require that a precise intermolecular interaction take place to the exclusion of others that could interfere with a desired measurement or affect a biologic system beyond the system in question. Until recently, empiricism was the sole and often laborious route to this specificity in diagnosis and treatment. In diagnosis, simple substances, such as sodium or glucose, could be measured readily and precisely by straightforward chemical methods. More complex, though more important, substances, such as peptides or protein hormones, were beyond chemical measurement and required tedious and often imprecise bioassay.

The route to drug development was through extensive screening of existing chemicals, natural substances, and bacterial fermentation broths and the use as biologic indicators of pathogens grown in vitro, reactive tissues, and whole animals. Screening assays required the sorting out of false positive results, and only after great effort could candidate compounds be identified. If one were lucky enough to know the structure of a physiologic agonist (such as epinephrine), then a medicinal chemist could synthesize a series of analogs (such as propranolol) that would, in turn, be evaluated by the same screening assays used to search for unknown compounds.

Three developments have permitted an escape from this kind of empiricism: rational drug design based on protein structure, an area covering both new protein design and ligand modeling; recombinant DNA technology, which has allowed an understanding of tissue-specific gene expression and modulation, as well as an examination of newly identified gene products and their functions; and methods for using the exquisite selectivity of the antibody-combining site as an analytic tool. This book highlights areas of cardiovascular medicine in which our understanding of the molecular and cellular biology of physiologic phenomena is expanding rapidly. In this introductory chapter, I endeavor to place these advances in the context of the medical problems the phenomena cause.

Hypertension and the Renin-Angiotensin System [*See Chapters 15–18*]

Renin was defined in the 19th century as a hypertensive agent produced by the kidney,[1] and its secretion consequent to impairment of renal blood flow was studied extensively in the early years of the 20th century.[2] By 1956, we knew that renin was a protease that generated angiotensin I,[3] a peptide of known sequence that was in turn converted to angiotensin II by another protease, angiotensin-converting enzyme.[4] Although angiotensin II was recognized as a powerful vasoconstrictor and hypertensive agent, it was difficult to define a clinical role for renin because the bioassays available were insensitive and cumbersome. The demonstration that angiotensin could act as an antigenic hapten and result in the production of highly specific antibodies rapidly led to the development of a radioimmunoassay for renin activity.[5,6] Studies in normal humans and patients with hypertension followed shortly thereafter.[7,8]

In the 1970s, tools for defining the role of renin in experimental physiology were limited to snake-venom peptides that also had the potential to enhance the activity of bradykinin. The purification of canine renin allowed for the development of a renin-specific antibody that could then be used as a highly selective pharmacological tool for inhibiting the activity of renin in experimental animals without influencing other homeostatic systems.[9,10] By the end of the 1970s, it could be stated unequivocally that renin had a major role in the maintenance of blood pressure in normal salt-depleted animals.

The year 1977 saw the report of the first successful exercise in rational drug design, which produced an inhibitor of angiotensin-converting enzyme (ACE). Ondetti and colleagues knew that ACE was a dipeptidyl-carboxypeptidase that removed two amino acids from the inactive prohormone angiotensin I to produce the active hormone angiotensin II.[11] They also knew that the structure of carboxypeptidase A (which removed only a single amino acid from its peptide substrates) had been determined by x-ray crystallography. Carboxypeptidase A and ACE both require a zinc atom for activity. By extrapolating from knowledge about the interaction of substrates with carboxypeptidase A and accounting for the greater distance in ACE between the zinc atom and the peptide cleavage site, Ondetti's group synthesized a series of carboxyalkanoyl and mercaptoalkanoyl derivatives of proline that mimicked the conformation of substrates for a dipeptidyl carboxypeptidase but proved to be potent inhibitors of ACE. One of these compounds, captopril, was the first of a family of drugs that has had an enormous impact on cardiovascular medicine.

Angiotensin-converting enzyme inhibitors have proved to be highly effective in the treatment of hypertension and congestive heart failure[12,13] and in improving long-term survival of patients after myocardial infarction.[14] A description of other efforts in rational drug design, an activity now widely practiced in academic as well as pharmaceutical laboratories, is beyond the scope of this chapter.[15,16] In brief, nuclear magnetic resonance has joined x-ray crystallography as another powerful tool for determining protein structure, with the added advantage that nuclear magnetic resonance permits a determination of structure in solution.[17] Furthermore, advances in the speed of computers and the design of sophisticated algorithms have refined methods for fitting ligands into protein-binding sites.[18] Although most drugs are still discovered by the older methods of screening and analogue development (including inhibitors of renin and the angiotensin II receptor),[19-21] I expect that rational drug design, with its inherent potential for greater specificity, will become the dominant method in the next century.

The success of ACE inhibitors in the treatment of hypertension did not immediately define a defect in the renin-angiotensin system as one of the causes of essential hypertension. Studies in rodent models showed that transgenic rats overexpressing a mouse renin gene were indeed hypertensive,[22] as were mice expressing both rat renin and rat angiotensinogen genes.[23] Recent studies have defined the mechanism of hypertension in these animals.[24] Studies in stroke-prone, spontaneously hypertensive rats have shown that a gene having a major effect on blood pressure mapped to a position on chromosome 10 closely linked to the gene for ACE[25] and, in the same model, that another gene (designated SA) on chromosome 1 might also be associated with hypertension[26] [*see Chapter 16*].

Of greater interest to research in human hypertension are genetic studies from two widely separated geographic areas that show a link between hypertension and the angiotensinogen gene[27] [*see Chapter 17*]. Because mutants of this gene manifested amino-acid-sequence variants of angiotensinogen that were associated with significant differences in plasma angiotensinogen concentrations, the presence of these mutant genes may indicate an inherited predisposition to essential hypertension. Various polymorphic variants of the angiotensin II type 1 receptor have also been implicated in human essential hypertension.[28]

We have long known that hypertension is a risk factor in coronary artery disease. Consequently, it was of considerable interest that homozygotes of a genetic variant of ACE (associated with higher circulating levels of the enzyme) were identified more frequently in patients with myocardial infarction than in controls.[29] This specific polymorphism of ACE was a potent risk factor in subjects otherwise considered to be at low risk according to commonly accepted criteria. Rapid progress in human genetic studies suggests that specific DNA probes soon will be available on which to base tests for the risk of developing hypertension or coronary artery disease.

Cardiac Hypertrophy and Failure [*See Chapters 12 and 13*]

Digitalis, a cardiac glycoside used to treat heart failure for more than 200 years, has a close toxic-therapeutic ratio and consequently is difficult to administer. Before 1970, digitalis dosages were determined by trial and error, and severe toxicity was often a consequence of overdose. Because of low plasma concentrations of the cardiac glycosides, chemical methods for determining their concentration were impractical. The development of a specific radioimmunoassay for the cardiac glycosides redefined the clinical pharmacologic action of these drugs.[30-32] The antiserum used in the immunoassay also yielded a purified antigen-binding fragment (Fab) that proved to be an antidote to digitalis intoxication.[33-35] Digoxin-specific Fab is now used widely in clinical practice.

A definition of the molecular and cellular mechanisms underlying cardiac arrhythmias [*see Chapter 14*], cardiac hypertrophy, and heart failure has proved more elusive. Rockman and colleagues showed that an increase in cardiac afterload is associated with a rapid and transient expression of an immediate early gene program in the heart (c-*fos*/c-*jun*/*junB*/*egr*1/*nur*77), and with upregulation of the atrial natriuretic factor (ANF) gene.[36] These investigators then demonstrated, in transgenic mice expressing a marker gene under control of the ANF promoter, that pressure-induced expression of atrial ANF was under the control of a set of regulatory *cis*-acting sequences that were distinct from those directing the atria-specific expression of ANF.[36] Tsutsui and associates showed that pressure loading increased the microtubule component of the cardiac muscle cell cytoskeleton, which, through inhibition of microtubule polymerization with colchicine, proved to be responsible for the contractile dysfunction observed.[37] More recently, coordination of nuclear and mitochondrial gene expression was observed during the development of cardiac hypertrophy in rats.[38] These observations taken together constitute early insights into the mechanisms responsible for the contractile abnormalities in hypertrophied cardiac muscle that lead to heart failure.

Although an understanding of the genetic programs of cardiac hypertrophy and failure in animal models is still at an early and incomplete stage, an inherited cause of cardiac hypertrophy has been defined in humans [*see Chapter 13*]. Specific missense mutations have been identified in the β cardiac myosin heavy chain in approximately 12 of 25 unrelated families with familial hypertrophic cardiomyopathy.[39-41] It is of great interest that the nature of the mutation appears to be related to prognosis. Patients with mutations that change the charge of the altered amino acid had significantly shortened life expectancies, whereas those with a mutation that did not change the charge had nearly normal life expectancies. The same kind of mutation was also identified in two of seven sporadic cases of hypertrophic cardiomyopathy, in children of parents who were genetically and phenotypically normal.[42] In one case, transmission of the mutation to an offspring occurred, indicating a germ-line mutation. A diagnostic test for this disease has been devised that is based on the detection of mutations in the β myosin heavy-chain gene in circulating lymphocytes.[43] This advance makes possible prenatal screening in affected families, as well as longitudinal study of patients prior to the development of clinical signs of the disease. The structural consequences of myosin missense mutations can also be demonstrated in cell culture.[44] When the normal α myosin heavy-chain gene is transfected into a test cell in vitro, arrays of thick filaments form that resemble normal muscle. However, when mutant α myosin heavy-chain genes are transfected into the same test cells, a disordered array of fibers is seen that resembles the histologic picture in hypertrophic cardiomyopathy. α-Tropomyosin and cardiac troponin T mutations also appear to cause hypertrophic cardiomyopathy.[45]

Thrombosis and Thrombolysis [*See Chapters 8–11*]

The first commercial product of genetic engineering to be used widely as a cardiovascular therapeutic derived from the cloning and expression of the tissue plasminogen activator (t-PA) gene.[46] Although debate continues on the merits of t-PA in comparison with those of streptokinase,[47,48] a recent comparative study seemed to indicate that t-PA has an advantage over streptokinase: the use of t-PA resulted in a modest increase in survival after myocardial infarction.[49,50] t-PA is a relatively fibrin-selective agent, and the results of the GUSTO study suggest that plasminogen activators having this property may lyse coronary thrombi more rapidly. An improvement in survival correlated in this study with more rapid and complete restoration of coronary blood flow.

The facility with which the techniques of genetic engineering permit the cloning and expression of new proteins, as well as the modification of known proteins, has led to considerable activity aimed at identifying plasminogen activators with properties superior to those of t-PA—that is, those with better pharmacokinetics, longer half-lives, or greater fibrin specificity. Examples of this work include studies with a highly fibrin-selective plasminogen activator from the vampire bat,[51,52] alterations in the amino acid sequence of t-PA that render it less susceptible to inhibition by plasminogen activator inhibitor–1,[53,54] hybrid proteins containing elements of t-PA and single-chain urokinase,[55] and fusion proteins containing a fibrin-specific antibody-combining site and the catalytic site of single-chain urokinase.[56] This last plasminogen activator, antibody-targeted urokinase, provides an example of how genetic engineering can be used to design a protein that does not exist in nature and furnish it with properties planned before its expression [*see Chapter 10*].

Genetic engineering also has made anticoagulants available from species such as the leech and tick.[57-59] Clinical trials show that a monoclonal antibody to platelet glycoprotein IIb-IIIa not only prevents thrombosis after angioplasty but also retards restenosis.[60] Although this antibody is very potent in preventing thrombosis by interfering with the ability of platelets to aggregate, synthetic peptide and peptidomimetic inhibitors of the glycoprotein IIb-IIIa receptor may have advantages over the antibody, both in ease of production and in control of pharmacokinetics.[61]

An innovative alternative to the administration of an anticoagulant is the restoration or enhancement of the endothelium's natural antithrombotic properties. One such approach is the introduction of the t-PA gene into endothelial cells to induce expression of the plasminogen activator in amounts higher than normal, which would thereby prevent thrombus formation.[62] A catheter has been used to transfect selected arterial segments with retroviral vectors containing the t-PA gene,[63] and intra-arterial stents have been covered with modified, antithrombotic endothelium.[64] Urokinase has been engineered so that it binds to the cell surface by a lipid anchor, thereby enhancing its ability to activate plasminogen.[65]

Arteriosclerosis [*See Chapters 2–7 and 20*]

Application of the techniques of molecular and cellular biology has led to an understanding of the specific mechanisms underlying several causes of human arteriosclerosis, has provided sophisticated animal models for the study of the disease, and has given insight into innovative potential treatments. Michael Brown and Joseph Goldstein received the Nobel Prize in 1985 for showing that a common inherited form of arteriosclerosis was caused by the absence (by virtue of many different mutations) of the low-density lipoprotein (LDL) receptor in homozygotes and by its inadequate expression in heterozygotes.[66] Because this form of the disease is caused by a monogenic defect, it is an ideal candidate for gene replacement therapy. Several promising experiments indicate that replacing the LDL receptor in humans may ultimately be feasible. Dichek and associates have stably transduced LDL receptors into skin fibroblasts of the Watanabe rabbit, which is subject to the same defect as people with inherited LDL-receptor deficiency.[67] Because the fibroblast takes up LDL for its own metabolic purposes only and does not participate in significant clearance of plasma LDL, a more appropriate target for receptor transduction would be the hepatocyte. Grossman and colleagues showed that the targeted delivery of LDL-receptor genes to the liver resulted in a significant alleviation of hypercholesterolemia in early clinical trials[68] [*see Chapter 7*].

An acute lesion related to arteriosclerosis is the arterial stenosis that occurs with distressing frequency after angioplasty. As discussed earlier, one of the few helpful clinical interventions has been administration of an antibody to the platelet glycoprotein IIb-IIIa receptor.[60] Simons and colleagues proposed an innovative approach to this lesion by showing that local application of an antisense oligonucleotide specific for the c-*myb* proto-oncogene inhibited proliferation of intimal arterial smooth muscle cells in an instrumented rat carotid artery.[69] Because the c-*myb* proto-oncogene has other important roles, particularly in the regulation of hematopoiesis, this approach is not likely to lead to a systemic therapy for arteriosclerosis until a gene is discovered that is selectively expressed in proliferating smooth muscle cells. Another gene inhibited by the introduction of antisense oligonucleotides is the one coding for cdk2 kinase.[70]

Genetic engineering techniques have provided a number of new animal models of arteriosclerosis, some of which closely mimic human disease and provide opportunities for detailed study. Deletion of the apolipoprotein E gene,[71,72] overexpression of the human apolipoprotein(a) gene,[73] and deletion of the gene coding for the LDL receptor[74] all lead to chronic arteriosclerosis in mice that is histologically indistinguishable from the human disease. Also, acute arterial lesions that resemble those seen after angioplasty have been caused by introduction into porcine artery of an expression vector plasmid encoding the platelet-derived growth factor (PDGF) B gene.[75] (PDGF has been implicated as a factor in smooth muscle cell migration and proliferation by the demonstration that antibodies to PDGF inhibit intimal proliferation after arterial injury.[76])

New Therapies [*See Chapters 6, 7, 10, 19, and 20*]

In the foregoing remarks, I have alluded to the use of genes as therapeutic agents in settings in which conventional pharmaceuticals are ineffective. Genes that are missing and thereby cause disease can be replaced (as in LDL-receptor deficiency), genes that contribute to disease can be repressed (inhibiting the gene coding for cdk2 kinase in experimental restenosis), or genes normally present can be augmented (overexpressing plasminogen activator genes in the prevention of experimental thrombosis). However, situations still exist in which neither drugs nor genes are sufficient, for example when an entire organ fails. Here, organ transplantation is an option. Chapter 19 details the problems and opportunities of cardiac transplantation, and Chapter 20 deals with the mechanisms underlying the most important long-term complication of this procedure, immune-mediated arteriosclerosis. As they are developed and refined further, these new therapies will join the precisely designed drugs of the future to provide physicians with treatment options where none exist today.

References

1. Tigerstedt RAA, Bergman PG: Niere und Kreislauf. *Skand Arch Physiol* 8:223, 1898
2. Goldblatt H: The renal origin of hypertension. *Physiol Rev* 27:120, 1947
3. Lentz KE, Skeggs LT Jr, Woods KR, et al: The amino acid composition of hypertensin II and its biochemical relationship to hypertensin I. *J Exp Med* 104:183, 1956
4. Skeggs LT Jr, Lentz KE, Kahn JR, et al: The amino acid sequence of hypertensin II. *J Exp Med* 104:193, 1956
5. Haber E, Page LB, Jacoby GA: Synthesis of antigenic branch-chain copolymers of angiotensin and poly-L-lysine. *Biochemistry* 4:693, 1965
6. Haber E, Koerner T, Page LB, et al: Application of a radioimmunoassay for angiotensin I to the physiologic measurements of plasma renin activity in normal human subjects. *J Clin Endocrinol* 29:1349, 1969
7. Oparil S, Vassaux C, Sanders CA, et al: Role of renin in acute postural homeostasis. *Circulation* 41:89, 1970
8. Laragh JH, Baer L, Brunner HR, et al: Renin, angiotensin and aldosterone system in pathogenesis and management of hypertensive vascular disease. *Am J Med* 52:633, 1972
9. Dzau VJ, Slater EE, Haber E: Complete purification of dog renal renin. *Biochemistry* 18:5224, 1979
10. Dzau VJ, Kopelman RI, Barger AC, et al: Renin-specific antibody for study of cardiovascular homeostasis. *Science* 207:1091, 1980
11. Ondetti MA, Rubin B, Cushman DW: Design of specific inhibitors of angiotensin-converting enzyme: new class of orally active antihypertensive agents. *Science* 196:441, 1977
12. Case DB, Atlas SA, Laragh JH, et al: Clinical experience with blockade of the renin-angiotensin-aldosterone system by an oral converting-enzyme inhibitor (SQ 14,442, captopril) in hypertensive patients. *Prog Cardiovasc Dis* 21:195, 1978

13. Dzau VJ, Colucci WS, Williams GH, et al: Sustained effectiveness of converting-enzyme inhibition in patients with severe congestive heart failure. *N Engl J Med* 302:1373, 1980
14. Pfeffer MA, Braunwald E, Moye LA, et al: Effect of captopril on mortality and morbidity in patients with left ventricular dysfunction after myocardial infarction: results of the Survival And Ventricular Enlargement trial: the SAVE investigators. *N Engl J Med* 327:669, 1992
15. Livingstone DJ: Pattern recognition methods in rational drug design. *Methods Enzymol* 203:613, 1991
16. Martin YC: Computer-assisted rational drug design. *Methods Enzymol* 203:587, 1991
17. de Vlieg J, van Gunsteren WF: Combined procedures of distance geometry and molecular dynamics for determining protein structure from nuclear magnetic resonance data. *Methods Enzymol* 202:268, 1991
18. Stoddard BL, Koshland DE Jr: Molecular recognition analyzed by docking simulations: the aspartate receptor and isocitrate dehydrogenase from *Escherichia coli*. *Proc Natl Acad Sci USA* 90:1146, 1993
19. Burton J, Cody RJ Jr, Herd JA, et al: Specific inhibition of renin by an angiotensinogen analog: studies in sodium depletion and renin-dependent hypertension. *Proc Natl Acad Sci USA* 77:5476, 1980
20. Kleinert HD, Rosenberg SH, Baker WR, et al: Discovery of a peptide-based renin inhibitor with oral bioavailability and efficacy. *Science* 257:1940, 1992
21. Wong PC, Price WA Jr, Chiu AT, et al: Nonpeptide angiotensin II receptor antagonists: studies with EXP9270 and DuP 753. *Hypertension* 15:823, 1990
22. Mullins JJ, Peters J, Ganten D: Fulminant hypertension in transgenic rats harbouring the mouse *Ren-2* gene. *Nature* 344:541, 1990
23. Ohkubo H, Kawakami H, Kakehi Y, et al: Generation of transgenic mice with elevated blood pressure by introduction of the rat renin and angiotensinogen genes. *Proc Natl Acad Sci USA* 87:5153, 1990
24. Moriguchi A, Brosnihan KB, Kumagai H, et al: Mechanisms of hypertension in transgenic rats expressing the mouse *Ren*-2 gene. *Am J Physiol* 266:R1273, 1994
25. Jacob HJ, Lindpaintner K, Lincoln SE, et al: Genetic mapping of a gene causing hypertension in the stroke-prone spontaneously hypertensive rat. *Cell* 67:213, 1991
26. Lindpaintner K, Hilbert P, Ganten D, et al: Molecular genetics of the SA-gene: cosegregation with hypertension and mapping to rat chromosome 1. *J Hypertens* 11:19, 1993
27. Jeunemaitre X, Soubrier F, Kotelevtsev YV, et al: Molecular basis of human hypertension: role of angiotensinogen. *Cell* 71:169, 1992
28. Bonnardeaux A, Davies E, Jeunemaitre X, et al: Angiotensin II type 1 receptor gene polymorphisms in human essential hypertension. *Hypertension* 24:63, 1994
29. Cambien F, Poirier O, Lecerf L, et al: Deletion polymorphism in the gene for angiotensin-converting enzyme is a potent risk factor for myocardial infarction. *Nature* 359:641, 1992
30. Smith TW, Butler VP Jr, Haber E: Determination of therapeutic and toxic serum digoxin concentrations by radioimmunoassay. *N Engl J Med* 281:1212, 1969
31. Smith TW, Haber E: Digoxin intoxication: the relationship of clinical presentation to serum digoxin concentration. *J Clin Invest* 49:2377, 1970
32. Beller GA, Smith TW, Abelmann WH, et al: Digitalis intoxication: a prospective clinical study with serum level correlations. *N Engl J Med* 284:989, 1971
33. Curd J, Smith TW, Jaton J-C, et al: The isolation of digoxin specific antibody and its use in reversing the effects of digoxin. *Proc Natl Acad Sci USA* 68:2401, 1971
34. Smith TW, Haber E, Yeatman L, et al: Reversal of advanced digoxin intoxication with Fab fragments of digoxin-specific antibodies. *N Engl J Med* 294:797, 1976
35. Antman EM, Wenger TL, Butler VP Jr, et al: Treatment of 150 cases of life-threatening digitalis intoxication with digoxin-specific Fab antibody fragments: final report of a multicenter study. *Circulation* 81:1744, 1990
36. Rockman HA, Ross RS, Harris AN, et al: Segregation of atrial-specific and inducible expression of an atrial natriuretic factor transgene in an in vivo murine model of cardiac hypertrophy. *Proc Natl Acad Sci USA* 88:8277, 1991
37. Tsutsui H, Ishihara K, Cooper G IV. Cytoskeletal role in the contractile dysfunction of hypertrophied myocardium. *Science* 260:682, 1993
38. Wiesner RJ, Aschenbrenner V, Ruegg JC, et al: Coordination of nuclear and mitochondrial gene expression during the development of cardiac hypertrophy in rats. *Am J Physiol* 267:C229, 1994
39. Geisterfer-Lowrance AA, Kass S, Tanigawa G, et al: A molecular basis for familial hypertrophic cardiomyopathy: a beta cardiac myosin heavy chain gene missense mutation. *Cell* 62:999, 1990

40. Tanigawa G, Jarcho JA, Kass S, et al: A molecular basis for familial hypertrophic cardiomyopathy: an alpha/beta cardiac myosin heavy chain hybrid gene. *Cell* 62:991, 1990
41. Watkins H, Rosenzweig A, Hwang DS, et al: Characteristics and prognostic implications of myosin missense mutations in familial hypertrophic cardiomyopathy. *N Engl J Med* 326:1108, 1992
42. Watkins H, Thierfelder L, Hwang DS, et al: Sporadic hypertrophic cardiomyopathy due to de novo myosin mutations. *J Clin Invest* 90:1666, 1992
43. Rosenzweig A, Watkins H, Hwang DS, et al: Preclinical diagnosis of familial hypertrophic cardiomyopathy by genetic analysis of blood lymphocytes. *N Engl J Med* 325:1753, 1991
44. Straceski AJ, Geisterfer-Lowrance A, Seidman CE, et al: Functional analysis of myosin missense mutations in familial hypertrophic cardiomyopathy. *Proc Natl Acad Sci USA* 91:589, 1994
45. Thierfelder L, Watkins H, MacRae C, et al: Alpha-tropomyosin and cardiac troponin T mutations cause familial hypertrophic cardiomyopathy: a disease of the sarcomere. *Cell* 77:701, 1994
46. Pennica D, Holmes WE, Kohr WJ, et al: Cloning and expression of human tissue-type plasminogen activator cDNA in *E. coli*. *Nature* 301:214, 1983
47. Gruppo Italiano per lo Studio della Sopravvivenza nell'Infarto miocardico: GISSI-2: a factorial randomised trial of alteplase versus streptokinase and heparin versus no heparin among 12,490 patients with acute myocardial infarction. *Lancet* 336:65, 1990
48. ISIS-3 (Third International Study of Infarct Survival) Collaborative Group: A randomised comparison of streptokinase vs tissue plasminogen activator vs anistreplase and of aspirin plus heparin vs aspirin alone among 41,299 cases of suspected acute myocardial infarction: ISIS-3. *Lancet* 339:753, 1992
49. The GUSTO Angiographic Investigators: The effects of tissue plasminogen activator, streptokinase, or both on coronary-artery patency, ventricular function, and survival after acute myocardial infarction. *N Engl J Med* 329:1615, 1993
50. The GUSTO Investigators: An international randomized trial comparing four thrombolytic strategies for acute myocardial infarction. *N Engl J Med* 329:673, 1993
51. Gardell SJ, Duong LT, Diehl RE, et al: Isolation, characterization, and cDNA cloning of a vampire bat salivary plasminogen activator. *J Biol Chem* 264:17947, 1989
52. Kratzschmar J, Haendler B, Bringmann P, et al: High-level secretion of the four salivary plasminogen activators from the vampire bat *Desmodus rotundus* by stably transfected baby hamster kidney cells. *Gene* 116:281, 1992
53. Madison EL, Goldsmith EJ, Gerard RD, et al: Serpin-resistant mutants of human tissue-type plasminogen activator. *Nature* 339:721, 1989
54. Madison EL, Goldsmith EJ, Gerard RD, et al: Amino acid residues that affect interaction of tissue-type plasminogen activator with plasminogen activator inhibitor 1. *Proc Natl Acad Sci U S A* 87:3530, 1990
55. Collen D, Nelles L, De Cock F, et al: $K_1K_2P_u$, a recombinant t-PA/u-PA chimera with increased thrombolytic potency, consisting of amino acids 1 to 3 and 87 to 274 of human tissue-type plasminogen activator (t-PA) and amino acids 138 to 411 of human single chain urokinase-type plasminogen activator (scu-PA): purification in centigram quantities and conditioning for use in man. *Thromb Res* 65:421, 1992
56. Runge MS, Quertermous T, Zavodny PJ, et al: A recombinant chimeric plasminogen activator with high affinity for fibrin has increased thrombolytic potency in vitro and in vivo. *Proc Natl Acad Sci USA* 88:10337, 1991
57. Harvey RP, Degryse E, Stefani L, et al: Cloning and expression of a cDNA coding for the anticoagulant hirudin from the bloodsucking leech, *Hirudo medicinalis*. *Proc Natl Acad Sci USA* 83:1084, 1986
58. Lefkovits J, Topol EJ: Direct thrombin inhibitors in cardiovascular medicine. *Circulation* 90:1522, 1994
59. Waxman L, Smith DE, Arcuri KE, et al: Tick anticoagulant peptide (TAP) is a novel inhibitor of blood coagulation factor Xa. *Science* 248:593, 1990
60. Topol EJ, Califf RM, Weisman HF, et al: Randomised trial of coronary intervention with antibody against platelet IIb/IIIa integrin for reduction of clinical restenosis: results at six months: the EPIC Investigators. *Lancet* 343: 881, 1994
61. Kouns WC, Kirchhofer D, Hadvary P, et al: Reversible conformational changes induced in glycoprotein IIb-IIIa by a potent and selective peptidomimetic inhibitor. *Blood* 80:2539, 1992
62. Jaklitsch MT, Biro S, Casscells W, et al: Transduced endothelial cells expressing high levels of tissue plasminogen activator have an unaltered phenotype in vitro. *J Cell Physiol* 154:207, 1993
63. Flugelman MY, Jaklitsch MT, Newman KD, et al: Low level in vivo gene transfer into the arterial wall through a perforated balloon catheter. *Circulation* 85:1110, 1992

64. Flugelman MY, Virmani R, Leon MB, et al: Genetically engineered endothelial cells remain adherent and viable after stent deployment and exposure to flow in vitro. *Circ Res* 70:348, 1992

65. Lee SW, Ellis V, Dichek DA, et al: Characterization of plasminogen activation by glycosylphosphatidylinositol-anchored urokinase. *J Biol Chem* 269:2411, 1994

66. Motulsky AG: The 1985 Nobel Prize in physiology or medicine. *Science* 231:126, 1986

67. Dichek DA, Bratthauer GL, Beg ZH, et al: Retroviral vector-mediated in vivo expression of low-density-lipoprotein receptors in the Watanabe heritable hyperlipidemic rabbit. *Somat Cell Mol Genet* 17:287, 1991

68. Grossman M, Raper SE, Kozarsky K, et al: Successful ex vivo gene therapy directed to liver in a patient with familial hypercholesterolaemia. *Nat Genet* 6:335, 1994

69. Simons M, Edelman ER, DeKeyser JL, et al: Antisense c-*myb* oligonucleotides inhibit intimal arterial smooth muscle cell accumulation in vivo. *Nature* 359:67, 1992

70. Morishita R, Gibbons GH, Ellison KE, et al: Intimal hyperplasia after vascular injury is inhibited by antisense cdk 2 kinase oligonucleotides. *J Clin Invest* 93:1458, 1994

71. Plump AS, Smith JD, Hayek T, et al: Severe hypercholesterolemia and atherosclerosis in apolipoprotein E-deficient mice created by homologous recombination in ES cells. *Cell* 71:343, 1992

72. Zhang SH, Reddick RL, Piedrahita JA, et al: Spontaneous hypercholesterolemia and arterial lesions in mice lacking apolipoprotein E. *Science* 258:468, 1992

73. Lawn RM, Wade DP, Hammer RE, et al: Atherogenesis in transgenic mice expressing human apolipoprotein(a). *Nature* 360:670, 1992

74. Ishibashi S, Goldstein JL, Brown MS, et al: Massive xanthomatosis and atherosclerosis in cholesterol-fed low density lipoprotein receptor-negative mice. *J Clin Invest* 93:1885, 1994

75. Nabel EG, Yang Z, Liptay S, et al: Recombinant platelet-derived growth factor B gene expression in porcine arteries induces intimal hyperplasia in vivo. *J Clin Invest* 91:1822, 1993

76. Ferns GA, Raines EW, Sprugel KH, et al: Inhibition of neointimal smooth muscle accumulation after angioplasty by an antibody to PDGF. *Science* 253:1129, 1991

CHAPTER 2

Arteriosclerosis, an Overview

Russell Ross, Ph.D.

Arteriosclerosis is a synonym for hardening of the arteries and the generic term for a group of diseases that affect different parts of the arterial tree, often leading to their occlusion. These diseases range from arteriolosclerosis, which results in degenerative changes and fibrosis in small arteries (arterioles), to atherosclerosis, the ubiquitous disease of medium- and large-sized muscular and elastic arteries that involves the coronary arteries, the aorta, the carotid and major arteries supplying the brain, and the arteries supplying the peripheral vasculature, particularly, the leg arteries, such as the iliac and superficial femoral arteries. As a consequence, atherosclerosis is the principal cause of mortality and morbidity in Western society; it results in myocardial infarction, cerebral infarction, aortic aneurysm, and peripheral vascular disease, the last leading to gangrene and loss of function of the extremities. It is responsible for 50 percent of all deaths in the United States and Western Europe, in contrast to cancer, which is responsible for approximately 23 percent of all deaths.[1]

The lesions that form in arteries subjected to angioplasty or bypass surgery principally represent a migratory, proliferative response of smooth muscle cells to the trauma associated with either the angioplasty catheter or the surgery at the perianastomotic sites of the bypass. The atherosclerotic lesions that form after cardiac transplantation in transplants that are eventually rejected represent a response to immune-induced injury that consists of massive accumulation of smooth muscle cells, monocyte-derived macrophages, and T cells. In contrast, the lesions that form after angioplasty or bypass surgery consist largely of smooth muscle cells, which with time also accumulate inflammatory cells. Mural thrombosis is often associated with the presence of these trauma-induced lesions as well. Lipids are generally not a common feature of these lesions because, in most cases, the patients have been receiving some form of lipid-lowering therapy.

Before the 1960s, the incidence of coronary artery disease in the United States was increasing. However, a reversal of this trend became evident in the mid-1960s and has been followed by a continuously progressive decline in the mortality from both coronary artery disease and cerebrovascular disease. Clinical investigations have demonstrated that, similar to findings in experimental animals, the lesions of atherosclerosis observed by angiography can be reversed clinically by aggressive management of hypercholesterolemia—for example, by reduction of lipid intake and by administration of lipid-lowering agents that increase cholesterol excretion, decrease cholesterol absorption, or interfere with the rate-limiting enzyme of cholesterol synthesis, HMG-CoA reductase. The lesions of atherosclerosis may possibly be reversed not only in the beginning stages of the disease but also, albeit slowly, in some forms of advanced lesions.[2]

The Lesions of Atherosclerosis

The lesions of atherosclerosis include a range of pathological alterations in the artery that have different gross and microscopic appearances. These alterations include fatty streaks, which are the earliest grossly detectable lesions; intermediate, or fibrofatty, lesions; and advanced or complicated lesions, called fibrous plaques.[3-6]

During their formation and progression, atherosclerotic lesions contain critical cellular elements of inflammation and associated fibrous connective tissue formation. They begin as a fatty streak, which consists of a collection of accumulated lipid in monocyte-derived macrophages, together with variable numbers of T cells. The progression from this earliest grossly detectable lesion to the advanced, complicated lesions of atherosclerosis (fibrous plaques) involves three fundamental cellular processes occurring at different points in lesion formation and progression. These processes include (1) continuing entry of monocytes/macrophages and proliferation of macrophages, smooth muscle cells, and possibly lymphocytes, (2) formation of an extensive fibrous connective tissue matrix by the accumulated smooth muscle cells, and (3) accumulation of intracellular and extracellular lipid, principally in the form of free and esterified cholesterol within macrophages and smooth muscle cells in the lesions.

Each form of the lesions characteristically occurs in medium or large muscular arteries, as well as in the major elastic artery, the aorta. They tend to begin at bifurcations and in the outflow tracks at these sites. When vessels such as the carotid, cerebral, or basilar arteries are involved, occlusive lesions may lead to a decrease in the oxygen supply to particular parts of the brain and thus to cerebrovascular disease and its sequela, stroke. When any of the major coronary arteries is involved, the lesions may lead to altered supply to the cardiac muscle and to myocardial infarction. When the peripheral leg arteries are involved, atherosclerosis can lead to gangrene or loss of function of the extremities. Involvement of the aorta may lead to the destruction of underlying elastic laminae and connective tissue and possibly to the formation of aneurysms.

The fatty streak is a ubiquitous lesion found in patients of all ages, even in infants.[7,8] The term fatty streak is derived from the gross appearance of the lesion, a relatively flat, yellow discoloration of the luminal surface of the artery that results from accumulation of lipid within the superficial intimal, or innermost, part of the arterial wall. Microscopically, the fatty streak consists of intracellular and extracellular deposits of lipid and lipoprotein particles. These deposits accumulate in scavenger cells, or macrophages, which are derived from peripheral blood monocytes. The monocytes become lipid-filled foam cells and are accompanied by variable numbers of T cells ($CD4^+$ and $CD8^+$). The fatty streaks may form at sites where preexisting accumulations of intimal smooth muscle cells or where few smooth muscle cells are found. When smooth muscle cells are present, some of them may also accumulate lipid and become foam cells within the fatty streak. Of importance is the recognition that from its composition of blood monocyte–derived macrophages and T cells, the fatty streak represents a particular form of chronic inflammatory response [*see Figure 1*]. Thus, the process of atherogenesis begins as a specialized form of inflammation, presumably in response to one or more sources of injury to the cells of the arterial wall.

The intermediate, or fibrofatty, lesion contains the same cellular elements as the fatty streak; however, the relative proportions of lipid-filled macrophages, T cells, and smooth muscle cells can vary from lesion to lesion. Generally, fibrofatty lesions attain a more complex appearance consisting of alternating layers of foam cells and smooth muscle cells with varying amounts of connective tissue [*see Figure 2*]. They may develop a core of lipid-rich material, suggesting that they represent the precursor of the better-defined advanced lesion of atherosclerosis, the fibrous plaque.

The fibrous plaque, or advanced, complicated lesion, has a characteristic morphology. Its surface is covered by a fibrous cap of varying density, consisting of several layers of smooth muscle cells surrounded by a relatively dense matrix of connective tissue that contains collagen, elastic fibers, and proteoglycans. The smooth muscle cells that make up the fibrous cap often take on an unusual appearance: they become very flattened and appear to lie in lacunalike spaces. These unusual-looking smooth muscle cells are surrounded by an onion skin–like, dense layer of basement membrane–type connective tissue. This layer is in turn surrounded by loose connective tissue that contains variable numbers of macrophages, which may or may not contain lipid, together with some T cells. The fibrous cap can vary in thickness and is usually less thick at the shoulders, or margins, of the lesion, where relatively large numbers of macrophages may be present. Beneath the fibrous cap lies a core of material that contains lipid-filled macrophages, necrotic cells, cell debris, extracellular lipid, and often, as the lesions become more advanced, calcification. The formation of the advanced lesions is usually associated with a continuing decrease in the thickness of the underlying media [*see Figure 3*]. The media of the artery constitutes the normal smooth muscle arterial wall that provides the tonus to the artery and diminishes the alterations in arterial blood flow between systole and dias-

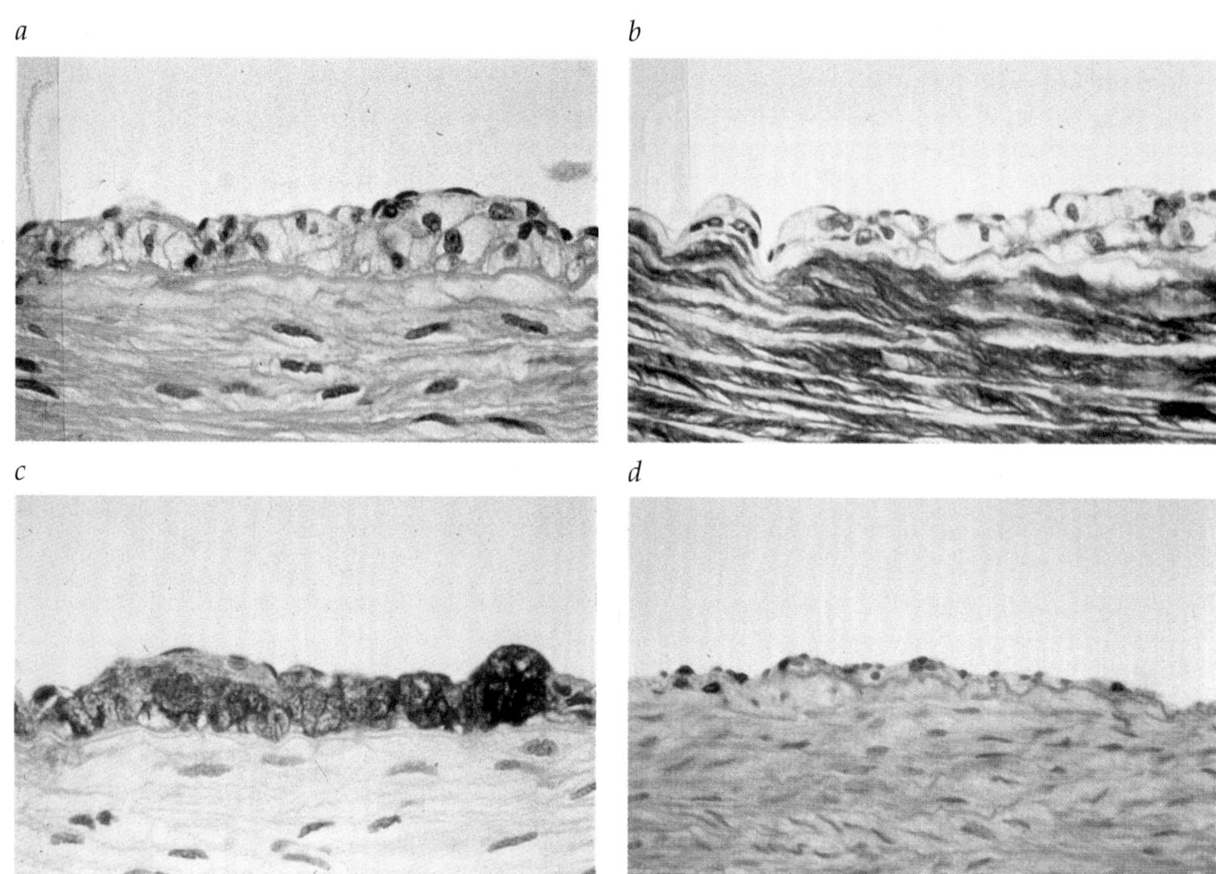

Figure 1 *Four stained sections of a fatty streak in a hyperlipidemic nonhuman primate are shown. (a) Hematoxylin (pink) and eosin (blue) stain demonstrates the foam cells that make up this fatty streak, which is one- to two-cell layers thick. (b) Peroxidase stain (black), using a monoclonal antibody (HHF-35) that recognizes smooth muscle α-actin and demonstrates positive staining of the medial smooth muscle cells and one or two smooth muscle cells between the foam cells in the lesion. Note that the foam cells are negative. (c) An adjacent section of tissue was stained using an immunoperoxidase technique with a monoclonal antibody (HAM-56) that is specific for monocyte-derived macrophages (black). All of the foam cells in this early fatty streak are derived from human peripheral blood monocytes. (d) This section is from a block of frozen tissue that was adjacent to the block from which the other three sections were taken. It was stained using an immunoperoxidase technique with a monoclonal antibody that recognizes $CD4^+$ T cells (brown). Note that several $CD4^+$ T cells are present within the lesion.*

tole. Presumably, the thinning of the media is partly a result of the migration of the smooth muscle cells of the expanding lesion from the media into the intima and the multiplication of the smooth muscle cells in the intima during lesion development and progression.

Examination at autopsy of individuals who experienced sudden death suggests that death was principally a result of thrombotic occlusion of the coronary arteries. Surprisingly, the lesions over which the thrombi form often occlude less than 50 percent of the artery's lumen. These findings suggest that the lesions of atherosclerosis that are potentially the most dangerous are not necessarily those that occlude 60 to 80 percent of the artery. Such markedly occlusive lesions appear to progress slowly, during which time the lesions gradually intrude into the lumen. In this process, compensatory dilation of the artery may occur. When this dilation does not occur, the patient begins to develop symptoms of angina, particularly on exertion. In contrast, patients who experienced sudden death are often found to have atherosclerotic lesions that may occlude no more than 40 percent of the lumen of the artery. Unlike the dense fibrotic lesions that occlude most of the arterial lumen found in patients with 60 to 80 percent occlusion, the lesions that occlude only 40 percent or less of the lumen appear to be fibrous plaques, in which the fibrous cap of connective tissue is less dense and may be poorly formed at the margins of the lesions, where fewer smooth muscle cells, less connective tissue matrix, and relatively large numbers of macrophages and T cells may exist. As the lesions progress, they become vascularized by endothelium-lined channels, or vasa vasora, which can become an important component in the advanced, complex lesions of atherosclerosis. In some cases, it has been suggested that these vasa vasora may become additional sites of hemorrhage when complex lesions undergo changes, such as ulceration

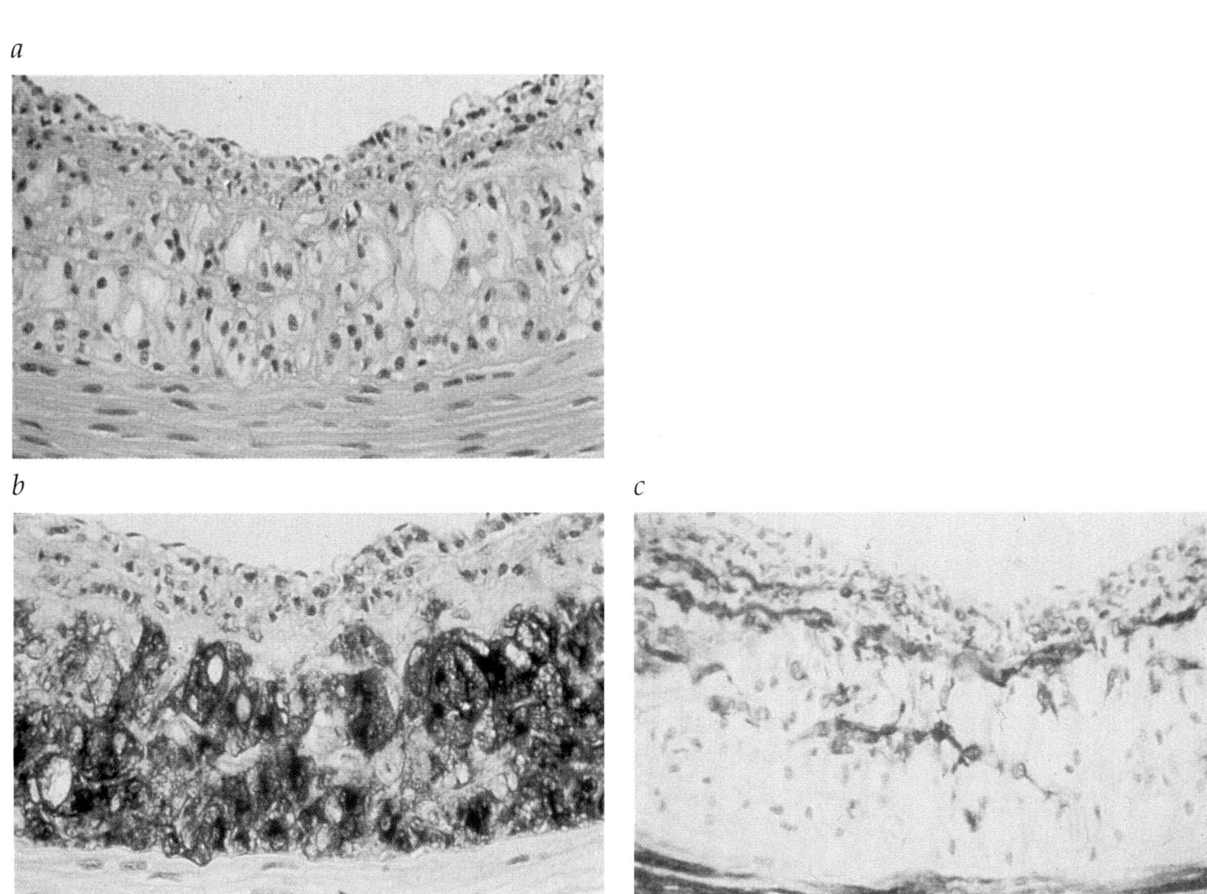

Figure 2 *An intermediate (fibrofatty) lesion from an atherosclerotic nonhuman primate is shown. This animal had been receiving a hypercholesterolemic diet long enough to develop intermediate lesions. Compare the increasing complexity of the lesion, with its multiple layers, with the fatty streak shown in Figure 1. (a) Hematoxylin-eosin staining, which demonstrates several layers of vacuolated macrophages and numerous cells. (b) Immunoperoxidase stain using a monoclonal antibody (HAM-56) against monocyte-derived macrophages (black). The several layers of foam cells are derived from macrophages. Numerous monocyte-derived macrophages that contain little to no lipid can be seen close to the lumen. (c) An adjacent section of tissue stained by immunoperoxidase with a monoclonal antibody against smooth muscle α-actin (HHF-35) is shown. Layers of smooth muscle cells (black) can be seen to alternate between the layers of foamy macrophages in this intermediate lesion.*

a

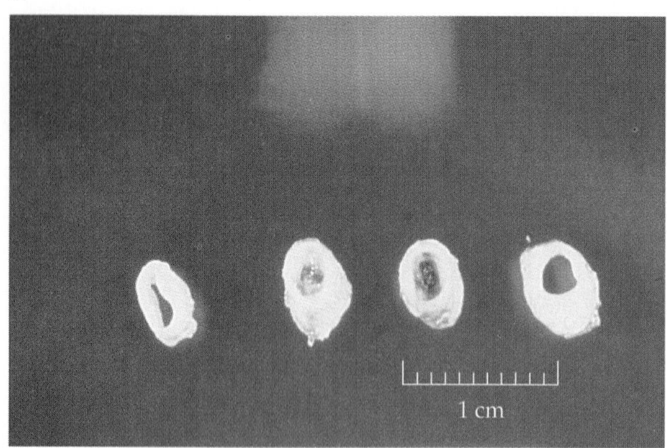

b c

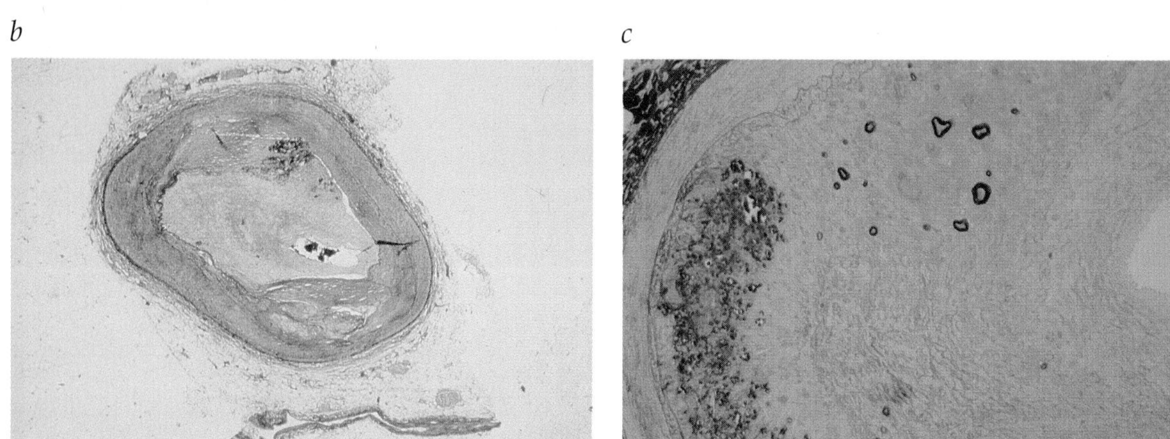

Figure 3 *(a) Several gross sections of a coronary artery obtained from an individual with advanced atherosclerosis who died of a myocardial infarct are shown. The thrombus that occludes the artery can be seen in the two center sections. The increased thickness of the arterial wall which results from atherosclerotic lesions is readily apparent. (b) In this micrograph of a section of one of the segments of the coronary arteries in (a), two advanced fibrous plaques (top and bottom) have formed in the artery, which has been occluded by a thrombus with a small lumen in the center. The thrombus has begun to organize. The fibrous caps that cover the fibrous plaques lie above areas of necrotic debris and a lipid-rich core. The thinned media beneath these advanced lesions is easily visible. (c) A segment of a fibrous plaque in an iliac artery from a hyperlipidemic nonhuman primate is shown. The decrease in lumen size resulting from the marked thickening of this fibrous plaque is apparent. Toward the lumen, the fibrous plaque is covered by a dense, fibrous cap consisting of numerous smooth muscle cells and large amounts of connective tissue. Below the fibrous cap lies an area rich in lipid, below which is an area of calcification that covers a markedly thinned media.*

or fissuring. Consequently, such lesions, particularly when they are located at bifurcations, may be more fragile in response to alterations in flow. In this case, tears, fissures, or ulcerations have been shown to occur at the relatively weak sites where the fibrous cap is thinner. Such alterations could lead to formation of thrombi or to hemorrhage into the necrotic core of the lesion; such a hemorrhage would be followed by the development of an acute thrombus that might occlude the artery[9] [*see Figure 4*].

The Response-to-Injury Hypothesis of Atherogenesis

In 1973, J.A. Glomset and I[10] proposed a hypothesis, based on the early ideas of Virchow[11] and others,[12] to explain the genesis of the lesions of atherosclerosis. We suggested that some form of injury to the artery wall might result in the formation of atherosclerotic lesions. Based on results of experiments designed to test this response-to-injury hypothesis, it has been modified and revised over the past 20 years. Those components of the hypothesis that could be disproved were removed or reformulated, and the hypothesis continues to be tested.[4-6,10,13,14] The present form of the hypothesis[6] states that each of the different risk factors known to be associated with an increased incidence of atherosclerosis directly or indirectly leads to specific changes in the lining cells of the artery (the endothelium) or to the underlying smooth muscle cells of the intima or media of the artery [*see Figure 5*].

One of the earliest changes in the artery that takes place—for example, in individuals with hypercholesterolemia—results from increased transport by endothelial cells of low-density lipoproteins (LDL), the principal cholesterol-carrying lipoprotein in the plasma, in the form of particles called liposomes.[15,16] While these lipids are transported into the artery, or later during exposure to macrophages or smooth muscle cells, the lipids may be modified by the endothelium.[17] Modifications that can take place include oxidation of LDLs and glycation of these lipoproteins. Glycation occurs when blood sugar is elevated, as in diabetes.[18] Both oxidation and glycation can lead to free radical formation. Oxidized lipoproteins can injure the overlying endothelium, the adjacent smooth muscle cells, or both.[19-23] Oxidized lipoproteins are chemotactic agents. It is likely that they act by inducing the endothelium to express cell-surface adhesive glycoproteins [*see Chapter 4*]. These glycoproteins interact with circulating leukocytes, such as monocytes and lymphocytes, resulting in their adhesion and entry into the artery wall.[22,23]

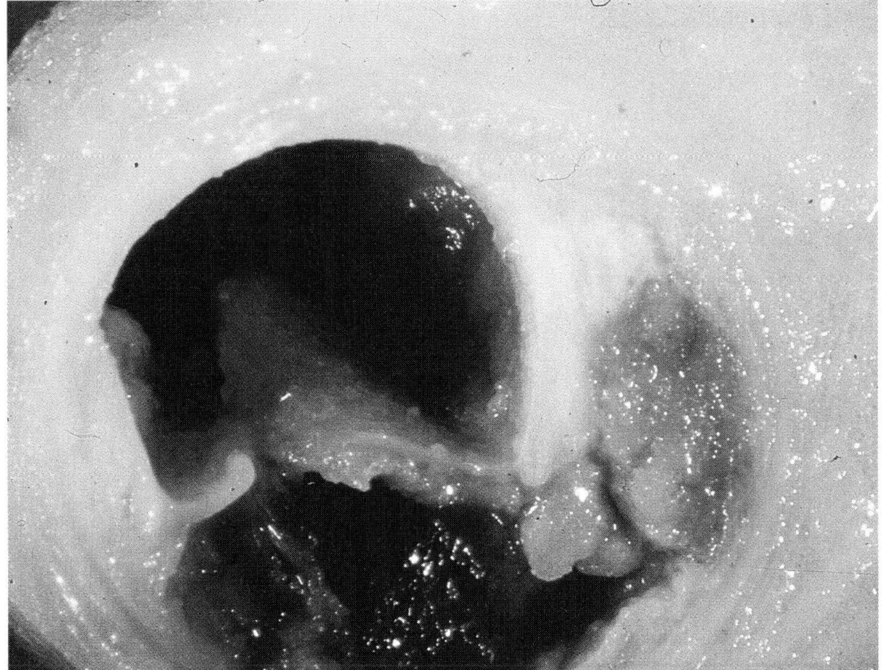

Figure 4 *Cross-section of a coronary artery in which an advanced atherosclerotic lesion (a fibrous plaque) has ruptured through one shoulder of the lesion. Thrombus occupies much of the lipid pool but has not yet extended into the lumen of the artery.*

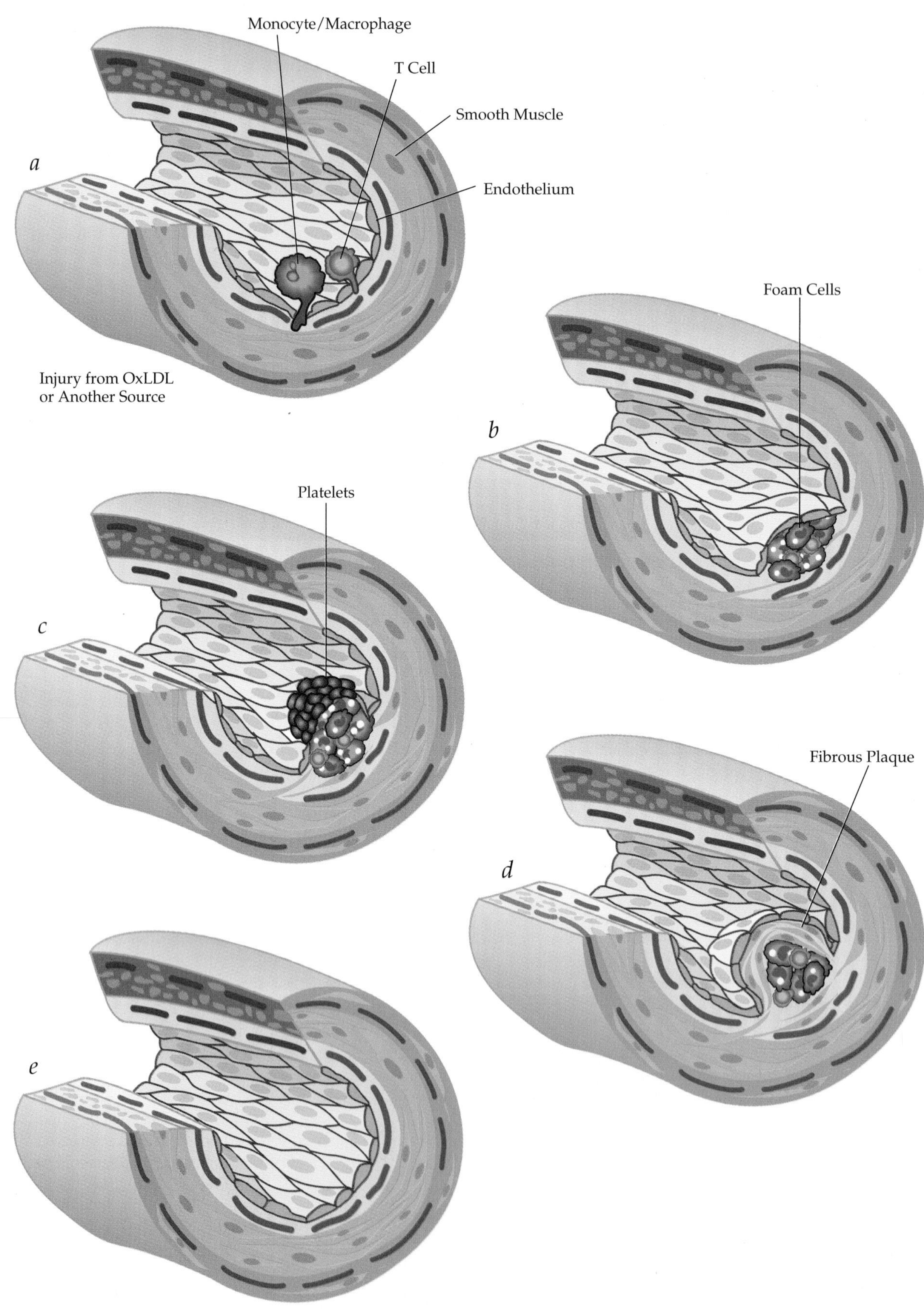
Monocyte/Macrophage
T Cell
Smooth Muscle
a
Endothelium
Injury from OxLDL
or Another Source
Foam Cells
b
Platelets
c
Fibrous Plaque
d
e

Studies of atherogenesis in experimental animals, including hypercholesterolemic rabbits,[24-26] swine,[27,28] nonhuman primates,[29-32] and, most recently, transgenic mice,[33] have demonstrated that the lesions of atherosclerosis begin with adherence of clusters of monocytes and lymphocytes, which migrate into the arterial wall in an inflammatory response, presumably in reaction to the local accumulation of such substances as modified lipoproteins [*see Figure 6*]. As the monocytes enter the artery, many become lipid-filled foam cells as a result of their capacity to act as scavenger cells and take up the modified lipids and lipoproteins that preceded them into the artery. When they are activated as macrophages, these cells express a series of genes that lead to the formation of cytokines and growth-stimulatory and growth-inhibitory molecules. Such molecules can stimulate the smooth muscle cells within the intima or beneath the accumulations of macrophages and T cells in the media to express new genes, change phenotype, migrate, or proliferate.

The accumulation of lipid-filled macrophages within the intima of the artery represents the first demonstrable lesion of atherosclerosis, the fatty streak. If the macrophages form cytokines and other growth-regulatory molecules, they may induce additional monocyte immigration as well as smooth muscle cell migration, proliferation, or both, leading to the enlargement of the fatty streaks, to the formation of intermediate lesions, and, ultimately, to the formation of the advanced lesions of atherosclerosis (fibrous plaques). Because one of the roles of the macrophage is to scavenge and clear material it has ingested, many of the macrophages, as they do in other sites of inflammation, may attempt to take the material they have scavenged to other parts of the mononuclear phagocytic system, such as the spleen, liver, lung, and lymph nodes. In so doing, some macrophages appear to exit back into the arterial circulation between the overlying endothelial cells.[25,30] At such sites, mural thrombi may form as a result of the adhesion and aggregation of circulating platelets on the surface of the existing macrophages [*see Figure 7*]. Platelets activated in such thrombi could serve as an additional source of potent growth-regulatory molecules. An intercellular network may develop within the lesions linking the

Figure 5 *Several different sources of injury to the endothelium (pink) can lead to endothelial cell dysfunction. (a) One of the parameters associated with endothelial cell dysfunction that results from exposure to agents such as oxLDL is increased adherence of monocytes/macrophages (blue) and T cells (green). These cells then migrate between the endothelium and localize subendothelially. (b) The macrophages become large foam cells because of lipid accumulation and, with the T cells and smooth muscle cells (orange), form a fatty streak. The fatty streak can then progress to an intermediate, fibrofatty lesion and ultimately to a fibrous plaque. (c) As the lesions accumulate more cells and the macrophages scavenge the lipid, some of the lipid-laden macrophages may migrate back into the bloodstream by pushing apart the endothelial cells. At sites such a branches and bifurcations, where the blood flow is irregular with eddy currents and back currents, the macrophages may become thrombogenic and lead to formation of platelet mural thrombi. Such thrombi can release many potent growth-regulatory molecules from the platelets that can join with those released into the artery wall by the activated macrophages and possibly by lesion smooth muscle cells. Platelet thrombi can also form at sites where endothelial dysjuction may have occurred. (d) Ultimately, the formation and release of numerous growth-regulatory molecules and cytokines establish a network between cells in the lesion, consisting of activated macrophages, smooth muscle, T cells, and endothelium, and lead to progression of the lesions of atherosclerosis to a fibrous plaque or advanced, complicated lesion. (e) Each of the stages of lesion formation is potentially reversible. Thus, lesion regression can occur if the injurious agents are removed, or when protective factors intervene to reverse the inflammatory and fibroproliferative processes.*

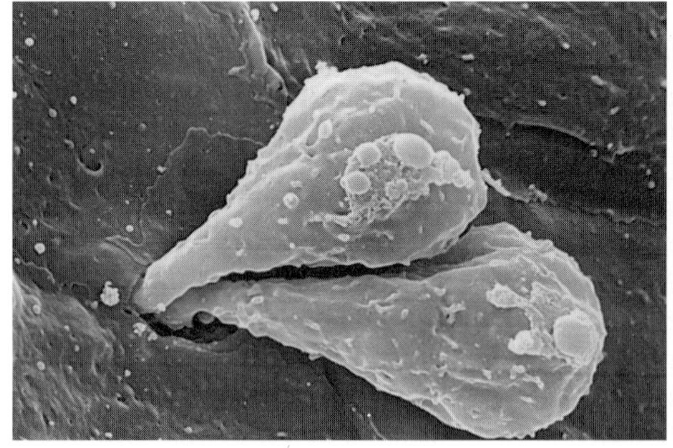

Figure 6 Two leukocytes, presumably circulating blood monocytes, have adhered to the surface of the endothelium. After adhering, they begin to probe until they find a site between endothelial cells through which they can send a process. The cellular processes may release enzymes at their leading edge, and their probing between endothelial cells may lead to separation of the endothelial cells at their junctional complexes. Once separation occurs, the migrating leukocytes are able to penetrate completely between the endothelial cells until they are localized subendothelially and eventually enter the intima of the artery wall.

monocyte-derived macrophages, T cells, smooth muscle cells, and endothelium; formation of this network may result in lesion expansion or, if sufficient amounts of growth-inhibitory molecules are formed, in lesion regression.

Thus, the response-to-injury hypothesis of atherogenesis suggests that injury resulting from factors associated with hyperlipidemia, hypertension, diabetes, cigarette smoking, or other, less common, risk factors (e.g., the elevated homocysteine level in homocystinuria[34]) leads to dysfunctional changes or more overt changes in the endothelium and the underlying smooth muscle cells. This injury leads to a specialized, chronic, inflammatory-fibroproliferative response that may culminate in the occlusive, advanced lesions of atherosclerosis, whose clinical sequelae can have disastrous consequences. Although such an inflammatory-fibroproliferative response is designed to be protective, if it becomes excessive, as may occur in untreated patients who are hyperlipidemic, hypertensive, or diabetic, this response becomes progressive atherosclerosis.[6]

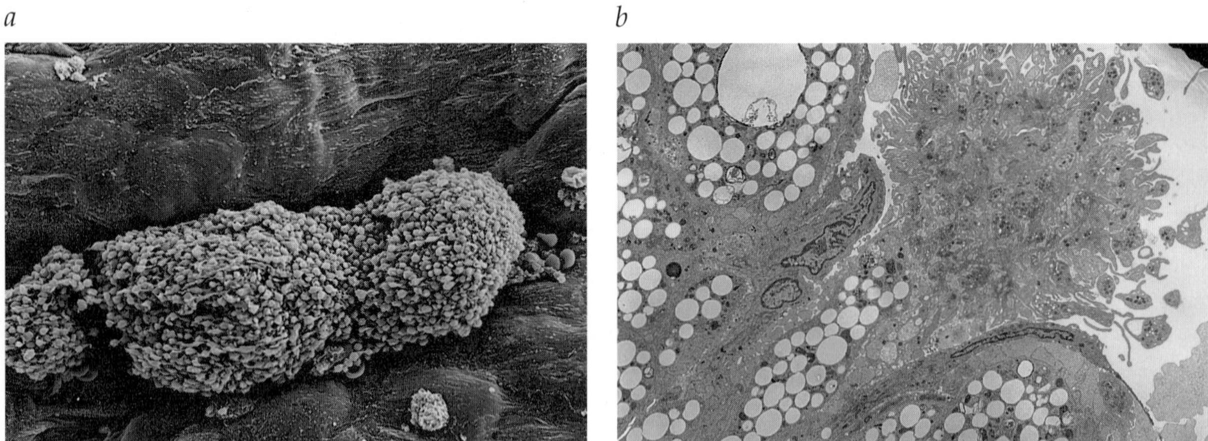

Figure 7 (a) Numerous platelet aggregates adhere to exposed macrophages associated with a fatty streak. Attached monocytes, presumably in the process of entry into the lesion, are present on the surface of the fatty streak. (b) Platelets adhere to an exposed macrophage from a fatty streak. The thrombi generally adhere to exposed foam cells and penetrate into the depth of a crevice in the fatty streak. Many of the platelets have undergone degranulation and released their contents.

Cellular Interactions and Gene Expression in Atherogenesis: Cytokines, Growth Factors, and Other Molecules

A series of growth-regulatory molecules, both stimulatory and inhibitory, cytokines, and other substances, including fatty acid derivatives (e.g., prostaglandins), and small, very active molecules (e.g., nitric oxide),[35,36] play potentially important roles in the function of endothelium, smooth muscle, macrophages, and T cells in the process of atherogenesis. These molecules can have numerous effects, depending on their environment, including stimulation or inhibition of DNA replication and cell proliferation; directed cell migration or chemotaxis; cell recruitment; and synthesis of connective tissue matrix macromolecules, such as collagens, proteoglycans, and elastic fiber proteins. The formation of numerous vasodilatory molecules, such as prostacyclin and nitric oxide, or vasocontrictive molecules, such as thromboxane A_2, angiotensin, and endothelin, can profoundly affect lesion formation as well as its clinical consequences. Figure 8 shows many of the molecules that may be formed by each of the cells involved in atherosclerosis. An understanding of the regulation of the gene expression of these molecules, as well as the roles played by each cell, will provide insight into new therapeutic strategies.

Endothelial Dysfunction

Normal endothelial cells play a key role in the prevention of atherogenesis.[37] A central component of the response-to-injury hypothesis suggests that interruption of endothelial function somehow stimulates a series of cellular and molecular events that elicit an inflammatory response and culminate in the lesions of atherosclerosis. Normal endothelium provides many physiologically important regulatory and protective functions, including

1. A nonthrombogenic surface.
2. A permeability barrier that controls the exchange of nutrients and determines which molecules from the plasma enter the arterial wall.
3. Control of arterial tone by formation of vasodilatory or vasoconstrictive substances.
4. Formation and secretion of growth-stimulatory and growth-inhibitory molecules and cytokines.
5. Formation and maintenance of the basement membrane collagen and proteoglycan on which the cells rest.
6. A nonadherent luminal surface that prevents leukocytes and platelets from sticking.
7. The capacity to modify substances, such as lipoproteins, as they are transported into the arterial wall. Two of the earliest indications of dysfunction in hypercholesterolemic animals are the increased entry of lipid and lipoproteinlike molecules into, and their localization in, the arterial wall. These molecules often have membranous structures, termed liposomes, associated with them; lipid and lipoproteinlike molecules are a prominent feature of human lesions as well.[15,16]

Endothelial cells are acutely sensitive to flow conditions, as demonstrated by their release of endothelium-derived relaxing factor or nitric oxide[35,36] in

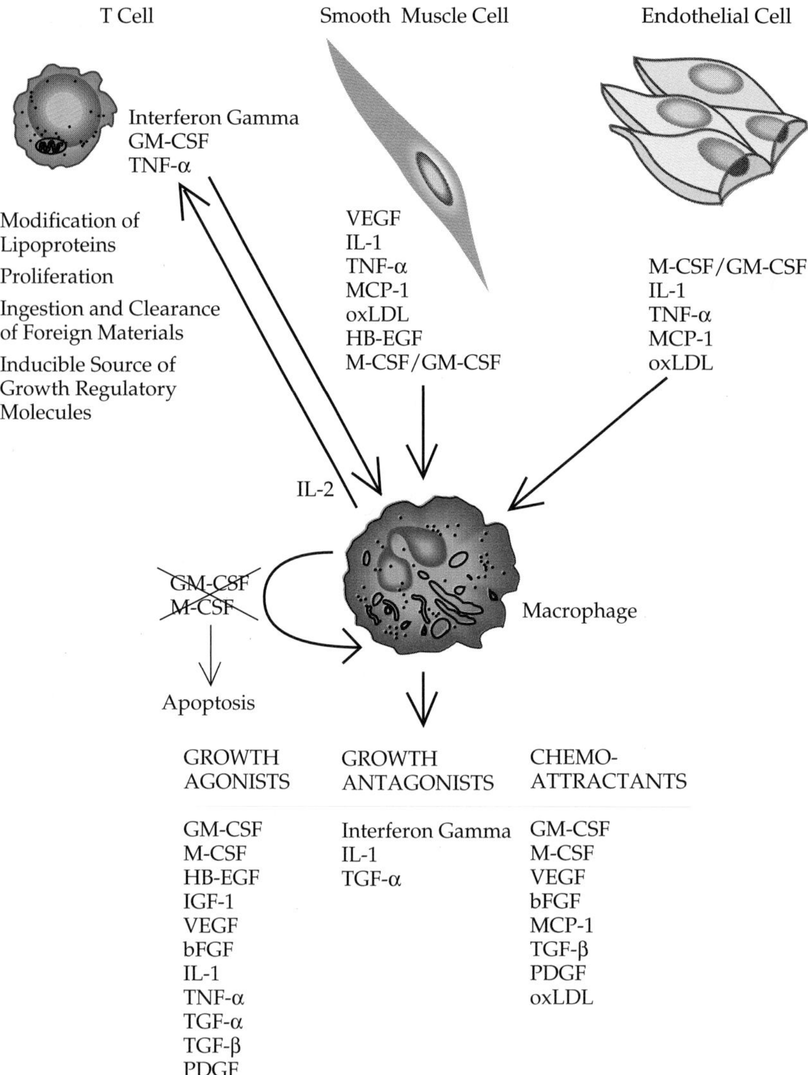

Figure 8 *This illustration shows the potential roles of the macrophage in atherogenesis. The reverse arrows between the T cell and the macrophage suggest that some form of immune response may occur during atherogenesis. Interactions between T cells and macrophages can result in proliferation of each of these cell types through IL-2 and CSFs, respectively. All of the cells with which the macrophages can interact, namely, T cells, smooth muscle cells, and endothelial cells, can present CSF to the macrophages to maintain cell viability and prevent apoptosis with consequent cell death. The cells may participate in further macrophage activation and replication. In addition, smooth muscle and endothelial cells can present antigens at their surfaces and secrete chemoattractants for macrophages, including MCP-1 and oxLDL, as well as factors that can alter macrophage metabolism, such as IL-1 or TNF-α. When the macrophages are activated, they can produce an extraordinary number of biologically relevant molecules, some of which are listed in the diagram in their capacity to induce or inhibit replication of endothelium, smooth muscle, or macrophages, and to make chemoattractants for each of these cell types.*

response to acute increases in blood flow. Similarly, vasoconstriction associated with disease has been partly attributed to reduced formation of nitric oxide by the affected artery.[36] Endothelin, a potent vasoconstrictor, can be released under conditions of decreased flow.[38] Endothelial cells susceptible to altered flow at bifurcations may respond physiologically during early phases of atherogenesis, whereas their capacity to respond may be markedly altered as lesions form, impinge on the lumen, and alter the flow of blood, further aggravating the process of atherogenesis.[39]

Endothelial cells respond to flow not only by releasing vasoactive molecules, but they also may contain shear stress–sensitive potassium channels,[40] they can be stimulated to deliver adenosine triphosphate–derived purines to the endothelial surface,[41] and they can respond to shear stress by expressing genes for growth factors, such as platelet-derived growth factor (PDGF)[42] and fibroblast growth factor.[43]

Leukocyte-Endothelium Interactions

Alterations in the homeostatic capacity of endothelium can lead to the formation of a series of adhesive cell-surface molecules. Such molecules include vascular cell adhesion molecule–1 (VCAM-1),[44] E-selectin, and P-selectin, which have appropriate ligands and receptors on monocytes and on T cells that can lead to increased adherence of these leukocytes,[45-47] as well as PECAM, a molecule that can induce platelet-endothelium adhesion and can aid in transmigration of leukocytes [*see Chapter 4*].[48] After they adhere, the cells spread, and if chemotactic molecules, such as oxidized LDL (oxLDL), colony-stimulating factors (CSFs), or monocyte chemotactic protein–1 (MCP-1) are generated by the endothelium, the leukocytes may enter the artery. Platelets may form microthrombi, aggregate, and release their contents. These and other adhesive and chemotactic molecules may be important in the earliest phases of the inflammatory response because one of the first changes observed in animals made hypercholesterolemic by diet is the adhesion and the spreading of leukocytes to endothelium in clusters throughout the arterial tree or the spreading of platelets at sites of endothelial separation.[6]

Monocyte-Lymphocyte Interactions

The presence of T cells, together with monocytes during atherogenesis, and the capacity of the macrophage to express and present antigens suggest that some form of immune response may be involved in the process of atherogenesis.[49,50] The nature of such antigens and the role of monocyte-lymphocyte interactions and their relation to the various risk factors associated with atherosclerosis are still poorly understood. Macrophages express high levels of human leukocyte antigen, which can also be expressed on endothelium and smooth muscle, but a definitive role of the immune response in atherogenesis in common atherosclerosis remains to be elucidated.[51]

Macrophage Function

Because at every stage of their formation and progression the lesions of atherosclerosis represent examples of a specialized type of chronic inflammatory-fibroproliferative response, it is not surprising that both macrophages and T cells are ubiquitous in all phases of atherogenesis.[52,53] The macrophages initially may exert their principal influence by acting as scavenger cells because of their capacity to phagocytose and remove noxious substances and debride the area. Ultimately, their role may shift so that they act as a source of potent growth-regulatory molecules and cytokines responsible for the proliferative response that results in the advanced atherosclerotic lesion. Thus, the macrophage appears to be the principal inflammatory cellular mediator of the process of atherogenesis. Results of early studies suggested that the major proliferative response in atherogenesis involved smooth muscle cells. However, it has become appreciated that not only do smooth muscle cells proliferate in the lesion, but that macrophages actively replicate their DNA and multiply in the lesions of atherosclerosis as well.[54,55] In fact, during some phases of atherogenesis, macrophage replication may be a more active process than is smooth muscle cell proliferation. Ultimately, the combination of macrophage accumulation and smooth muscle cell proliferation leads to the culminating fibroproliferative advanced lesion, which is the fibrous plaque, or complicated lesion. In part, the development of the advanced lesion may depend on the expression of growth-stimulatory and chemotactic molecules generated by activated monocyte-derived macrophages, and possibly by smooth muscle cells as well. Studies of smooth muscle turnover in lesions suggest that the turnover rates are relatively low, consonant with a low-grade chronic proliferative response that may require years to result in a lesion of significant size.[56]

Macrophages can phagocytose oxLDL via their scavenger receptors as well as via a putative oxLDL receptor on their surfaces.[57,58] Macrophages can oxidize LDL by forming a number of oxygen intermediates. The importance of oxLDL as a component of the process of atherogenesis was first appreciated in a study of genetically hyperlipidemic rabbits in which the potent antioxidant probucol was able to diminish the size of atherosclerotic lesions.[59,60] This same antioxidant has also been successfully used in hyperlipidemic nonhuman primates to diminish the process of atherogenesis.[61] Interestingly, the antioxidant appears to have the greatest effect by decreasing the monocyte/macrophage component of the lesions.[62]

Depending on how they are stimulated, macrophages can form numerous growth factors, including PDGF, heparin-binding epidermal growth factor–like growth factor (HB-EGF), macrophage colony-stimulating factor (M-CSF), granulocyte-macrophage colony-stimulating factor (GM-CSF), interleukin-1 (IL-1), tumor necrosis factor–α (TNF-α), the connective tissue–forming molecule and growth inhibitor, transforming growth factor–β (TGF-β), interleukin-2 (IL-2), and numerous others [*see Figure 8*]. Several of these molecules are chemoattractants, some are growth inhibitory, and others are growth stimulatory. TGF-β, a potent molecule, may have an important role in the induction of smooth muscle cells to form the large amount of connective tissue matrix commonly associated with the advanced lesions of atherosclerosis.[63]

T cells can form three relatively important molecules: interferon gamma, which could play a critical role in the activation of macrophages; GM-CSF, which may help maintain macrophage stability and possibly stimulate replication; and TNF-α, which can play a role in the activation of macrophages.

Macrophage–Smooth Muscle Interactions

Macrophages may play a key role in the induction of smooth muscle proliferation and connective tissue formation. However, smooth muscle cells may in turn express genes that can profoundly affect macrophages, including M-CSF and GM-CSF, which could result in monocyte-derived macrophage proliferation within the lesions.[64] Smooth muscle cells can provide cytokines, which can induce further macrophage activation. Smooth muscle cells can also provide chemotactic factors, such as monocyte chemotactic protein–1 or oxidized LDL, which can induce macrophage migration and activation.

Smooth Muscle Function

Normally, smooth muscle cells control the tone of the artery within the media via their intercellular and connective tissue attachments. Because smooth muscle cells within the lesions are more widely separated than is typically the case, they may no longer have the same capacity to modify vessel tone. Lack of contractile effectiveness may also result in part from a diminution of the intercellular contractile apparatus and from its disorganization in these abornormal smooth muscle cells. Smooth muscle cells can also form a number of growth-stimulatory molecules, including basic fibroblast growth factor (bFGF), insulinlike growth factor–1 (IGF-1), TGF-β, PDGF-A chain, and CSF.[6] At least three factors can induce smooth muscle cells to stimulate themselves in an autocrine fashion. IL-1, TNF-α, and TGF-β can each induce smooth muscle cells to proliferate. However, this proliferation does not result from the capacity of any of these agents to act directly as a mitogen on the smooth muscle cells, but in fact they each may do so via their capacities to induce expression of the gene that codes for PDGF-A chain and stimulate PDGF-AA synthesis and secretion. The secreted PDGF stimulates smooth muscle cells in an autocrine manner that could result in their further replication within the lesions. The capacity of smooth muscle cells to respond in this way to IL-1, TNF-α, or TGF-β has been clearly demonstrated in arterial smooth muscle cells in vitro.[65,66]

Smooth muscle cells actively respond to vasoconstrictive or vasodilatory agents, such as endothelin, catecholamines, angiotensin II, prostaglandin E (PGE), prostacyclin (PGI_2), neuropeptides, leukotrienes, and nitric oxide. Normally, nitric oxide constantly regulates arterial tone by prevention of vasoconstriction. If nitric oxide production is reduced, vasoconstrictive molecules are able to act without opposition.

Smooth muscle cells are critical in the formation of connective tissue matrix. The stability of atherosclerotic lesions and their capacity to resist rheologic forces that may result in fissuring, ulceration, or thrombosis depend on the extent of matrix formation and turnover. The control of the phenotypic state and the capacity of smooth muscle to contract, migrate, or synthesize growth-regulatory and vasoactive molecules are key elements in the regulation of the response of smooth muscle cells to atherogenic agents.[6,67-69]

Restenosis after Angioplasty and after Bypass Surgery

As many as 50 percent of arteries treated by angioplasty and 30 to 40 percent of coronary arteries that undergo bypass restenose, either at the site of a preexisting atherosclerotic lesion after angioplasty or at the perianastomotic site where the normal bypass artery or vein is tied into the coronary artery.[70] The restenosed tissue contains both migratory and proliferative smooth muscle cells as well as macrophage infiltrates at the site of trauma induced by movement of the angioplasty catheter or by the surgical manipulation of the artery during bypass surgery.[71]

Thus far, few animal models of restenosis exist that accurately reflect clinical problems in humans. Most experimental studies in animals have been performed by subjecting a normal rat carotid artery to balloon angioplasty. Consequently, the response to injury is that of a normal artery rather than that of an artery with an atherosclerotic lesion. Although much has been learned about the growth factors involved in this model and of the importance of smooth muscle migration and proliferation, it is possible that lesion cells, which are phenotypically different from normal smooth muscle cells, may respond differently to these events. Thus, different models are being developed in rabbits and in nonhuman primates that are based on the responses of arteries with preexisting, advanced lesions of atherosclerosis.

After balloon angioplasty in a normal rat carotid artery, three phases of cellular activity apparently occur. The first of these occurs within the medial smooth muscle cells, which are injured by the markedly expanded balloon. This injury to the media leads to the release of basic fibroblast growth factor from the injured medial smooth muscle cells, which is accompanied by a wave of medial smooth muscle replication within the first 48 hours.[72] These events are followed by the second phase of activity, a wave of migration of smooth muscle cells from the media into the intima of the artery or within the preexisting intima between days 3 and 5. The third phase consists of further proliferation of these intimal smooth muscle cells over the next 10 days. PDGF has been shown to be involved in the medial-to-intimal migration of smooth muscle cells in the rat carotid artery injury model.[73] The various growth-regulatory molecules responsible for the third phase, the process of intimal proliferation, remain to be determined. Such elucidation would require an animal model in which a preexisting, advanced atherosclerotic lesion (similar to an advanced human lesion) is treated by angioplasty.

Whether or not restenosis will occur after angioplasty or bypass surgery may be partly based on the characteristics of the cells within the atherosclerotic lesions. Experimental data suggest that cells from advanced human atherosclerotic lesions grown in culture behave as senescent cells; that is, they undergo very few doublings.[74] If this were to be the case in vivo, these cells would be less responsive to the growth-regulatory molecules that may be released during angioplasty or bypass surgery. Conversely, if the lesion is fairly young and not much smooth muscle cell replication has occurred during lesion genesis, and if sufficient doublings remain available to these cells, they may be able to respond to the released growth factors and may induce a lesion that results in restenosis. By use of atherectomy catheters, tissue has been obtained from human lesions of atherosclerosis and from restenotic lesions.[75,76] The data obtained from cells derived from these tissues suggest that the processes of smooth muscle migration and proliferation are indeed important in this phenomenon and that some of the same growth-regulatory molecules and cytokines involved in the process of atherogenesis are also involved in restenosis.

Future Directions

Our knowledge of the cells involved in atherogenesis, the genes expressed by these cells, their potential interactions, and the factors that activate them is rapidly unfolding, thereby presenting numerous opportunities to develop modalities that interfere with specific cell adhesions, chemotaxis, proliferation, and gene expression. Factors that lead to endothelial dysfunction can be inhibited through the use of low-molecular-weight inhibitors, peptidomimetics, antisense molecules, humanized monoclonal antibodies, and other approaches with high specificity; these new developments suggest that the time is rapidly approaching when atherosclerosis, which is responsible for 50 percent of deaths in America and Europe, will be preventable and reversible.

References

1. Working Group of Arteriosclerosis: Report of the Working Group of Arteriosclerosis of the National Heart, Lung, and Blood Institute, Vols 1 and 2. Government Printing Office, Washington DC, 1981, Dept. of Health, Education, and Welfare publications no. 81-2034 and 82-2035
2. Brown BG, Albers JJ, Fisher LD, et al: Regression of coronary artery disease as a result of intensive lipid-lowering therapy in men with high apolipoprotein B. *N Engl J Med* 323:1289, 1990
3. World Health Organization Report of a Study Group: Classification of atherosclerotic lesions. *WHO Tech Rep* Serv 143:1, 1985
4. Ross R, Glomset JA: The pathogenesis of atherosclerosis. *N Engl J Med* 295:369, 420, 1976
5. Ross R: The pathogenesis of atherosclerosis: an update. *N Engl J Med* 314:488, 1986
6. Ross R: The pathogenesis of atherosclerosis: a perspective for the 1990s. *Nature* 362:801, 1993
7. Stary HC: Evolution and progression of atherosclerotic lesions in coronary arteries of children and young adults. *Arteriosclerosis* 9 (suppl I):I19, 1989
8. McGill HC Jr: Persistent problems in the pathogenesis of atherosclerosis. *Arteriosclerosis* 4:443, 1984
9. Davies MJ, Thomas A: Thrombosis and acute coronary-artery lesions in sudden cardiac ischemic death. *N Engl J Med* 310:1137, 1984
10. Ross R, Glomset JA: Atherosclerosis and the arterial smooth muscle cell. *Science* 180:1332, 1973
11. Virchow R: Phlogose und thrombose im gefassystem. *Gesammelte Abhandlungen zur Wissenschaftlichen Medizin.* Meidinger Sohn and Company, Frankfurt-am-Main, 1856, p 458
12. French JE: Atherosclerosis in relation to the structure and function of the arterial intima, with special reference to the endothelium. *Int Rev Exp Pathol* 5:253, 1966
13. Ross R, Harker LA: Hyperlipidemia and atherosclerosis. *Science* 193:1094, 1976
14. Ross R: George Lyman Duff memorial lecture: Atherosclerosis—a problem of the biology of arterial wall cells and their interactions with blood components. *Arteriosclerosis* 1:293, 1981

15. Simionescu N, Vasile E, Lupu F, et al: Prelesional events in atherogenesis: accumulation of extracellular cholesterol-rich liposomes in the arterial intima and cardiac valves of the hyperlipidemic rabbit. *Am J Pathol* 123:109, 1986
16. Mora R, Lupu F, Simionescu N: Prelesional events in atherogenesis: colocalization of apolipoprotein B, unesterified cholesterol and extracellular phospholipid liposomes in the aorta of hyperlipidemic rabbit. *Atherosclerosis* 67:143, 1987
17. Henriksen T, Mahoney EM, Steinberg D: Enhanced macrophage degradation of low density lipoprotein previously incubated with cultured endothelial cells: recognition by receptors for acetylated low density lipoproteins. *Proc Natl Acad Sci USA* 78:6499, 1981
18. Vlassara H, Brownlee M, Cerami A: High-affinity-receptor-mediated uptake and degradation of glucose-modified proteins: a potential mechanism for the removal of senescent macromolecules. *Proc Natl Acad Sci USA* 82:5588, 1985
19. Cathcart MK, Morel DW, Chisolm GM: Monocytes and neutrophils oxidize low-density lipoprotein making it cytotoxic. *J Leukoc Biol* 38:341, 1985
20. Rosenfeld ME, Palinski W, Ylä-Herttuala S, et al: Macrophages, endothelial cells, and lipoprotein oxidation in the pathogenesis of atherosclerosis. *Toxicol Pathol* 18:560, 1990
21. Berliner JA, Territo MC, Sevanian A, et al: Minimally modified low density lipoprotein stimulates monocyte endothelial interactions. *J Clin Invest* 85:1260, 1990
22. Steinbrecher UP, Zhang HF, Lougheed M: Role of oxidatively modified LDL in atherosclerosis. *Free Radic Biol Med* 9:155, 1990
23. Steinberg, D: Antioxidants and atherosclerosis: a current assessment. *Circulation* 84:1420, 1991
24. Rosenfeld ME, Tsukada T, Gown AM, et al: Fatty streak initiation in Watanabe heritable hyperlipemic and comparably hypercholesterolemic fat-fed rabbits. *Arteriosclerosis* 7:9, 1987
25. Rosenfeld ME, Tsukada T, Chait A, *et al*: Fatty streak expansion and maturation in Watanabe heritable hyperlipemic and comparably hypercholesterolemic fat-fed rabbits. *Arteriosclerosis* 7:24, 1987
26. Poole JCF, Florey HW: Changes in the endothelium of the aorta and the behaviour of macrophages in experimental atheroma of rabbits. *J Pathol* 75:245, 1958
27. Gerrity RG, Naito HK, Richardson M, et al: Dietary induced atherogenesis in swine: morphology of the intima in prelesion stages. *Am J Pathol* 95:775, 1979
28. Florentin RA, Nam SC, Daoud AS, et al: Dietary-induced atherosclerosis in miniature swine. *Exp Mol Pathol* 8:263, 1968
29. Faggiotto A, Ross R, Harker L: Studies of hypercholesterolemia in the nonhuman primate: I. Changes that lead to fatty streak formation. *Arteriosclerosis* 4:323, 1984
30. Faggiotto A, Ross R: Studies of hypercholesterolemia in the nonhuman primate: II. Fatty streak conversion to fibrous plaque. *Arteriosclerosis* 4:341, 1984
31. Masuda J, Ross R: Atherogenesis during low level hypercholesterolemia in the nonhuman primate: I. Fatty streak formation. *Arteriosclerosis* 10:164, 1990
32. Masuda J, Ross R: Atherogenesis during low level hypercholesterolemia in the nonhuman primate: II. Fatty streak conversion to fibrous plaque. *Arteriosclerosis* 10:178, 1990
33. Nakashima Y, Plump AS, Raines EW, et al: ApoE-deficient mice develop lesions of all phases of atherosclerosis throughout the arterial tree. *Arterioscler Thromb* 14:133, 1994
34. Harker LA, Ross R, Slichter SJ, et al: Homocysteine-induced arteriosclerosis: the role of endothelial cell injury and platelet response in its genesis. *J Clin Invest* 58:731, 1976
35. Furchgott RF: Role of endothelium in responses of vascular smooth muscle. *Circ Res* 53: 557, 1983
36. Lüscher TF: Imbalance of endothelium-derived relaxing and contracting factors: a new concept in hypertension? *Am J Hypertens* 3:317, 1990
37. DiCorleto PE, Soyombo AA: The role of the endothelium in atherogenesis. *Curr Opin Lipidol* 4:364, 1993
38. Yanagisawa M, Kurihara H, Kimura S, et al: A novel potent vasoconstrictor peptide produced by vascular endothelial cells. *Nature* 332:411, 1988
39. Glagov S, Weisenberg E, Zarins CK, et al: Compensatory enlargement of human atherosclerotic coronary arteries. *N Engl J Med* 316:1371, 1987
40. Olesen S-P, Clapham DE, Davies PF: Haemodynamic shear stress activates a K^{2+} current in vascular endothelial cells. *Nature* 221:168, 1988
41. Dull RO, Davies PF: Flow modulation of agonist (ATP)-response (Ca^{2+}) coupling in vascular endothelial cells. *Am J Physiol* 261:H149, 1991
42. Resnick W, Collins T, Atkinson W, et al: Platelet-derived growth factor B chain promoter contains a *cis*-acting fluid shear-stress-responsive element. *Proc Natl Acad Sci USA* 90:4591, 1993

43. Langille BL: Blood flow-induced remodeling of arteries in health and disease. *Cardiovasc Pathol* 1:245, 1992

44. O'Brien KD, Allen MD, McDonald TO, et al: Vascular cell adhesion molecule-1 is expressed in human coronary atherosclerotic plaques: implications for the mode of progression of advanced coronary atherosclerosis. *J Clin Invest* 92:945, 1993

45. Springer TA: Adhesion receptors of the immune system. *Nature* 346:425, 1990

46. Cybulsky MI, Gimbrone MA Jr: Endothelial expression of a mononuclear leukocyte adhesion molecule during atherogenesis. *Science* 251:788, 1991

47. Carlos TM, Harlan JM: Membrane proteins involved in phagocyte adherence to endothelium. *Immunol Rev* 114:5, 1990

48. Muller WA, Weigl SA, Deng X, Phillips DM: PECAM-1 is required for transendothelial migration of leukocytes. *J Exp Med* 178:449, 1993

49. Libby P, Hansson GK: Involvement of the immune system in human atherogenesis: current knowledge and unanswered questions. *Lab Invest* 64:5, 1991

50. Hansson GK, Holm J, Jonasson L: Detection of activated T lymphocytes in the human atherosclerotic plaque. *Am J Pathol* 135:169, 1989

51. Hansson GK, Jonasson L, Seifert PS, et al: Immune mechanisms in atherosclerosis. *Arteriosclerosis* 9:567, 1989

52. Gown AM, Tsukada T, Ross R: Human atherosclerosis: II. Immunocytochemical analysis of the cellular composition of human atherosclerotic lesions. *Am J Pathol* 125:191, 1986

53. Jonasson L, Holm J, Skalli O, et al: Regional accumulations of T cells, macrophages, and smooth muscle cells in the human atherosclerotic plaque. *Arteriosclerosis* 6:131, 1986

54. Rosenfeld ME, Ross R: Macrophage and smooth muscle cell proliferation in atherosclerotic lesions of WHHL and comparably hypercholesterolemic fat-fed rabbits. *Arteriosclerosis* 10:680, 1990

55. Gordon D, Reidy MA, Benditt EP, et al: Cell proliferation in human coronary arteries. *Proc Natl Acad Sci USA* 87:4600, 1990

56. Gordon D: Cell proliferation in human arteries. *Cardiovasc Pathol* 1:259, 1992

57. Goldstein JL, Ho YK, Basu SK, et al: Binding site of macrophages that mediates uptake and degradation of actylated low density lipoprotein, producing massive cholesterol deposition. *Proc Natl Acad Sci USA* 76:333, 1979

58. Parthasarathy S, Printz DJ, Boyd D, *et al*: Macrophage oxidation of low density lipoprotein generates a modified form recognized by the scavenger receptor. *Arteriosclerosis* 6:505, 1986

59. Carew TE, Schwenke DC, Steinberg D: Antiatherogenic effect of probucol unrelated to its hypocholesterolemic effect: evidence that antioxidants in vivo can selectively inhibit low density lipoprotein degradation in macrophage-rich fatty streaks and slow the progression of atherosclerosis in the Watanabe heritable hyperlidemic rabbit. *Proc Natl Acad Sci USA* 84:7725, 1987

60. Kita T, Nagano Y, Yokode M, et al: Probucol prevents the progression of atherosclerosis in Watanabe heritable hyperlipidemic rabbit, an animal model for familial hypercholesterolemia. *Proc Natl Acad Sci USA* 84:5928, 1987

61. Sasahara M, Raines EW, Chait A, et al: Inhibition of hypercholesterolemia-induced atherosclerosis in the nonhuman primate by probucol: I. Is the extent of atherosclerosis related to resistance of LDL to oxidation? *J Clin Invest* 94:155, 1994

62. Chang MY, Sasahara M, Raines EW, et al: Inhibition of hypercholesterolemia-induced atherosclerosis in *Macaca nemestrina* by probucol: II. Quantitative immunohistochemical analysis of aortic lesions. (submitted)

63. Roberts AB, Sporn MB: The transforming growth factor-βs. *Handbook of Experimental Pharmacology: Peptide Growth Factors and Their Receptors I.* Sporn MB, Roberts AB, Eds. Springer-Verlag, Berlin, 1990, p 419

64. Rosenfeld MD, Ylä-Herttuala S, Lipton BA, et al: Macrophage colony-stimulating factor mRNA and protein in atherosclerotic lesions of rabbits and humans. *Am J Pathol* 140:291, 1992

65. Raines EW, Dower SK, Ross R: IL-1 mitogenic activity for fibroblasts and smooth muscle cells is due to PDGF-AA. *Science* 243:393, 1989

66. Battegay EJ, Raines EW, Seifert RA, et al: TGF-β induces bimodal proliferation of connective tissue cells via complex control of an autocrine PDGF loop. *Cell* 63:515, 1990

67. Fuster V, Badimon L, Badimon JJ, et al: The pathogenesis of coronary artery disease and the acute coronary syndromes. *N Engl J Med* 326:242, 1992

68. Campbell GR, Campbell JH, Manderson JA, et al: Arterial smooth muscle. A multifunctional mesenchymal cell. *Arch Pathol Lab Med* 112:977, 1988

69. Thyberg J, Hedin U, Sjölund M, et al: Regulation of differentiated properties and proliferation of arterial smooth muscle cells. *Arteriosclerosis* 10:966, 1990

70. Ferrell M, Fuster V, Gold HK, et al: A dilemma for the 1990s: choosing appropriate experimental animal model for the prevention of restenosis. *Circulation* 85:1630, 1992

71. Anderson PG: Restenosis: Animal models and morphometric techniques in studies of the vascular response to injury. *Cardiovasc Pathol* 1:263, 1992

72. Lindner V, Reidy MA: Proliferation of smooth muscle cells after vascular injury is inhibited by an antibody against basic fibroblast growth factor. *Proc Natl Acad Sci USA* 88:3739, 1991

73. Ferns GAA, Raines EW, Sprugel KH, et al: Inhibition of neointimal smooth muscle accumulation after angioplasty by an antibody to PDGF. *Science* 253:1129, 1991

74. Ross R, Wight TN, Strandness E, et al: Human atherosclerosis: cell constitution and characteristics of advanced lesions of the superficial femoral artery (part 1). *Am J Pathol* 114:79, 1984

75. Dartsch PC, Bauriedel G, Schinko I, et al: Cell constitution and characteristics of human atherosclerotic plaques selectively removed by percutaneous atherectomy. *Atherosclerosis* 80:149, 1989

76. Nikol S, Isner JM, Pickering JG, et al: Expression of transforming growth factor-β1 is increased in human vascular restenosis lesions. *J Clin Invest* 90:1582, 1992

Acknowledgments

This work is supported by National Heart, Lung, and Blood Institute grant HL18645 and an unrestricted grant for cardiovascular research from Bristol-Myers Squibb Company.

Figure 4 From "Arterial Plaque and Thrombus Formation," by N.Woolf and M.J. Davies, in *Scientific American Science & Medicine* 1:38,1994. Used by permission.

Figures 5, 8 Dana Burns-Pizer. Adapted from "The Pathogenesis of Athersclerosis: A perspective for the 1990s," by R. Ross, in *Nature* 362:801,1993. Used by permission.

Figure 6 From *The Gallery of the Pathogenesis of Atherosclerosis*, by R. Ross. Bristol-Myers Squibb Pharamceutical Research Institure, Princeton, 1991. Used by permission.

Figure 7 From "Studies of Hypercholesterolemia in the Nonhuman Primate: II. Fatty Streak Conversion to Fibrous Plaque," by A. Faggiotto and R. Ross, in *Arteriosclerosis* 4:391,1984. Used by permission.

CHAPTER 3

Lipoprotein Receptors and Atherosclerosis

Monty Krieger, Ph.D.

The circulatory system sustains the life of individual cells and integrates the metabolism of cells in different tissues so that diverse cellular functions are properly coordinated. The intercellular transport of critical cellular components must be well regulated because its disruption can lead to disease, such as aberrant lipid transport and atherosclerosis. The intercellular transport of lipids, including cholesterol, cholesteryl esters, triglycerides, certain vitamins, and even some drugs, through the aqueous circulatory system is dependent on the packaging of these hydrophobic molecules into water-soluble carriers called lipoproteins. There are four major classes of mammalian lipoproteins, three of which have been named on the basis of their differing buoyant densities[1]: low-density lipoprotein (LDL), the principal cholesterol transporter in human plasma; high-density lipoprotein (HDL); very low density lipoprotein (VLDL), principally a triglyceride carrier synthesized by the liver; and chylomicron, a dietary triglyceride carrier synthesized in the intestines.

These lipoproteins have different protein and lipid compositions, sizes, and physiologic and pathophysiological activities [*see Table 1*]. For example, there is a direct correlation of risk of coronary artery disease with high plasma LDL concentrations and an inverse correlation with high plasma HDL concentrations.[2,3] LDL is composed of a core of approximately 1,500 cholesteryl ester molecules and an outer phospholipid and cholesterol monolayer shell containing a single copy of a very large protein called apolipoprotein B-100 [*see Figure 1*]. Lipoprotein production not only requires the assembly of apolipoproteins, triglycerides, cholesterol, cholesteryl esters, and phospholipids within the secretory apparatus of hepatic and other cells but

Table 1 Properties of Human Lipoproteins

Property	*LDL*	*HDL*	*VLDL*	*Chylomicron*
Density (g/ml)	1.019–1.063	1.063–1.21	0.93–1.006	0.93
Diameter (nm)	18–25	5–12	30–80	75–1,200
Approximate mass (kd)	2,300	175–360	$10–80 \times 10^3$	$50–1,000 \times 10^3$
Composition (wt%)				
Cholesterol	6–8	3–5	4–8	1–3
Cholesteryl esters	42–50	13–20	12–22	2–4
Protein	18–22	40–55	6–10	1–2
Phospholipids	18–24	26–35	15–20	3–7
Triglycerides	4–8	2–7	45–65	80–95
Major apolipoproteins	B	A-I, A-II, E	B, E, CI, CII, CIII	A-I, A-IV, B, CI, CIII, E

also involves the extracellular modification and interconversion of lipoproteins, including the transfer of apolipoprotein and lipid components.[4] For example, after hepatic secretion of VLDL, it is converted to intermediate-density lipoprotein (IDL) and eventually to LDL. A number of key enzymes participate in these transformations, including lipoprotein lipase (LPL), lecithin:cholesterol acyltransferase (LCAT), and cholesteryl ester transfer protein (CETP).

For effective cholesterol transport and cellular cholesterol homeostasis to occur, lipoproteins must be targeted to appropriate tissues so that they can either deliver or remove cholesterol. This targeting must be regulated to ensure that intercellular cholesterol transport is coordinated with intracellular cholesterol biosynthesis (virtually all cells can synthesize cholesterol from acetyl coenzyme A). This chapter focuses on the physiologic and pathophysiological targeting and delivery of LDL to cells via two cell surface receptors: the LDL receptor and the class A macrophage scavenger receptor. The LDL receptor has been shown to play a critical role in mediating cellular delivery of LDL cholesterol, in regulating plasma LDL levels, and thus in determining the development of hypercholesterolemia and atherosclerosis.[3,5,6] Macrophage scavenger receptors have been implicated both in the deposition of lipoprotein cholesterol in artery walls during the formation of atherosclerotic plaques and in other clinically relevant functions.[7]

LDL Receptor Pathway

LDL receptor activity was initially discovered in cultured cells, and its physiologic role in vivo was demonstrated using genetic and pharmacological techniques.[3] A key method for studying the LDL receptor (and essentially all other receptor systems) is radioactively tagging the receptor's ligand, in this case LDL. A variety of methods can then be used to examine how the tagged LDL binds to its receptors on the surfaces of cells and how it is subsequently internalized and catabolized by the cells, both in cultured cells and in whole animals.[8] In addition, the cellular location of either LDL or its receptor can be visualized using standard light or electron microscopy, by employing specific antibodies, or by other techniques.

When increasing amounts of LDL are incubated with normal cultured human fibroblasts for a fixed amount of time, it is possible to observe and measure the amounts of LDL bound to the cells' surfaces, the subsequent cellular internalization and catabolism of the LDL, and the effects of LDL on cellular cholesterol metabolism[3,5] [*see Figure 2*]. This process is called the receptor-mediated endocytosis of LDL, or the LDL receptor pathway [*see Figure 3*]. There are three key characteristics of the LDL receptor pathway: (1) Binding to receptors on the cell surfaces at physiologic pH (approximately 7.4) is saturable (approximately 20,000 to 50,000 receptors/cell) and very tight (high-affinity binding) [*see Figure 2*]. The ligand concentration at which there is 50 percent of maximal binding (the dissociation constant, K_d) is approximately 1 nM; thus, very low concentrations of LDL in the extracellular fluid can be efficiently bound. (2) Binding is highly specific, and only LDL and one or two closely related lipoproteins can bind to LDL receptors—not HDL, insulin, albumin, or any other of the myriad of proteins in plasma and interstitial fluids. High-affinity and high-specificity ligand binding is a hallmark of most cell surface receptors, including those for LDL, insulin, growth hormone, and many others.[2]

The LDL receptor is a mosaic of five distinct protein domains [*see Figure 4*] that appear in a variety of other proteins.[3,9] These include the epidermal growth factor (EGF) precursor and several complement components

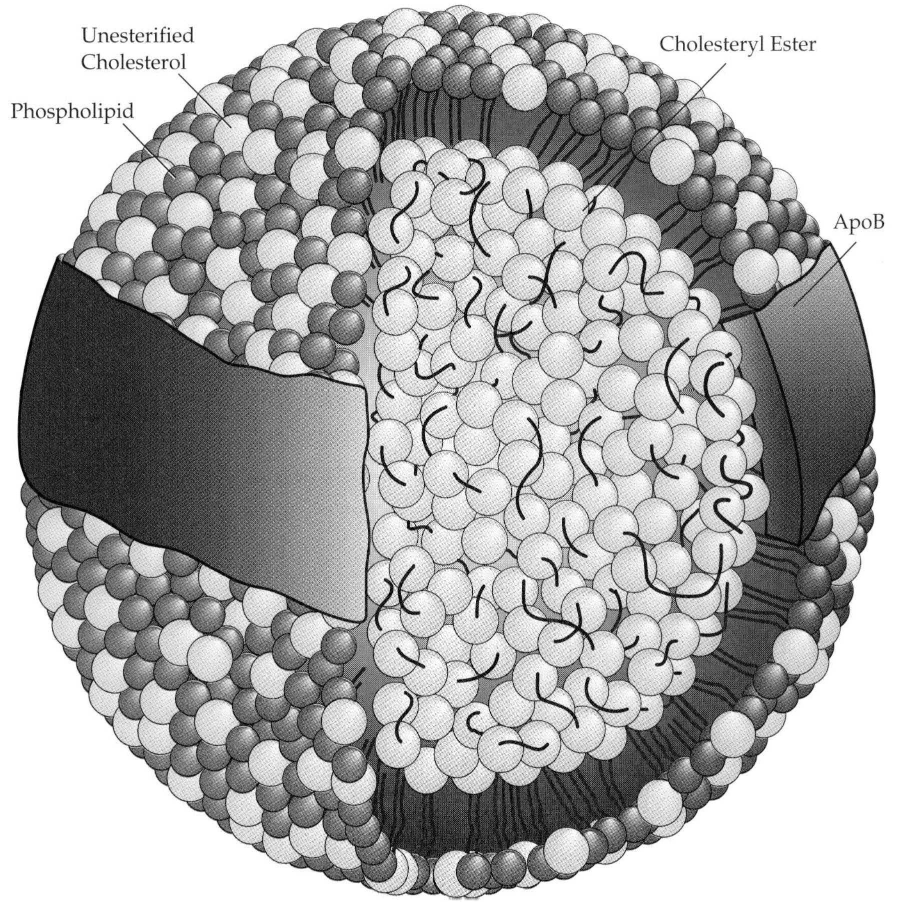

Figure 1 *Low-density lipoprotein (LDL) is a complex spherical particle with a mass of approximately 2.5 × 10*^{6} *daltons. It consists of a hydrophobic core containing approximately 1,500 cholesteryl ester molecules and an amphipathic lipid monolayer shell of unesterified cholesterol and phospholipid in which the protein apolipoprotein B-100 (approximately 513 kilodaltons) is embedded. Apolipoprotein B-100 is responsible for binding native LDL to LDL receptors and for binding chemically modified LDL to macrophage scavenger receptors.*

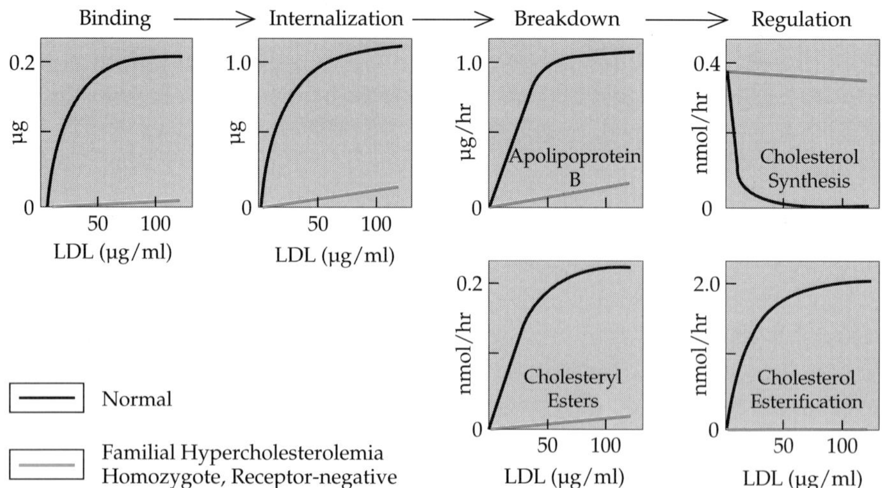

Figure 2 *Concentration dependence of LDL and cholesterol metabolism in cultured human fibroblasts from normal individuals (black line) and familial hypercholesterolemia (FH) homozygotes (blue line). Incubation of the cells with increasing concentrations of LDL results in high-affinity and saturable surface binding, followed by internalization, degradation (breakdown) of the protein and cholesteryl esters of LDL, and release of LDL cholesterol into the metabolic pool of the cell. This increased release of cholesterol results in the suppression of HMG-CoA reductase activity, and thus cholesterol biosynthesis, and LDL receptor synthesis, and in an increase in cholesterol esterification for storage (ACAT activity).*

(e.g., component C9). LDL binds to a group of complement-related, cysteine-rich domains at the extracellular N-terminal of the receptor. The addition to serine and threonine of O-linked oligosaccharide chains on the extracellular portion of the receptor near the plasma membrane protects the receptor from cleavage by proteases.[10,11] (3) Even before LDL binds, its receptors cluster in special patches on the surfaces of cells called coated pits.[5] These patches have a polygonal cytoplasmic protein coating comprising a protein called clathrin and a complex of associated proteins. A short sequence of amino acids in the receptor's C-terminal cytoplasmic domain is responsible for the receptor's clustering into coated pits. The LDL receptors and bound LDL particles enter cells when the coated pits invaginate and pinch off of the plasma membrane, forming coated endocytic vesicles [*see Figure 3*]. The vesicles lose their coats and form endocytic vesicles called endosomes. The luminal contents of the endosomes are acidified by proton pumps, and the consequent low pH causes the dissociation of LDL from its receptors. Dissociation frees the receptors to recycle back to the cell surface so that they can mediate additional rounds of LDL endocytosis. As a consequence, a relatively small number of LDL receptors can mediate the internalization of a large number of LDL particles. After dissociation, the LDL is transferred to the lumen of the cellular lysosomes, organelles containing numerous hydrolytic enzymes. These enzymes disassemble the LDL particles, hydrolyzing protein to individual amino acids, triglycerides to glycerol and fatty acids, and cholesteryl esters to fatty acids and unesterified cholesterol. The cholesterol is then able to enter the metabolically active pool of cholesterol within the cell and in so doing, satisfy the cell's requirements for this important sterol and regulate cellular lipoprotein and sterol metabolism.

Regulation

A critical feature of the LDL receptor pathway is the coordinated regulation of LDL endocytosis and cholesterol synthesis and storage so that cellular cholesterol homeostasis is maintained.[3,6,12] When cellular cholesterol requirements increase, such as during membrane biosynthesis in cell division, adrenal corticotropic hormone–induced steroid synthesis in the adrenal cortex, or increased hepatic bile acid synthesis, cholesterol biosynthesis and import of LDL cholesterol increase, and the conversion

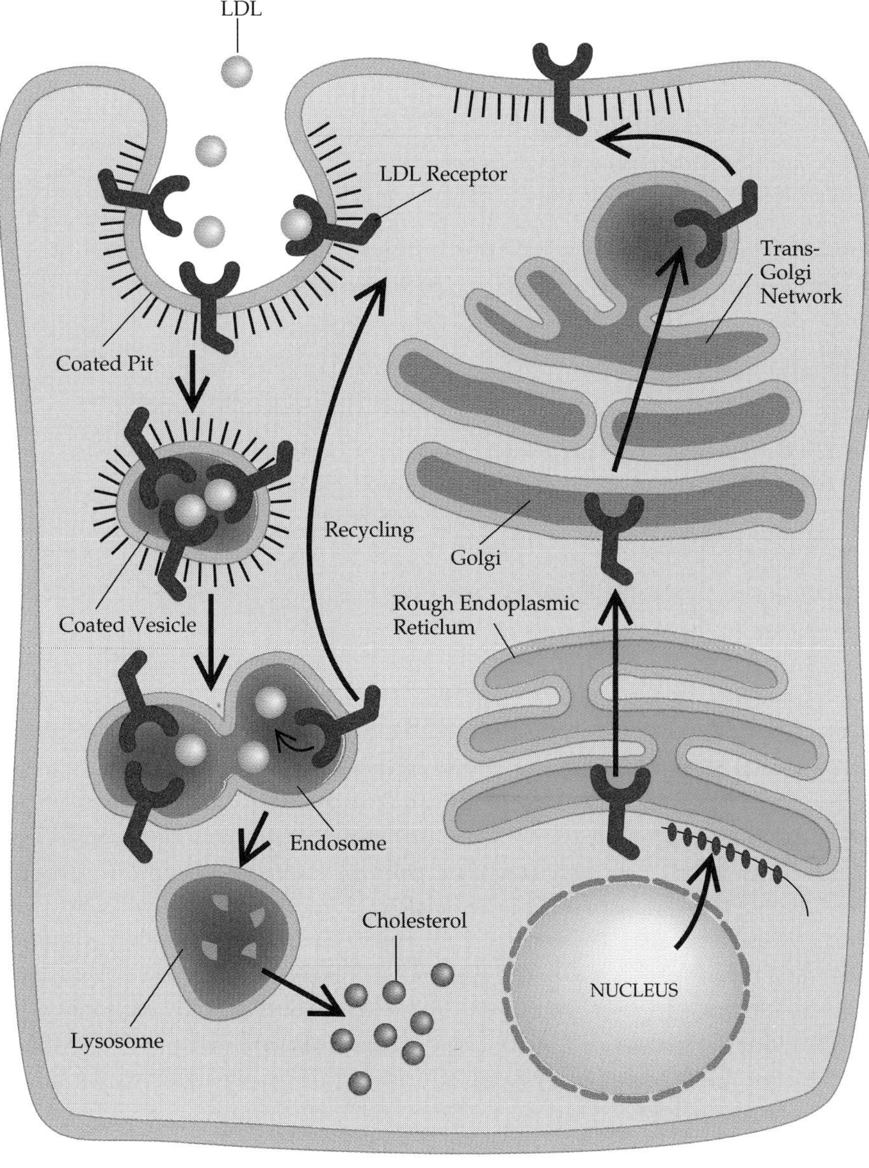

Figure 3 *LDL receptors are synthesized as integral membrane proteins in the rough endoplasmic reticulum, where they are covalently modified by asparagine-linked and serine/threonine-linked glycosylation. The receptors are transported to the Golgi apparatus and the trans-Golgi network for additional processing of their polysaccharide chains and sorting to the cell surface. Receptor-mediated endocytosis of LDL occurs via a coated pit–coated vesicle mediated pathway. In brief, after high-affinity binding of ligands to the receptor occurs, invagination of cell surface coated pits that contain the receptor-ligand complex results in the formation of coated endocytic vesicles. These are converted to endosomes. The low pH in the lumen of the endosome induces receptor-ligand dissociation, after which the receptors recycle to the cell surface and the LDL is delivered to lysosomes for enzymatic digestion. This digestion leads to the release of cholesterol from the LDL [see Figure 1] and its subsequent entry into the metabolic pool of the cell. As a consequence, LDL receptor and cholesterol synthesis is suppressed and cholesterol storage as cholesteryl esters is stimulated.*

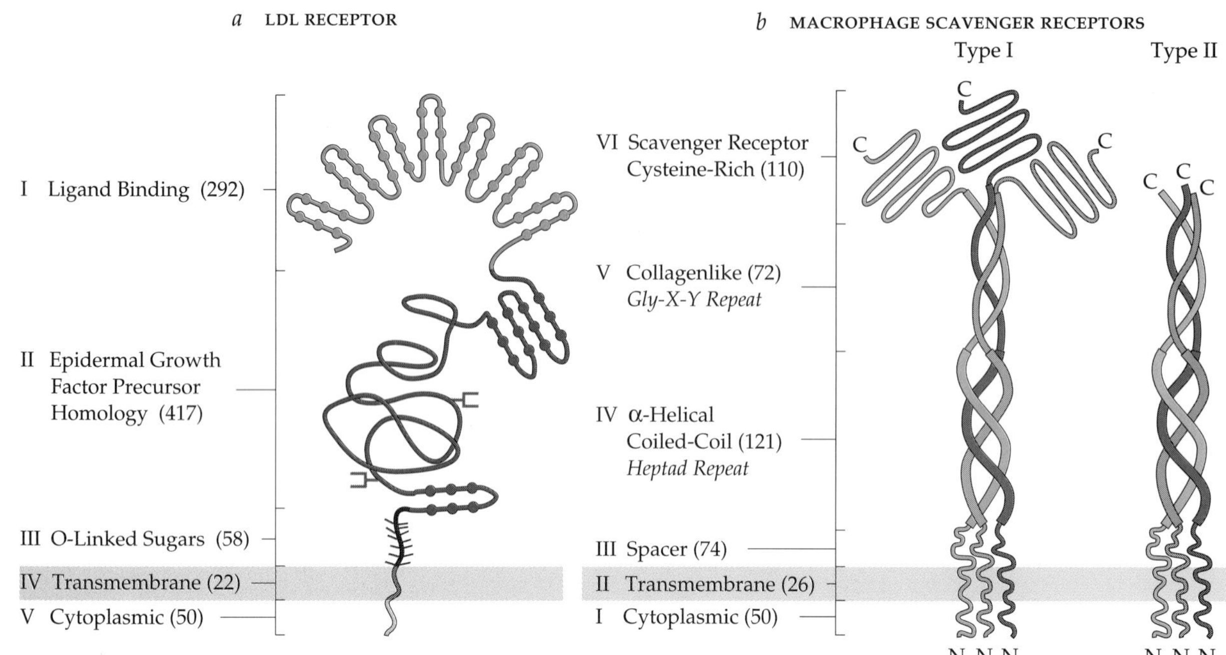

Figure 4 *(a) The human LDL receptor is a 839-amino-acid, mosaic, integral membrane glycoprotein composed of five distinct domains, including a cytoplasmic C-terminal domain (50 amino acids) with its coated pit clustering signal; a single transmembrane (TM) domain (22 residues); a juxtamembrane, O-linked sugar domain (58 residues); an N-glycosylated epidermal growth factor (EGF) precursor domain (417 residues); and, at the N-terminal, a group of seven cysteine-rich domains (292 residues) that serve as the LDL binding site. A single receptor polypeptide chain is represented here; however, experiments suggest that the functional receptor on the surface of cells may actually be a homodimer. (b) The type I and II macrophage scavenger receptors are composed of six domains.*[39,40,42] *The first five domains of both types of receptor are identical. They are the (I) N-terminal cytoplasmic domain (50 residues); (II) TM domain (26 residues); (III) spacer domain (74 residues); (IV) α-helical coiled-coil domain (121 residues), comprising heptad repeats with aliphatic amino acids in the first and fourth positions; and (V) collagenlike domain comprising 24 (or 23) Gly-X-Y repeats (72 residues). The number of amino acids in each domain of the bovine type I receptor are indicated in parentheses. The sixth (C-terminal) domain in the type I scavenger receptor contains an eight-residue hinge followed by a 102-amino-acid scavenger receptor, cysteine-rich (SRCR) domain. Domain VI of the type II receptor is a short peptide of six to 17 residues, depending on the species. This model assumes that the α-helical coiled coil of domain IV forms a single, triple-stranded, left-handed superhelix that merges with the right-handed, collagenlike triple helix of domain V to form a single, long, fibrous stalk. Here, the α-helical coiled-coil and collagenous domains are overwound to emphasize their helical quaternary structures.*

of metabolically active cholesterol to its storage form, cholesteryl ester, decreases. Conversely, when adequate levels of cholesterol accumulate in cells, cholesterol synthesis and import are suppressed and cholesterol storage via esterification is induced. The control of cholesterol import is achieved by varying the rate of synthesis of LDL receptors, which, in turn, determines the steady-state levels of LDL receptors. The control of cholesterol synthesis is mediated by the transcriptional regulation of several of the enzymes in the cholesterol biosynthetic pathway, especially the rate-controlling enzyme 3-hydroxy-3-methylglutaryl coenzyme A (HMG-CoA) reductase and also by the cholesterol-dependent degradation of this enzyme. Conversion of cholesterol to cholesteryl ester is catalyzed by the enzyme acyl coenzyme A:cholesterol acyltransferase (ACAT). The detailed molecular mechanisms by which cells detect and respond to cellular cholesterol levels are not yet well defined. Nevertheless, pharmacological manipulation of LDL receptor expression on the basis of regulation of cellular sterol metabolism is currently one of the principal treatments of hypercholesterolemia. These drugs include HMG-CoA reductase inhibitors and bile acid sequestrants.

Familial Hypercholesterolemia—An LDL Receptor-Deficiency Disease

The strongest evidence for the physiologic significance of the LDL receptor pathway in lipoprotein metabolism and atherosclerosis comes from studies of familial hypercholesterolemia (FH).[3] FH is an autosomal codominant genetic disease that arises because of mutations in the LDL receptor gene. FH is one of the most common genetic diseases, with an incidence of approximately one in 500 for the heterozygous form (one defective LDL receptor allele) and one in 10^6 for the homozygous form (both LDL receptor genes defective). FH is characterized by elevated concentrations of plasma LDL (twofold to threefold in heterozygotes and more than sixfold in homozygotes), cholesterol deposition as arcus lipoides corneae and xanthomas, and premature atherosclerosis. The age at onset of symptoms of coronary artery disease (angina pectoris, myocardial infarction, and sudden death) in homozygotes is proportional to the residual level of LDL receptor activity and usually occurs between the ages of 5 and 30 years. Homozygotes rarely survive past age 30. The risk and age at onset of coronary artery disease are substantially higher in heterozygotes than in unaffected individuals. For example, the mean age of death for heterozygotes in one study was 55 years for males and 64 years for females.[13]

Many different kinds of mutations in the LDL receptor genes of FH patients have been described.[3] These mutations result in four broad categories of defective LDL receptors: (1) no detectable synthesis of LDL receptors (null alleles), (2) precursor forms of the receptors are synthesized in the endoplasmic reticulum [*see Figure 3*] but are not transported normally to the Golgi apparatus and then to the cell surface (transport-defective alleles), (3) defective receptors are transported to the cell surface but either cannot bind lipoprotein or, once internalized, cannot release the bound lipoprotein in the low pH environment of endosomes (binding-deficient alleles), and (4) defective receptors cannot cluster into coated pits because of mutations in their cytoplasmic domain clustering signal (internalization-defective alleles). In addition to the mutant alleles in FH patients, many well-defined mutations have been introduced into the cloned human LDL receptor.[14] Also, rabbits[15,16] and monkeys[17] with LDL receptor gene mutations and FH-like characteristics have been discovered and used extensively to study atherosclerosis. Additional mutants with defects in the LDL receptor gene (*ldlA* locus) or other genes required for normal LDL receptor function (*ldlB* to *ldlI* loci) have been generated by treating cultured mammalian cells with mutagens and isolating LDL receptor–defective cells.[18-20] These mutant cell lines have been used for detailed analyses of the structure of LDL receptors[14] and to define gene products and functions required for the synthesis and function of LDL receptors and other membrane proteins.

Analysis of lipoprotein metabolism in FH patients, of cells cultured from these patients, and of animal models of FH has unequivocally established two key facts: (1) LDL receptors are not essential—intracellular cholesterol synthesis can supply adequate amounts of this sterol for survival in the absence of normal LDL import—and (2) the level of expression of LDL receptors plays a critical role in determining the amounts of LDL in the circulation. The lower the LDL receptor activity, the higher the plasma LDL level.

Receptor-Based Therapies

Because increases in LDL receptor activity, particularly in the liver, where approximately 70 percent of all LDL receptor activity is expressed, result in decreases in plasma LDL levels, pharmacological manipulation of the LDL receptor pathway in the liver provides a powerful approach for treating patients with hypercholesterolemia.[3,6] Currently, two classes of drugs, separately or in combination, are used to induce hepatic LDL receptor activity and lower circulating LDL and thus plasma cholesterol levels [*see Figure 5*]. One class comprises anion-exchange bile acid sequestrant resins,

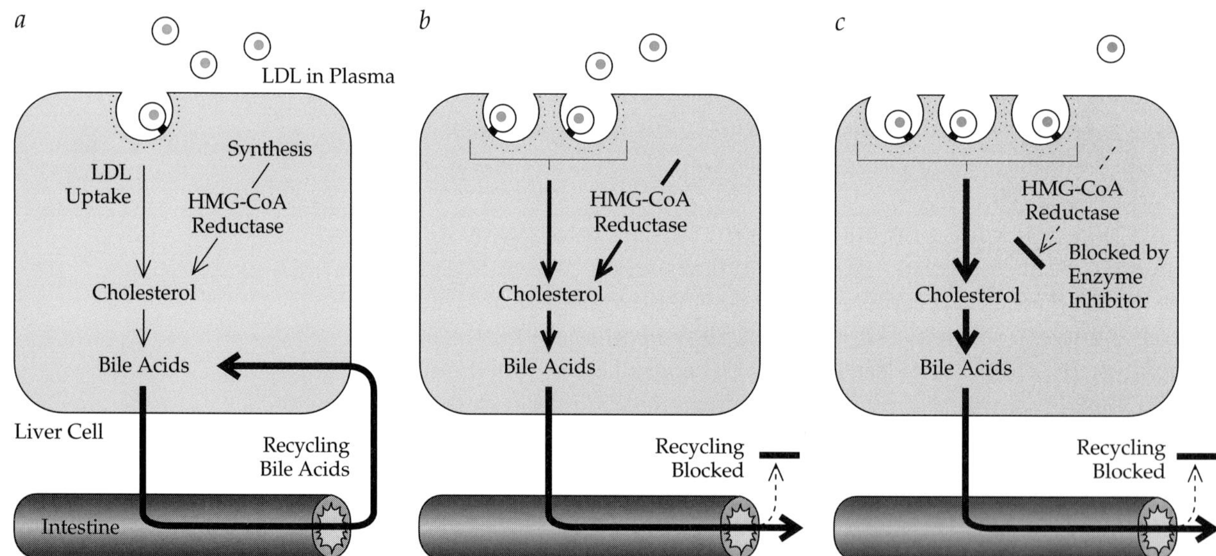

Figure 5 *The effects of bile acid sequestrant and cholesterol biosynthesis inhibitor therapy on LDL receptor activity and plasma LDL levels are shown. The levels of metabolically active cholesterol in cells coordinately regulate cholesterol synthesis via HMG-CoA reductase and cholesterol import via LDL receptors. (a) In hepatocytes, cholesterol is normally converted at a relatively slow rate to bile acids to replace the relatively small fraction of the total bile acids not recovered from the lumen of the intestine by enterohepatic circulation. (b) Bile acid sequestrant resins, such as cholestyramine, block the enterohepatic circulation of bile acids, resulting in an increased conversion of cholesterol to bile acids, a reduction of cellular cholesterol, and a compensatory stimulation of LDL receptor synthesis and activity and HMG-CoA reductase activity to maintain cholesterol homeostasis. The increase in LDL receptor activity increases the rate of removal of LDL from the circulation and thus lowers plasma LDL levels. (c) Combined bile acid sequestrant and HMG-CoA reductase inhibitor therapy dramatically decreases hepatic cholesterol levels by stimulating conversion of cholesterol to bile acids and reducing cholesterol synthesis. This situation then leads to even greater stimulation of LDL receptor synthesis and activity and more substantial reductions in plasma LDL concentrations.*

such as colestipol and cholestyramine [*see Figure 5b*]. These nonabsorbable polymers are given orally and interfere with the enterohepatic circulation by binding to bile acids in the lumen of the intestines, and the complexes are excreted. As a consequence, conversion of hepatic cholesterol to bile acids is stimulated to replenish the bile acid pool, and this stimulation lowers the hepatic cholesterol pool. The hepatocytes respond to this lowering by increasing LDL receptor and cholesterol synthesis. Increased hepatic LDL receptor synthesis results in an increased rate of removal of LDL from the circulation and lower plasma cholesterol levels. The second class of drugs, HMG-CoA reductase inhibitors such as lovastatin and pravastatin, also lower plasma cholesterol by decreasing hepatic cholesterol pools and thereby increasing hepatic LDL receptor levels. They act by binding tightly to HMG-CoA reductase, thus inhibiting cholesterol biosynthesis. When combined, bile acid sequestrants and HMG-CoA reductase inhibitors work synergistically to increase LDL receptor activity and lower plasma cholesterol [*see Figure 5c*]. A somewhat different approach, which may provide future therapeutic strategies, is the development of drugs that can increase cellular LDL receptor activity either by directly stimulating the expression of the receptor's gene or perhaps by decreasing the normal degradation of receptors (half-life in cells is approximately 16 to 24 hours[21,22]).

Homozygous FH patients do not respond well to bile acid sequestrant and HMG-CoA reductase inhibitor treatment, because these patients have no functional LDL receptors to stimulate. Liver transplantation has been used to successfully restore hepatic LDL receptor activity in a homozygous FH patient, and LDL receptor gene therapy approaches are currently being developed [*see Chapter 7*].

Macrophage Scavenger Receptor

One of the earliest known stages of atherosclerotic plaque formation is the attachment of blood monocytes to the endothelium, followed by migration of the monocytes across the endothelium into the subendothelial space.[2,23-26] There the monocytes differentiate into macrophages, and, when hypercholesterolemia is present, the macrophages begin to accumulate massive amounts of lipoprotein cholesterol. The cholesterol is stored in the cytoplasm as cholesteryl ester–rich, foamlike fat droplets that give these cells their distinctive foamy microscopic appearance and their name, macrophage foam cells. As the plaque develops, vascular smooth muscle cells are stimulated to proliferate and are also converted into foam cells. Although the correlation of plasma LDL levels and atherosclerosis suggested the possibility that LDL receptors mediate the uptake of LDL cholesterol into macrophages, several lines of evidence indicate that the LDL receptor pathway is neither required for nor probably involved in cholesterol accumulation during foam cell development.[2,3,25] For example, in FH patients, plaque formation is accelerated despite the absence of LDL receptor activity. Also, cultured macrophages exhibit relatively low levels of LDL receptor activity, and the cholesterol feedback regulation of receptor activity prevents LDL receptor–mediated accumulation of massive amounts of cholesterol. Thus, one or more additional mechanisms for lipoprotein uptake by macrophages are required to account for plaque formation.

One of the most attractive models for lipoprotein/cholesterol accumulation in macrophages is the scavenger receptor model.[2,3,25,26] Macrophages, but not their monocyte precursors, express a receptor activity that mediates the endocytosis of chemically modified LDL and the consequent conversion of cultured macrophages into foamlike cells. One receptor responsible for this activity (there may be several) is called the macrophage scavenger receptor because of its distinctive ligand-binding properties.[2,7,27] Unlike LDL receptors, scavenger receptors are not inactivated by any known natural mutations; thus, their potential role in atherogenesis has not been established with certainty. Nevertheless, the identification of a scavenger receptor ligand, oxidized LDL (oxLDL), in plaques[25,28,29] and the discovery that the antioxidant probucol can inhibit plaque formation in an animal model of atherosclerosis[30,31] have focused attention on scavenger receptors in atherogenesis.

Distinctive Broad Ligand-Binding Specificity

Macrophage scavenger receptors are similar to other cell surface endocytic receptors in that they bind their ligands tightly (high-affinity binding); however, they differ markedly from most other well-characterized receptors in that they can bind a wide variety of different ligands.[2,7,25,27,32-37] Thus, they exhibit broad (or low) ligand specificity rather than the high specificity that is a hallmark of most receptors. Scavenger receptor ligands include certain types of (1) chemically modified proteins, such as acetylated LDL (acLDL) or oxLDL and maleylated bovine serum albumin, but not their unmodified counterparts, (2) four-stranded polyribonucleotides, including poly I and poly G, (3) natural and modified polysaccharides, such as carrageenin and dextran sulfate, and (4) other molecules, such as polyvinyl sulfate, asbestos, bacterial lipopolysaccharide (endotoxin), and lipoteichoic acid. Some of these ligands (e.g., acLDL and polyvinyl sulfate) do not occur naturally and are certainly not biologically relevant. They presumably bind to scavenger receptors because of the fortuitous similarity of their structures to those of physiologically relevant ligands such as oxLDL and endotoxin. The only obvious feature common to all of these molecules or macromolecular complexes is that they are polyanionic. However, many polyanions, including poly (D-glutamic acid), poly C, poly A, and chondroitin sulfate, are not ligands.[2] The broad, but circumscribed, binding specificity of scavenger receptors suggests that, in addition to their putative role in atherosclerosis, they probably participate in other macrophage functions.

Predicted Quaternary Structure

Biochemical and molecular genetic analysis has established that there are two trimeric isoforms of the class A macrophage scavenger receptors, designated type I and type II.[38-40] The genes for both forms have been cloned from bovine,[39,40] murine,[41,42] human,[43] and rabbit[44] cDNA libraries. Similar to the LDL receptor, the scavenger receptors are mosaics of six protein domains; however, there are no similarities in the sequences or classes of domains between LDL receptors and scavenger receptors [*see Figure 4*]. Scavenger receptors are predicted to form elongated homotrimeric integral membrane proteins. The subunits assemble into disulfide cross-linked trimers and are hydroxylated on proline and lysine and glycosylated in the endoplasmic reticulum of the cell before transport to the cell surface via the Golgi apparatus.[45] Each trimer comprises six distinctive protein domains: I, N-terminal cytoplasmic; II, transmembrane; III, spacer; IV, α-helical coiled coil (with two distinctive subdomains, IVa and IVb); V, collagenous; and VI, C-terminal. Type II scavenger receptors are identical to type I receptors, except for their C-terminals. There, the 110 amino acid, scavenger receptor cysteine-rich (SRCR) domain in type I receptors is replaced by a short (6 to 17 amino acid) C-terminal in the type II receptors.[40,42] Despite its truncated C-terminal, the type II receptor exhibits high ligand affinity and broad ligand-binding specificity similar to those of the type I receptor[40,46,47]; however, there are several key exceptions.[42] Thus, the SRCR domain is not required for the characteristic broad ligand specificity.

The presence of the SRCR domain at the extracellular C-terminal of the type I scavenger receptor was not surprising, because cell surface receptors often contain many different types of cysteine-rich domains, which have been classified into several families or superfamilies.[48,49] Examples of such domains include the EGF-like and complement C9–like domains in the LDL receptor and immunoglobulinlike domains. These domains can withstand the rigors of the extracellular environment, are well suited for a variety of biochemical activities, and are readily juxtaposed to other classes of domains for the assembly of complex mosaic proteins. Unexpectedly, the scavenger receptors' SRCR domains helped define a previously unrecognized, ancient, and highly conserved family of cysteine-rich protein domains.[26,41] At least eight classes of cell surface and secreted proteins containing from one to 11 SRCR domains per polypeptide chain have been described.[50] The cysteines in these SRCR domains apparently form intramolecular disulfide bonds that presumably participate in their folding and their stabilization. It seems likely that SRCR domains fold into globular structures; however, this has not yet been established experimentally. Most of the SRCR-containing mammalian proteins identified to date are associated directly or indirectly with the immune system and host defense, a finding reminiscent of the frequent appearance of immunogobulinlike domains in proteins of the immune system.[51,52]

All known type I and type II macrophage scavenger receptor ligands are polyanions, although not all polyanions are ligands. Site-specific mutagenesis and other experiments[53-55] provide strong support for the prediction that the positively charged collagenous domains of these receptors compose the receptors' ligand-binding sites and are both necessary and sufficient to impart their broad ligand-binding specificity. In addition, charge repulsion by at least some of the evolutionarily conserved negatively charged residues in the collagenous domains may play a key role in differentiating between polyanions that can bind and those that cannot.[7] In the type I and type II scavenger receptors, the collagenous domains apparently provide selectively sticky surfaces that function as a kind of molecular flypaper for the high-affinity binding of certain polyanions.[7,26] The macrophage scavenger receptors were the first integral membrane proteins containing a collagenous domain to be described.

Scavenger Receptor Functions

The broad, but circumscribed, binding specificity of macrophage scavenger receptors suggests that these receptors may participate in many functions in addition to their putative role in atherosclerosis.[7] Macrophages play a part in host defense and development and in the pathogenesis of several diseases.[56] A characteristic of macrophage function is the binding, internalization, and often lysis of many endogenous and foreign substances. These include pathogens, such as bacteria and protozoans and dying or dead cells that arise during development and aging.[56-58] Macrophages sometimes recognize pathogens as foreign because they have been coated by antibodies or complement. Macrophages can also directly recognize pathogens; such direct binding of foreign substances (nonself) is an important tool used to defend the body.[56,59]

It has been proposed that receptors with broad binding specificity might be used to discriminate directly between self and nonself and may have arisen early in the evolution of host defense systems.[59] Macrophage scavenger receptors may play such a role in host defense. For example, at least some bacterial cell surface components, including some forms of bacterial endotoxin (lipid IV_A and reLPS) and lipoteichoic acid bind to scavenger receptors, and endotoxin is cleared from the circulation in vivo by scavenger receptors.[37,42,60] Thus, scavenger receptors presumably help protect the body from endotoxin or lipoteichoic acid–induced shock during bacterial sepsis and may participate in the clearance of whole bacteria from tissues and the circulation. Scavenger receptors can also bind via their collagenous domains to crocidolite asbestos, raising the possibility that they may play a role in the physiologic and pathological interactions of inhaled asbestos and other particles with alveolar macrophages.[47] In addition, these receptors may participate in development,[58] and recent studies suggest that they may play a role in macrophage adhesion.[61]

Collagenous Domains and Host Defense

The distinctive binding properties of short collagenous domains may contribute not only to the potential host defense functions of scavenger receptors but also to the host defense functions of other proteins with such domains, including complement component C1q, the mannose binding protein, conglutinin, bovine serum lectin, and lung surfactant apoproteins A and D.[7,62,63] All of these proteins are thought to be involved in clearing the extracellular space of debris and pathogenic material. Indeed, the collagenous domain of C1q can bind a distinctive set of polyanions that is similar but not identical to the set of scavenger receptor ligands.[53] These proteins with specialized short collagenous domains define one of at least two broad functional categories of proteins containing collagenous domains: host defense collagens (D-collagens) and extracellular matrix (structural) collagens (S-collagens).[7,53]

D-collagens may have evolved to perform host defense functions before the development of the humoral immune system. In this regard, a novel class C, type I macrophage-specific scavenger receptor (SR-CI) has been reported in fruit fly (*Drosophila melanogaster*) embryonic macrophages.[58,64] The binding properties of SR-CI are strikingly similar to those of mammalian class A, type I and II scavenger receptors (SR-AI and SR-AII), but there are no primary sequence similarities between SR-A and SR-C (i.e., SR-C does not contain a collagenous domain).[64] The presence of scavenger receptors on mammalian and invertebrate macrophages suggests that this class of receptor mediates critical, well-conserved functions, possibly pattern recognition, and raises the possibility that they may have appeared early in the evolution of host defense mechanisms.[58] Because macrophages play an important role in the recognition of apototic cells during the course of development and aging,[57,58] it is possible that scavenger receptors may also be involved in this crucial developmental process. The application of the genetic techniques available in *Drosophila* should provide a powerful new approach for studying scavenger receptor function.

Other Scavenger Receptors

A third type of class A macrophage-specific scavenger receptor (SR-AIII, also known as MARCO), which comprises both collagenous and SRCR domains, was recently discovered and shown to bind to modified LDL and bacteria.[65] In addition to class A and class C scavenger receptors, a structurally distinct class of scavenger receptors, class B (SR-B), has been identified.[66,67] SR-Bs are members of the CD36 superfamily of proteins and include CD36 itself and SR-BI. They do not exhibit the broad polyanion binding specificity of class A and C receptors. Cultured endothelial cells and some endothelial cells in vivo exhibit scavengerlike receptors that differ from the type I and type II class A molecules,[44,68,69] and an Fc receptor, FcγRII-B2, has been shown to recognize oxLDL.[70] Two other groups of cell surface proteins with multiple ligand-binding properties that differ substantially from SR-A, SR-B, and SR-C are the LDL receptor–related protein (LRP)[71] and certain β_2 integrins.[72] These and additional cases of scavengerlike binding activities, which have been reported but not yet fully characterized, have recently been reviewed.[55,71]

Other Lipoprotein Receptors

In addition to the genes for the LDL and scavenger receptors, genes for two other lipoprotein receptors have been cloned. These are LRP,[71] a putative lipoprotein remnant receptor, and a VLDL receptor.[73] Both of these receptors are structurally related to the LDL receptor. Unexpectedly, the class B scavenger receptor SR-BI can bind native as well as modified LDL and is expressed primarily, but not exclusively, in fat tissue.[67] SR-BI may play a critical role in lipid metabolism. A detailed description of these receptors is beyond the scope of this chapter.

Conclusion

Tremendous strides have been made in identifying and characterizing lipoprotein receptors and their roles in lipid metabolism and atherosclerosis. Analysis of the LDL receptor pathway has provided key insights into both the regulation of LDL and cholesterol metabolism and the design of effective pharmacological therapies for hypercholesterolemia. Additional molecular, cellular, genetic, and pharmacological studies of lipoprotein receptors should continue to elucidate the mechanisms underlying atherosclerosis and provide new therapeutic and preventive approaches to this widespread and devastating disease. Analysis of the cell and molecular biology of the LDL receptor pathway has already led to breakthroughs in the treatment of hypercholesterolemia, and there are now high expectations for macrophage scavenger receptor studies as well.

References

1. Havel RJ, Kane, JP: Structure and metabolism of plasma lipoproteins. *The Metabolic Basis of Inherited Disease,* 6th ed. Scriver CR, Beaudet AL, Sly WS, Valle D, Eds. McGraw-Hill, New York, 1989, p 1129
2. Brown MS, Goldstein JL: Lipoprotein metabolism in the macrophage: implications for cholesterol deposition in atherosclerosis. *Annu Rev Biochem* 52:223, 1983
3. Goldstein JL, Brown MS: Familial hypercholesterolemia. *The Metabolic Basis of Inherited Disease,* 6th ed. Scriver CR, Beaudet AL, Sly WS, Valle D, Eds. McGraw-Hill, New York, 1989, p 1215
4. Zannis VI, Kardassis E, Zanni EE: Genetic mutations affecting human lipoproteins, their receptors and their enzymes. *Adv Hum Genet* 21:145, 1993
5. Goldstein JL, Brown MS, Anderson RG, et al: Receptor-mediated endocytosis: concepts emerging from the LDL receptor system. *Annu Rev Cell Biol* 1:1, 1985
6. Brown MS, Goldstein JL: How LDL receptors influence cholesterol and atherosclerosis. *Sci Am* 251:58, 1984
7. Krieger M, Acton S, Ashkenas J, et al: Molecular flypaper, host defense, and atherosclerosis: structure, binding properties, and functions of macrophage scavenger receptors. *J Biol Chem* 268:4569, 1993
8. Goldstein JL, Basu SK, Brown MS: Receptor-mediated endocytosis of low-density lipoprotein in cultured cells. *Methods Enzymol* 98:241, 1983
9. Yamamoto T, Davis CG, Brown MS, et al: The human LDL receptor: a cysteine-rich protein with multiple Alu sequences in its mRNA. *Cell* 39:27, 1984
10. Kingsley DM, Kozarsky KF, Hobbie L, Krieger M: Reversible defects in O-linked glycosylation and LDL receptor expression in a UDP-Gal/UDP-GalNAc 4-epimerase deficient mutant. *Cell* 44:749, 1986
11. Kozarsky K, Kingsley D, and Krieger M: Use of a mutant cell line to study the kinetics and function of O-linked glycosylation of low density lipoprotein receptors. *Proc Natl Acad Sci USA* 85:4335, 1988
12. Brown MS, Goldstein JL: A receptor-mediated pathway for cholesterol homeostasis. *Science* 232:34, 1986
13. Heiberg A: The risk of atherosclerotic vascular disease in subjects with xanthomatosis. *Acta Med Scand* 198:249, 1975
14. Hobbs HH, Russell DW, Brown MS, Goldstein JL: The LDL receptor locus in familial hypercholesterolemia: mutational analysis of a membrane protein. *Annu Rev Genet* 24:133, 1990
15. Tanzawa K, Shimada Y, Kuroda M, et al: WHHL-rabbit: a low density lipoprotein receptor-deficient animal model for familial hypercholesterolemia. *FEBS Lett* 118:81, 1980

16. Yamamoto T, Bishop RW, Brown MS, et al: Deletion in cysteine-rich region of LDL receptor impedes transport to cell surface in WHHL rabbit. *Science* 232:1230, 1986

17. Hummel M, Li ZG, Pfaffinger D, et al: Familial hypercholesterolemia in a rhesus monkey pedigree: molecular basis of low density lipoprotein receptor deficiency. *Proc Natl Acad Sci USA* 87:3122, 1990

18. Krieger M, Kingsley DM, Sege R, et al: Genetic analysis of receptor-mediated endocytosis.*Trends Biochem Sci* 10:447, 1985

19. Malmstrom K, Krieger M: Use of radiation suicide to isolate constitutive and temperature-sensitive conditional Chinese hamster ovary cell mutants with defects in the endocytosis of low density lipoprotein. *J Biol Chem* 266:24025, 1991

20. Hobbie L, Fisher A, Lee S, et al: Isolation of three classes of conditional-lethal Chinese hamster ovary cell mutants with temperature-dependent defects in LDL receptor stability and intracellular membrane transport. *J Biol Chem* 269:20958, 1994

21. Tolleshaug H, Goldstein JL, Schneider WJ, Brown MS: Posttranslational processing of the LDL receptor and its genetic disruption in familial hypercholesterolemia. *Cell* 30:715, 1982

22. Kozarsky KF, Brush HA, Krieger M: Unusual forms of low density lipoprotein receptors in hamster cell mutants with defects in the receptor structural gene. *J Cell Biol* 102:1567, 1986

23. Gerrity RG: The role of the monocyte in atherogenesis: I. Transition of blood-borne monocytes into foam cells in fatty lesions. *Am J Pathol* 103:181, 1981

24. Ross R: The pathogenesis of atherosclerosis an update. *N Eng J Med* 314:488, 1986

25. Steinberg D, Parthasarathy S, Carew TE, et al: Beyond cholesterol. Modifications of low-density lipoprotein that increase its atherogenecity. *N Engl J Med* 320:915, 1989

26. Krieger M: Molecular flypaper and atherosclerosis: structure of the macrophage scavenger receptor. *Trends Biochem Sci* 17:141, 1992

27. Goldstein JL, Ho YK, Basu SK, Brown MS: Binding site on macrophages that mediates uptake and degradation of acetylated low density lipoprotein, producing massive cholesterol deposition. *Proc Natl Acad Sci USA* 76:333, 1979

28. Haberland ME, Fong D, Cheng L: Malondialdehyde-altered protein occurs in atheroma of Watanabe heritable hyperlipidemic rabbits. *Science* 241:215, 1988

29. Yla HS, Rosenfeld ME, Parthasarathy S, et al: Gene expression in macrophage-rich human atherosclerotic lesions: 15-lipoxygenase and acetyl low density lipoprotein receptor messenger RNA colocalize with oxidation specific lipid-protein adducts. *J Clin Invest* 87:1146, 1991

30. Kita T, Nagano Y, Yokode M, et al: Probucol prevents the progression of atherosclerosis in Watanabe heritable hyperlipidemic rabbit, an animal model for familial hypercholesterolemia. *Proc Natl Acad Sci USA* 84:5928, 1987

31. Carew TE, Schwenke DC, Steinberg D: Antiatherogenic effect of probucol unrelated to its hypercholesterolemic effect: evidence that antioxidants in vivo can selectively inhibit low density lipoprotein degradation in macrophage-rich fatty streaks and slow the progression of atherosclerosis in the Watanabe heritable hyperlipidemic rabbit. *Proc Natl Acad Sci USA* 84:7725, 1987

32. Brown MS, Basu SK, Falck JR, et al: The scavenger cell pathway for lipoprotein degradation: specificity of the binding site that mediates the uptake of negatively-charged LDL by macrophages. *J Supramol Struct* 13:67, 1980

33. Haberland ME, Olch CL, Folgelman AM: Role of lysines in mediating interaction of modified low density lipoproteins with the scavenger receptor of human monocyte macrophages. *J Biol Chem* 259:11305, 1984

34. Kamps JA, Kruijt JK, Kuiper J, et al: Characterization of the interaction of acetylated LDL and oxidatively modified LDL with human liver parenchymal and Kupffer cells in culture. *Arterioscler Thromb* 12:1079, 1992

35. Steinbrecher UP, Parthasarathy S, Leake DS, et al: Modification of low density lipoprotein by endothelial cells involves lipid peroxidation and degradation of low density lipoprotein phospholipids. *Proc Natl Acad Sci USA* 81:3883, 1984

36. Pearson AM, Rich A, Krieger M: Polynucleotide binding to macrophage scavenger receptors depends on the formation of base-quartet-stabilized four-stranded helices. *J Biol Chem* 268:3546, 1993

37. Hampton RY, Golenbock DT, Penman M, et al: Recognition and plasma clearance of endotoxin by scavenger receptors. *Nature* 353:342, 1991

38. Kodama T, Reddy P, Kishimoto C, Krieger M: Purification and characterization of a bovine acetyl low density lipoprotein receptor. *Proc Natl Acad Sci U S A* 85:9238, 1988

39. Kodama T, Freeman M, Rohrer L, et al: Type I macrophage scavenger receptor contains alpha-helical and collagen-like coiled coils. *Nature* 343:531, 1990

40. Rohrer L, Freeman M, Kodama T, et al: Coiled-coil fibrous domains mediate ligand binding by macrophage scavenger receptor type II. *Nature* 343:570, 1990

41. Freeman M, Ashkenas J, Rees DJ, et al: An ancient, highly conserved family of cysteine-rich protein domains revealed by cloning type I and type II murine macrophage scavenger receptors. *Proc Natl Acad* Sci *USA* 87:8810, 1990

42. Ashkenas J, Pennman M, Vasile E, et al: Structure and high and low affinity ligand binding properties of murin type I and type II macrophage scavenger receptors. *J Lipid Res* 34:983, 1993

43. Matsumoto A, Naito M, Itakura H, et al: Human macrophage scavenger receptors: primary structure, expression, and localization in atherosclerotic lesions. *Proc Natl Acad Sci USA* 87:9133, 1990

44. Bickel PE, Freeman MW: Rabbit aortic smooth muscle cells express inducible macrophage scavenger receptor messenger RNA that is absent from endothelial cells. *J Clin Invest* 90:1450, 1992

45. Penman M, Lux A, Freedman NJ, et al: The type I and type II bovine scavenger receptors expressed in Chinese hamster ovary cells are trimeric proteins with collagenous triple helical domains comprising noncovalently associated monomers and Cys83-disulfide-linked dimers. *J Biol Chem* 266:23985, 1991

46. Freeman M, Ekkel Y, Rohrer L, et al: Expression of type I and type II bovine scavenger receptors in Chinese hamster ovary cells: lipid droplet accumulation and nonreciprocal cross competition by acetylated and oxidized low density lipoprotein. *Proc Natl Acad Sci USA* 88:4931, 1991

47. Resnick D, Freedman NJ, Xu S, Krieger M: Secreted extracellular domains of macrophage scavenger receptors form elongated trimers which specifically bind crocidolite asbestos. *J Biol Chem* 268:3538, 1993

48. Doolittle RF: The genealogy of some recently evolved vertebrate proteins. *Trends Biochem Sci* 10:233, 1985

49. Krieger M: The LDL receptor pathway. *Molecular Structures of Receptors*. Rossow PW, Strosberg AD, Eds. Ellis Herwood Ltd., New York, 1986, p 210

50. Resnick D, Pearson A, and Krieger M: The SRCR superfamily: a family reminiscent of the Ig superfamily. *Trends Biochem Sci* 19:5, 1994.

51. Hunkapiller T, Hood L: Diversity of the immunoglobulin gene superfamily. *Adv Immunol* 44:1, 1989

52. Williams AF, Barclay AN: The immunoglobulin superfamily domains for cell surface recognition. *Annu Rev Immunol* 6:381, 1988

53. Acton S, Resnick D, Freeman M, et al: The collagenous domains of macrophage scavenger receptors and complement component C1q mediate their similar, but not identical, binding specificities for polyanionic ligands. *J Biol Chem* 268:3530, 1993

54. Doi T, Higashino K, Kurihara Y, et al: Charged collagen structure mediates the recognition of negatively charged macromolecules by macrophage scavenger receptors. *J Biol Chem* 268:2126, 1993

55. Krieger M: Type I and type II macrophage scavenger receptors. *Lipoproteins in Health and Disease*. Betteridge DJ, Illingworth DR, Shepherd J, Eds. Edward Arnold, London (in press)

56. Gordon S, Perry VH, Rabinowitz S, et al: Plasma membrane receptors of the mononuclear phagocyte system. *J Cell Sci Suppl* 9:1, 1988

57. Abrams JM, White K, Fessler LI, Steller H: Programmed cell death during *Drosophila* embryogenesis. *Development* 117:29, 1993

58. Abrams JM, Lux A, Steller H, Krieger M: Macrophages in *Drosophila* embryos and L2 cells exhibit scavenger receptor-mediated endocytosis. *Proc Natl Acad Sci USA* 89:10375, 1992

59. Janeway CA: The immune system evolved to discriminate infectious nonself from noninfectious self. *Immunology Today* 13:11, 1992

60. Dunne DW, Resnick D, Greenberg J, et al: The type I macrophage scavenger receptor binds to Gram-positive bacteria and recognizes lipoteichoic acid. *Proc Natl Acad Sci USA* 91:1863, 1994

61. Fraser I, Hughes D, Gordon S: Divalent cation-independent macrophage adhesion inhibited by monoclonal antibody to murine scavenger receptor. *Nature* 364:43, 1993

62. Thiel S, Reid KBM: Structures and functions associated with the group of mammalian lectins containing collagen-like sequences. *FEBS Lett* 250:79, 1989

63. Sastry K, Ezekowitz RA: Collectins: pattern recognition molecules involved in first line host defense. *Curr Opin Immunol* 5:59, 1993

64. Pearson A, Lux A, Krieger M: Expression cloning of dSR-CI, a macrophage-specific scavenger receptor from *Drosophila melanogaster*. *Proc Natl Acad Sci USA* (in press)

65. Elomaa O, Kangas M, Sahlberg C, et al: Cloning of a novel bacteria-binding receptor structurally related to scavenger receptors and expressed in a subset of macrophages. *Cell* 80:603, 1995

66. Endemann G, Stanton LW, Madden KS, et al: CD36 is a receptor for oxidized low density lipoprotein. *J Biol Chem* 268:11811, 1993

67. Acton SL, Scherer PE, Lodish HF, et al: Expression cloning of SR-B1, a CD36-related class B scavenger receptor. *J Biol Chem* 269:21003, 1994

68. van Berkel TJ, De Rijke YB, Kruijt JK: Different fate in vivo of oxidatively modified low density lipoprotein and acetylated low density lipoprotein in rats: recognition by various scavenger receptors on Kupffer and endothelial liver cells. *J Biol Chem* 266:2282, 1991

69. Via D, Fanslow A, Dresel HA, et al: Identification and density dependent regulation of the Ac-LDL receptor in normal and transformed bovine aortic endothelial cells (BAEC) (abstract). *FASEB J* 6:A371, 1992

70. Stanton LW, White RT, Bryant CM, et al: A macrophage Fc receptor of IgG is also a receptor for oxidized low density lipoprotein. *J Biol Chem* 267:22446, 1992

71. Krieger M, Herz J: Structures and functions of multiligand lipoprotein receptors: macrophage scavenger receptors and LDL receptor-related protein (LRP). *Annu Rev Biochem* 63:601, 1994

72. Davis GG: The Mac-1 and p150,95 beta 2 integrins bind denatured proteins to mediate leukocyte cell-substrate adhesion. *Exp Cell Res* 200:242, 1992

73. Takahashi S, Kawarabayasi Y, Nakai T, et al: Rabbit very low density lipoprotein receptor: a low density lipoprotein receptor-like protein with distinct ligand specificity. *Proc Natl Acad Sci USA* 89:9252, 1992

Acknowledgments

I thank my many colleagues for their contributions to the work from our laboratory, which was supported by grants from the National Institutes of Health and Arris Pharmaceutical Corporation.

Figures 1, 5 Talar Agasyan. Adapted from "How LDL Receptors Influence Cholesterol and Atherosclerosis," by M. S. Brown, J. L. Goldstein, in *Scientific American* 251:58, 1984 with the advice of J. Chatterton. Used by permission.

Figures 2, 4 Talar Agasyan, Tom Moore. Adapted from "Familial Hypercholesterolemia," by J. L. Goldstein, M. S. Brown, A. L. Beaudet, W.S. Sly, D. Valle. McGraw-Hill, New York, 1989 and "Molecular Flypaper, Host Defense, and Atherosclerosis: Structure, Binding Properties, and Functions of Macrophage Scavenger Receptors," by M. Krieger, S. Acton, J. Ashkenas, et al, in *Journal of Biological Chemistry* 268:4569, 1993. Used by permission.

Figure 3 Dana Burns-Pizer.

Table 1 Adapted from "Structure and Metabolism of Plasma Lipoproteins," by R. J. Havel, J.P. Kane, in *The Metabolic Basis of Inherited Disease*, 6th ed., edited by C. R. Scriver, A. L. Beaudet, W. S. Sly, D. Valle. McGraw-Hill, New York, 1989; and "Genetic Mutations Affecting Human Lipoproteins, Their Receptors and Their Enzymes 145-319," by V. I. Zannis, E. Kardassis, E. E. Zanni, in *Advances in Human Genetics* 21:145, 1993. Used by permission.

CHAPTER 4

Vascular Endothelium in Health and Disease

Michael A. Gimbrone, Jr., M.D.

The entire circulatory system is lined by a continuous, single-cell-thick layer—the vascular endothelium. For more than a century, pathologists have noted its involvement in cardiovascular disease processes such as atherosclerosis,[1] but a working knowledge of the underlying mechanisms has been developed only recently, largely through the application of modern cellular and molecular biologic techniques.[2] We now appreciate that this microscopic membrane is, in fact, a multifunctional organ, the health of which is essential to normal vascular physiology and the dysfunction of which can be a critical factor in the pathogenesis of vascular disease.[3-7]

In health, vascular endothelium comprises a container for blood and forms the biologic interface between circulating blood elements and all of the various tissues of the body. It is strategically situated to monitor systemic as well as locally generated stimuli and to alter its own functional state adaptively. This adaptive process typically proceeds without notice, contributing to normal homeostasis. However, nonadaptive changes in endothelial structure and function, provoked by pathophysiological stimuli, can result in localized, acute and chronic alterations in the interactions with the cellular and macromolecular components of circulating blood and the blood vessel wall. These alterations include enhanced permeability to (and subsequent oxidative modification of) plasma lipoproteins, hyperadhesiveness for blood leukocytes, and functional imbalances in local pro- and antithrombotic factors, growth stimulators and inhibitors, and vasoactive (dilator, constrictor) substances. These manifestations, collectively termed *endothelial dysfunction*, play an important role in the initiation, progression,

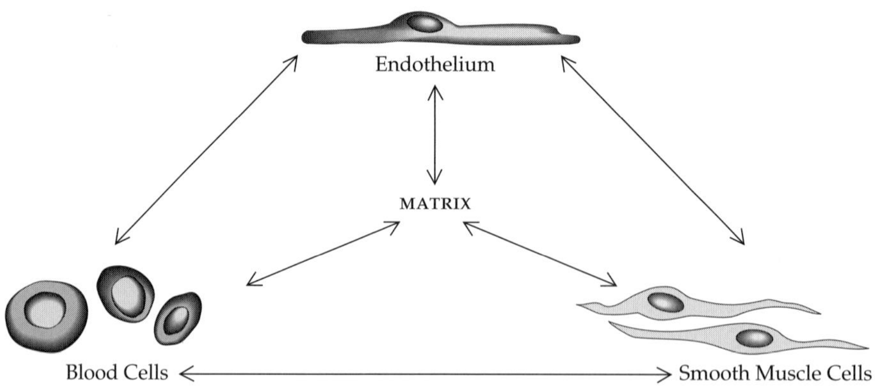

Figure 1 *A conceptual schematic of the multiple, reciprocal interactions that can occur among endothelium, smooth muscle, and blood cells and the potential modulating influence of the extracellular matrix.*

and clinical complications of various inflammatory and degenerative vascular diseases.

This chapter highlights recent progress in our understanding of the roles of vascular endothelium in the pathogenesis of atherosclerotic lesions, as well as their thrombotic, inflammatory, and vasospastic complications. It also discusses how insights gained from basic research in endothelial biology may help direct the development of novel diagnostic and therapeutic strategies in coronary artery disease.

Organization of the Vascular Endothelium

Because of its anatomic location, vascular endothelium is a biologically significant interface: it defines intra- and extravascular compartments, serves as a selectively permeable barrier, and provides a continuous nonthrombogenic lining for the cardiovascular system. Its location is also a key factor in its dynamic, reciprocal interactions with other cells, both in the circulating blood and within the vessel wall [*see Figure 1*]. Thus, endothelial cells, situated at the vessel wall–blood interface, can speak outward to platelets and leukocytes or inward to smooth muscle cells. This intercellular communication can occur at close range (e.g., via endothelium-derived vasorelaxor substances acting on adjacent vascular smooth muscle cells) or at a distance (e.g., endothelium-derived colony-stimulating factors acting on hematopoietic precursors in the bone marrow). In addition, each of the cellular components in these interactions may be subject to modulating influences exerted by extracellular matrix components, many of which are biosynthesized by vascular endothelium. Another functionally important consequence of endothelium's location is its ability to monitor, integrate and transduce bloodborne signals, thus making it a form of sensory organ. As detailed later in this chapter, this property extends beyond the realm of soluble stimuli (e.g., hormones, cytokines, and bacterial products) to the biotransduction of various types of mechanical forces generated by pulsatile blood flow (e.g., fluid shear stresses, wall tension, and intraluminal pressure).

A second important aspect of the structural organization of endothelium is its broad luminal surface area. Endothelium is the body's most extensive simple epithelium, its aggregate area totaling several thousand square meters.[8] This essentially continuous expanse of living cell membrane can function as a vast solid-phase reactor, a highly selective affinity chromatography column, or a relatively nonspecific adsorptive sponge. These surface-related activities are especially enhanced in the microcirculation, where the ratio of the surface of the endothelial container to the volume of contained blood reaches a maximum. The realization that the walls of this in vivo blood container can actively participate in the biochemical reactions of blood constituents represents a significant conceptual advance.[9] Equally important, from the pathophysiological standpoint, is that the key surface-related functions of vascular endothelium can be dynamically modulated, thus making the luminal endothelial surface a locus of physiologic regulation and pathological alteration.[10]

Another relevant aspect of endothelial organization is its regional specialization. Despite its apparent morphological simplicity and relative homogeneity, there is increasing evidence that the vascular endothelial lining does exhibit site-to-site variations that may have important physiologic and pathophysiological implications. These differences are manifested in properties such as permeability to macromolecules, secretion of biosynthetic products, and responsiveness to various exogenous stimuli.[11] Interestingly, the question of regional specializations extends down to the level of the individual endothelial cell. For example, ultrastructural techniques have demonstrated the existence of so-called microdomains in the luminal surface membrane of endothelial cells that appear to have characteristic patterns in different tissues.[5] In addition, despite its thin configuration, each vascular endothelial cell appears to have a clearly definable apical or luminal surface, which faces the bloodstream, and a basal or abluminal surface, which contacts the subendothelial connective tissues, each outfitted with its own distinct complement of intrinsic proteins.[12]

Taken together, these basic principles of endothelial organization—its interface location, dynamic surface properties, and regional specializations—have important implications for the vital functions of this tissue in health and disease.

Vital Functions of Endothelium: Dynamic Balances

Prothrombotic-Antithrombotic Balance

Blood normally does not clot inside its endothelial container. This failure of endothelium to activate the coagulation cascade, or to promote platelet adhesion, has been termed nonthrombogenicity. For many years, this vital function was considered simply a passive form of insulation, attributable to ill-defined physicochemical properties of the luminal endothelial surface. With the discovery that the vascular wall and, in particular, endothelial cells[13,14] could synthesize a unique arachidonate metabolite prostacyclin (PGI_2), which proved to be an extraordinarily potent inhibitor of platelet aggregation, a more active antithrombotic role for endothelium became apparent. In addition to its major influence on platelet function, endothelium also plays a pivotal role in the coagulation and fibrinolytic systems.[4] Many of these functions appear to be antithrombotic. For example, several of the body's natural anticoagulant mechanisms,[15,16] including the heparin-antithrombin, protein C–thrombomodulin, and tissue plasminogen activator mechanisms, are endothelium associated. The molecular components of these antithrombotic mechanisms are considered in Chapter 8 and Chapter 11.

In contrast to its antithrombotic functions, the endothelial cell also appears capable of active prothrombotic behavior. It synthesizes adhesive cofactors for platelets, such as von Willebrand factor, fibronectin, and thrombospondin; it synthesizes clotting factors, such as factor V; and it can be activated by various pathophysiological stimuli to express tissue factor, a trigger for the fibrin-generating coagulation cascade.[17] The endothelial cell also generates an inhibitor of the fibrinolytic pathway (plasminogen activator inhibitor–1), which can reduce the rate of fibrin breakdown.

Thus, the endothelial cell appears capable of playing multiple roles, both prothrombotic and antithrombotic, that are relevant to the maintenance of normal blood fluidity, stopping hemorrhage at sites of vascular injury, and pathological thrombosis. These endothelium-dependent mechanisms contribute to a dynamic physiologic antagonism, or balance, that can significantly influence the status of local hemostatic activity [*see Figure 2*].

Vasoconstrictor-Vasodilator Balance

The maintenance of cardiovascular tone traditionally has been viewed as a function of the vascular smooth muscle cell, responding primarily to sympathetic and parasympathetic nerve stimulation or to circulating hormones (e.g., products of the renin-angiotensin system). In 1980, the discovery by Furchgott and Zawadzki[18] of a potent endothelium-derived relaxing factor (EDRF) pointed to a significant role for the endothelial cell in the local regulation of vascular tone. The elucidation of the chemical nature of EDRF as endogenous nitric oxide, its metabolic pathway of generation via one or more nitric oxide synthases, and the cellular mechanisms of its action that result in vasodilation has added a new dimension to our understanding of the role of cell-cell interactions in the regulation of vascular functions.[19] Together with prostacyclin, which also has a potent vasorelaxor effect (via different mechanisms of generation and target cell action), nitric oxide and other related

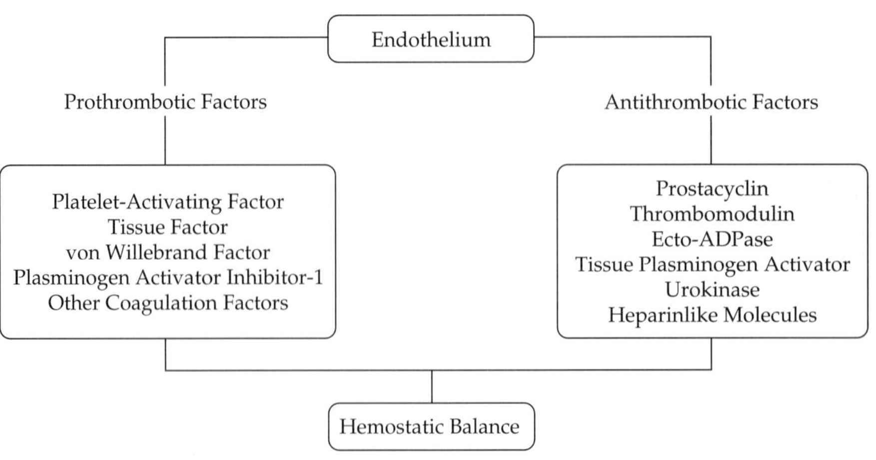

Figure 2 *Various endothelium-derived prothrombotic and antithrombotic factors and functions contribute to a dynamic physiologic antagonism that determines the prothrombotic-antithrombotic balance.*

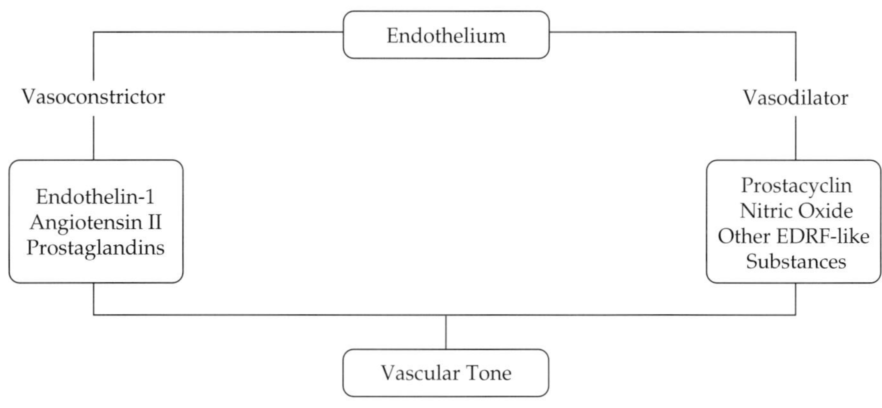

Figure 3 *Various endothelium-generated vasoconstrictors and vasodilators contribute to the local regulation of vascular tone through their effects on smooth muscle contractility.*

compounds constitute a class of natural endothelium-derived antihypertensive substances.

Balancing the action of these endothelium-derived vasorelaxors are various endothelium-derived substances that have vasoconstrictor activity [*see Figure 3*]. These substances include angiotensin II, generated at the luminal endothelial surface by angiotensin-converting enzyme; platelet-derived growth factor, which is secreted by endothelial cells and can act as a smooth muscle contractile agonist; and the novel vasoconstrictor substance endothelin-1.[20-22] The 18-amino-acid endothelin-1 peptide is generated by the proteolytic cleavage of a larger precursor, so-called big endothelin, and resembles the lethal toxin in the venom of certain snakes whose bite can induce coronary vasospasm. Endothelin-1 is reported to be the most potent endogenous vasoconstrictor known.[22] Understanding the production of these endothelium-derived vasoconstrictor substances and their mechanisms of target cell action may help elucidate the normal regulation of vascular tone, as well as suggest new strategies for antihypertensive therapies.

Endothelial Dysfunction: Stimuli and Consequences

Early interest in the endothelium's role in vascular diseases such as atherosclerosis was focused on morphologically detectable forms of cell damage, such as surface blebbing, intercellular gaps, and frank desquamation.[23] These physical alterations in the endothelial lining were envisioned as necessary precursors for platelet and leukocyte interaction with the vessel wall, as the initial step in a response-to-injury process—an adaptive response the pathologic extension of which could result in vascular disease.[24] With the appreciation that the endothelial cell is a dynamic, interactive element that supports multiple vital functions, it became apparent that the functional status of the vascular lining may be as important as its anatomic integrity. The term endothelial dysfunction was introduced to connote phenotypic modulation in response to a nonadaptive functional state.[6] This modulation might entail the loss of nonthrombogenic surface properties (as manifested by increased platelet adherence and/or triggering of intrinsic or extrinsic coagulation pathways) or a serious imbalance between endothelium-dependent procoagulant and anticoagulant mechanisms. The result conceivably could be manifested as an acute, localized thrombotic event, a more chronic thrombotic tendency, or disease of the vessel wall itself (as in atherosclerosis).[4] Other manifestations of endothelial dysfunction might involve decreased production of vasorelaxor substances, such as EDRF, with a resultant vasospastic tendency as is observed in diseases such as atherosclerosis, hypertension, and diabetes.[21] Another pathophysiologically important change in endothelial phenotype is its modulation to a proinflammatory state, with upregulation of cell surface adhesion molecules and chemoattractant factors that promote leukocyte recruitment and activation.[25] These molecular changes are directly relevant to acute and chronic inflammatory processes, immunologic reactions, and atherogenesis.

Various stimuli of endothelial dysfunction have been identified, including immunoregulatory substances such as tumor necrosis factor and interleukin-1, viral infection and transformation, bacterial toxins, cholesterol, and oxidatively modified lipoprotein.[7] At a molecular level, perhaps the best studied paradigm is the activation of endothelial cells by inflammatory cytokines, such as tumor necrosis factor and interleukin-1, and bacterial products, such as lipopolysaccharide (endotoxin).[26,27] This process involves a coordinated sequence of events, initiated by cell surface receptor activation, that culminates in a pattern of gene expression that typically is characteristic for a particular cytokine or mixture of cytokines. At the level of the nucleus, a number of these stimuli converge into final common pathways of transcriptional regulatory factors, such as the endothelial nuclear factor-κB system.[28]

In addition to these soluble cytokine stimuli, biomechanical forces generated by the pulsatile flow of blood through the branched arterial tree, such as oscillating wall shear stresses and cyclic stretching, can also influence endothelial functions.[29] Certain of these biomechanically induced effects appear to involve the modulation of endothelial gene expression at the transcriptional level. Recently, a shear stress response element was discovered in the platelet-derived growth factor (PDGF) B-chain gene that appears to be involved in these processes. This *cis*-acting transcriptional element was shown by deletion analysis to be necessary for shear-induced activation of the PDGF B-chain gene and, interestingly, is also present in the promoters of several other shear-inducible endothelial genes.[30] Experimental analysis of the transduction mechanisms that link externally applied forces to genetic regulatory events within the nucleus may provide new insights into the endothelial activation process. The ability to interrupt, block, or pharmacologically antagonize the various activation cascades involved in mediating the response of endothelium to both biochemical and biophysical stimuli offers exciting new opportunities for therapeutic interventions in vascular disease.

Endothelium-Dependent Mechanisms of Leukocyte Recruitment in Atherogenesis

Discovery of an Athero-ELAM

Perhaps the earliest morphologically detectable cellular event in atherogenesis is the adherence of circulating blood monocytes to the intact endothelial surface of large arteries.[31-33] These adherent cells then migrate across the endothelium into the intima, where they tend to accumulate, undergo limited replication, and become transformed into lipid-laden foam cells. Once present in the intima, in addition to accumulating cholesterol esters (the lipid hallmark of the early fatty streak lesion), this differentiating monocyte/macrophage population can promote lesion progression through the local generation of cytokines (e.g., interleukin-1 or tumor necrosis factor); growth factors (e.g., PDGF, fibroblast growth factor, or heparin-binding epidermal growth factor–like growth factor), various procoagulant and fibrinolytic components; eicosanoids; and toxic oxygen products.[2] Recently, considerable attention has also been focused on the presence, in more developed lesions, of T cells that have the capacity to generate other cytokines (e.g., interferon gamma or interleukin-4), through both immune- and nonimmune-triggered pathways. These cell-derived products add further complexity to the local cytokine milieu and the potential activation states of vessel wall cells (endothelium and smooth muscle) and other components of the developing atherosclerotic lesion.[34]

The localized, leukocyte-selective nature of this mononuclear cell recruitment process suggests that endothelium-dependent adhesion mechanisms analogous to those recently described in acute and chronic inflammation might be responsible.[35] This observation led to a working hypothesis, first suggested by M. I. Cybulsky and me,[36] that these localized mononuclear leukocyte–endothelium interactions reflect specific molecular changes in the adhesive properties of the endothelial surface, involving inducible endothelial-leukocyte adhesion molecules (ELAMs) expressed in atherosclerotic lesions (athero-ELAMs). According to this hypothesis, a candidate athero-ELAM should (1) support mononuclear (but not necessarily polymorphonuclear) leukocyte adhesion, (2) be inducibly expressed on the endothelial surface, and (3) be detectable in early atherosclerotic lesions (or in areas with a predilection for developing lesions).

The experimental search for molecules satisfying these criteria was undertaken in the rabbit, a species in which dietary and genetic models of atherosclerosis are well described.[36] Initially, leukocyte-endothelium interactions were examined in vitro, with cultured normal endothelial cells from rabbit aorta. Treatment of these endothelial cell monolayers with the nonspecific activator bacterial endotoxin resulted in a hyperadhesive surface change that was detectable on incubation with blood monocytes and monocytelike cell lines. This change in endothelial surface adhesion was dependent on protein synthesis and was detectable after a lag of one to two hours, reached a maximum within six to 12 hours, and then remained manifest for at least 96 hours. Murine monoclonal antibodies produced to these endotoxin-activated rabbit endothelial cells detected various inducible surface antigens. Some of these antigens exhibited a temporal profile similar to that of the adhesive endothelial surface change for blood leukocytes. In adhesion assays, pretreatment of activated endothelial cell monolayers with saturating concentrations of one of these monoclonal antibodies, designated Rb1/9, significantly inhibited mononuclear leukocyte attachment. Comparative studies with different types of blood leukocytes showed that this inhibition was selective for mononuclear, but not polymorphonuclear, leukocyte attach-

Table 1 Adhesion Molecules Implicated in Mononuclear Leukocyte Interactions with Activated Vascular Endothelium

*Molecule**	*Type*	*Ligand*	*Function*
L-selectin ligand	?Mucinlike glycoprotein	L-selectin (CD62L)	Rolling
P-selectin (CD62P)	Selectin family	Sialyl-Lewis^{x} (CD15s); others	Rolling
E-selectin (CD62E)	Selectin family	Sialyl-Lewis^{x} (CD15s); others	Rolling
VCAM-1 (CD106)	Immunoglobulin family	VLA-4 (CD49d/CD29)	Stable arrest
ICAM-1 (CD54)	Immunoglobulin family	LFA1; Mac-1 (CD11a,b/CD18)	Spreading
PECAM-1 (CD31)	Immunoglobulin family	PECAM-1 (CD31)	Transmigration

*Standardized international nomenclature indicated in parentheses.

ment. These in vitro studies thus identified an inducible molecule that could selectively support mononuclear leukocyte adhesion to activated arterial endothelial cells, thereby satisfying two of the experimental criteria for an athero-ELAM.

The expression of this inducible, mononuclear-leukocyte-selective adhesion molecule was then examined during experimental atherogenesis.[36] In rabbits fed a one percent cholesterol diet and in Watanabe heritable hyperlipidemic (WHHL) rabbits, which are congenitally deficient in low-density lipoprotein (LDL) receptors and have severe hypercholesterolemia [*see also Chapter 2, Chapter 3, and Chapter 7*], specific immunohistochemical staining with monoclonal antibody Rb1/9 was localized to aortic endothelium covering foam cell–rich intimal lesions. Staining was also evident at various stages of lesion development, ranging from focal regions with very small intimal accumulations of foam cells to near-circumferential lesions with abundant foam cells. Often, staining extended beyond the edges of intimal lesions; however, in the same hypercholesterolemic animals, endothelium in adjacent, uninvolved regions of the aorta did not stain. These in vivo immunohistochemical observations thus satisfied the third experimental criterion for an athero-ELAM, its expression by endothelium during early lesion formation and progression.

Characterization of the Athero-ELAM

Molecular characterization of this rabbit athero-ELAM, through a combination of immunochemical and molecular cloning approaches, revealed its homology to a human leukocyte adhesion molecule, intercellular adhesion molecule-110 (INCAM-110).This molecule was previously identified as an inducible endothelial receptor for lymphocytes[37] and was expression cloned from a cytokine-induced endothelial library as vascular cell adhesion molecule-1 (VCAM-1)[38] [*see Table 1*].[39] This cytokine-activated gene is a member of the immunoglobulin superfamily and is expressed on the surface of human and rabbit vascular endothelium in at least two molecular forms, presumably derived by alternative splicing.[40] Both forms can interact with a heterodimeric integrin receptor, termed very late antigen-4 (VLA-4) or $\alpha_4\beta_1$, a member of the β_1 subfamily of integrins which is differentially expressed on certain leukocytes, including blood monocytes and lymphocytes, but not on polymorphonuclear leukocytes.[41,42] This matching of endothelium-expressed VCAM-1 with mononuclear leukocyte-expressed VLA-4 therefore provides a functional ligand-receptor pair that can mediate a selective adhesion event [*see Figure 4*].

Interestingly, when the rabbit aorta in a dietary model of atherogenesis is carefully examined,[43] endothelial expression of VCAM-1 is detectable before mononuclear leukocyte recruitment into the arterial wall. Because one of the earliest changes during atherogenesis in cholesterol-fed animal models appears to be the focal accumulation and oxidative modification of LDL in the intima,[44,45] it is reasonable to hypothesize that oxidatively modified LDL, or one of its components, might be an initial stimulus for VCAM-1 induction in this setting. Recent in vitro studies with lysophosphatidylcholine, a component of oxidized LDL (and β-VLDL, another atherogenic lipoprotein in the rabbit), have shown that this material can selectively upregulate VCAM-1 expression in rabbit aortic endothelial cells.[46] Conceivably, this phospholipid could act alone or in combination with cytokines generated locally by activated vessel wall cells or migrating leukocytes to upregulate ELAMs and thus contribute to localized mononuclear leukocyte recruitment.

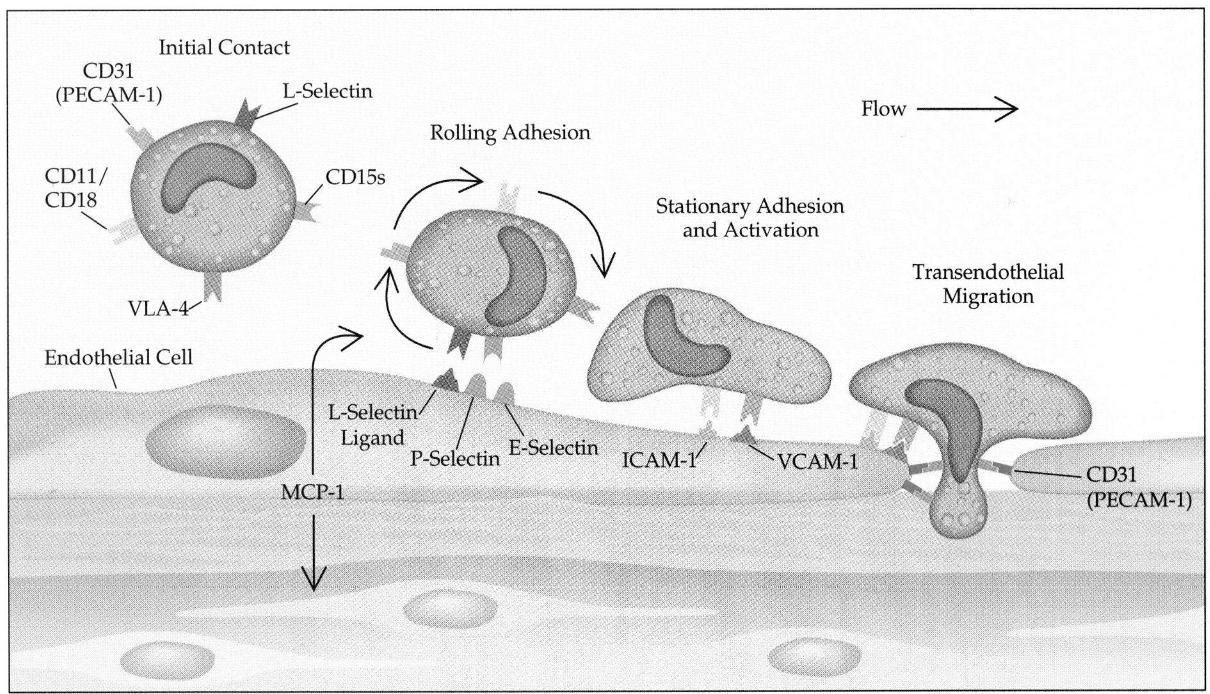

Figure 4 *In the current working concept of circulating blood mononuclear leukocyte adhesion to activated vascular endothelium, a multistep process is thought to involve the sequential interaction of different classes of adhesion receptors with their respective ligands, as well as the localized secretion of chemoattractant substances, such as monocyte chemoattractant protein-1 (MCP-1).*

In addition to an adhesive interaction between VCAM-1 and VLA-4, other endothelium-dependent mechanisms are also potentially relevant to mononuclear leukocyte (monocyte, lymphocyte) recruitment in atherogenesis [*see Figure 4 and Table 1*]. These include: intercellular adhesion molecule–1 (ICAM-1), a widely expressed member of the immunoglobulin superfamily that is also upregulated in vascular endothelium as a chronic ELAM (delayed, prolonged expression) and can interact with various components of the CD11/CD18 integrin complex[17]; P-selectin and E-selectin, acute ELAMs (rapid, transient expression) that can interact with sialyl-Lewis^x (CD15s) and related carbohydrate ligands[47,48]; and an inducible endothelial receptor for L-selectin (LAM-1), a ligand constitutively present on blood leukocyte surfaces.[49] Interestingly, although all of these receptor-ligand pairs have been implicated in monocyte-endothelium adhesion, only VCAM-1–VLA-4 has the potential to mediate mononuclear leukocyte, but not polymorphonuclear leukocyte, interactions. In addition, PECAM-1 (CD31), an adhesion molecule expressed by endothelial cells near their intercellular junctions, appears to interact in a homotypic fashion with the same molecule expressed on circulating mononuclear leukocytes, facilitating their penetration into the intima. Two other cytokine-induced, secretory products of endothelium also appear to be involved. Monocyte chemoattractant protein–1 (MCP-1), a monocyte-selective chemoattractant, has been implicated in endothelial transmigration by monocytes,[50] and macrophage-colony stimulating factor (M-CSF), a cytokine, can promote activation and maturation of monocytes and macrophages.[51] Recent immunohistochemical studies have localized the expression of these molecules at various stages of development of atherosclerotic lesions in experimental animals and, in some instances, in humans.[52-55] The relative contributions of these various mechanisms of leukocyte recruitment to the atherogenic process constitute an important area of ongoing study that has pathogenic as well as therapeutic implications.

Pathophysiological Implications and Potential Clinical Applications of the Athero-ELAM

The identification of an inducible mononuclear leukocyte–selective adhesion molecule (i.e., VCAM-1) that is expressed in developing atherosclerotic lesions in the hypercholesterolemic rabbit has several conceptual as well as practical implications. First, its observation provides evidence that endothelial activation/dysfunction is occurring early in the atherosclerotic process. It suggests that the net balance of local pathophysiological stimuli has elicited a pattern of response in the endothelium that is manifested by this change in surface phenotype. Second, endothelial VCAM-1 selectively interacting with its leukocyte ligand, VLA-4, is a molecular event in mononuclear leukocyte recruitment that may be susceptible to some form of anti-adhesion therapeutic intervention. Such therapy might take the form of a low-molecular-weight adhesion receptor blocker or a molecular genetic strategy targeted on the transcriptional or translational expression of endothelial VCAM-1. Third, characterization of the expression of VCAM-1 or other athero-ELAMs in human atherosclerotic lesions may provide novel markers for the early stages of this complex disease process, potentially of use in both diagnosis and treatment. These markers could find clinical applications in (1) noninvasive imaging of early lesions via labeled monoclonal antibodies, (2) differential analysis of the pattern of endothelial activation antigens as an indicator of the stage of underlying vessel wall disease, and (3) selective targeting to early atherosclerotic lesions of a conventional therapeutic agent or specifically engineered genetic construct for gene therapy. Clearly, the successful application of such diagnostic and therapeutic strategies will require better understanding of the basic mechanisms of endothelial activation in the context of human atherosclerotic vascular disease.

Vascular Endothelium as an Integrator of the Local Pathophysiological Milieu

As the examples in this chapter illustrate, the endothelial lining of the cardiovascular system is a dynamically mutable interface that can exhibit a spectrum of adaptive changes. Indeed, various members of its vast repertoire of autacoids, growth factors, and vasoactive, hemostatic, and fibrinolytic substances often contribute to agonist-antagonist balances that have important implications for the function of the vascular lining, adjacent vascular cells, and interacting blood constituents. By virtue of its unique anatomic position, the endothelium also plays an important role in the local transduction and integration of diverse biologic stimuli, including circulating hormones and bacterial products, locally generated cytokines, and even biomechanical forces. Thus, in an important sense, the phenotype of an endothelial cell is a reflection of the local pathophysiological milieu. As our knowledge of the stimuli and consequences of dysfunctional endothelial phenotypes increases, so will our working concepts of the pathogenesis of atherosclerosis. Hopefully, this insight will provide a rational basis for innovative diagnostic and therapeutic interventions in human coronary artery disease in the near future.

References

1. Virchow R: Der ateromatose Prozess der Arterien. *Wien Med Wochenschr* 6:825, 1856
2. Ross R: The pathogenesis of atherosclerosis: a perspective for the 1990's. *Nature* 362:801, 1993
3. Gimbrone MA Jr: Culture of vascular endothelium. *Prog Hemost Thromb* 3:1, 1976
4. Gimbrone MA Jr, Ed. *Vascular Endothelium in Hemostasis and Thrombosis*: Churchill Livingstone, Edinburgh, 1986
5. Simionescu N, Simionescu M, Eds. *Endothelial Cell Biology in Health and Disease*. Plenum Press, New York, 1988
6. Gimbrone MA Jr: Endothelial dysfunction and atherosclerosis. *J Card Surg* 4:180, 1989
7. Simionescu N, Simionescu M, Eds: *Endothelial Cell Dysfunctions*. Plenum Press, New York, 1992
8. Krogh A: *The Anatomy and Physiology of Capillaries*. Yale University Press, New Haven, 1929, p 22
9. Gimbrone MA Jr. Vascular endothelium: nature's blood-compatible container. *Ann NY Acad Sci* 516:5,1987
10. Bevilacqua MP, Gimbrone MA Jr: Inducible endothelial functions in inflammation and coagulation. *Semin Thromb Hemost* 13:425, 1987
11. Fishman AP: Endothelium: a distributed organ of diverse capabilities. *Ann NY Acad Sci* 401:1,1982

12. Muller WA, Gimbrone MA Jr: Plasmalemmal proteins of cultured vascular endothelial cells exhibit apical-based polarity: analysis by surface-selective iodination. *J Cell Biol* 103:2389, 1986
13. Moncada S, Herman AG, Higgs EA, et al: Differential formation of prostacyclin (PGX or PGI_2) by layers of the arterial wall. *Thromb Res* 11:323, 1977
14. Weksler BB, Marcus AJ, Jaff EA: Synthesis of prostaglandin I_2 (prostacyclin) by cultured human and bovine endothelial cells. *Proc Natl Acad Sci USA* 74:3922, 1977
15. Rosenberg RD, Rosenberg JS: Natural anticoagulant mechanisms. *J Clin Invest* 74:1, 1984
16. Esmon CT: The regulation of natural anticoagulant pathways. *Science* 235:1348, 1987
17. Bevilacqua MP, Pober JS, Wheeler ME, et al: Interleukin 1 (IL-1) activation of vascular endothelium: effects on procoagulant activity and leukoctye adhesion. *Am J Pathol* 121:394, 1985
18. Furchgott RF, Zawadzki JV: The obligatory role of endothelial cells in the relaxation of arterial smooth muscle by acetylcholine. *Nature* 288:373, 1980
19. Dinerman JL, Lowenstein CJ, Snyder SH: Molecular mechanisms of nitric oxide regulation: potential relevance to cardiovascular disease. *Circ Res* 73:217, 1993
20. Berk BC, Alexander RW, Brock TA, et al: Vasoconstriction: a new activity for platelet-derived growth factor. *Science* 232:87, 1986
21. Luscher TF, Vanhouette PM: *The Endothelium: Modulator of Cardiovascular Function.* Boca Raton, FL, CRC Press, 1990, p 1
22. Masaki T: Role of endothelin in mechanisms of local blood pressure control. *J Hypertens* 8(suppl 7):S107, 1990
23. French JE: Atherosclerosis in relation to the structure and function of the arterial intima, with special reference to the endothelium. *Int Rev Exp Pathol* 5:253, 1966
24. Ross R: Atherosclerosis: a defense mechanism gone awry (Rous-Whipple Award Lecture). *Am J Pathol* 143:987, 1993
25. Cybulsky MI, Gimbrone MA Jr: Endothelial leukocyte adhesion molecules in acute inflammation and atherogenesis. *Endothelial Cell Dysfunctions.* Simionescu N, Simionescu M, Eds. Plenum Press, New York, 1992, p 129
26. Pober JS: Cytokine-mediated activation of vascular endolethium: physiology and pathology. *Am J Pathol* 133:426, 1988
27. Pober JS, Cotran RC: Cytokines and endothelial cell biology. *Physiol Rev* 70:427, 1990
28. Collins TC: Endothelial nuclear factor-κB and the initiation of the atherosclerotic lesion. *Lab Invest* 68:499, 1993
29. Davies PF, Tripathi SC: Mechanical stress mechanisms and the cell: an endothelial paradigm. *Circ Res* 72:239, 1993
30. Resnick N, Collins T, Atkinson W, et al: Platelet-derived growth factor B chain promoter contains a *cis*-acting fluid shear-stress-responsive element. *Proc Natl Acad Sci USA* 90:4591, 1993
31. Gerrity RG, Naito HK, Richardson M, et al: Dietary induced atherogenesis in swine. *Am J Pathol* 113:341, 1979
32. Joris T, Nunnari JJ, Krolikowski FJ, et al: Studies on the pathogenesis of atherosclerosis: I. Adhesion and emigration of mononuclear cells in the aorta of hypercholesterolemic rats. *Am J Pathol* 113:341, 1993
33. Faggiotto A, Ross R, Herker L: Studies of hypercholesterolemia in the nonhuman primates: I. Changes that lead to fatty streak formation. *Arteriosclerosis* 4:323, 1984
34. Libby P, Hannson GK: Involvement of the immune system in human atherogenesis: current knowledge and unanswered questions. *Lab Invest* 64:5, 1991
35. Springer TA: Adhesion receptors of the immune system. *Nature* 346:425, 1990
36. Cybulsky MI, Gimbrone MA Jr: Endothelial expression of a mononuclear leukocyte adhesion molecule during atherogenesis. *Science* 251:788, 1991
37. Rice GE, Munro JM, Bevilacqua MP: Inducible cell adhesion molecule 110 (INCAM-110) is an endothelial receptor for lymphocytes: a CD11/CD18-independent adhesion mechanism. *J Exp Med* 171:1369, 1990
38. Osborn LC, Hession C, Tizard R, et al: Direct expression cloning of vascular cell adhesion molecule 1, a cytokine-induced endothelial protein that binds to lymphocytes. *Cell* 59:1203, 1989
39. Schlossman SF, Boumsell L, Gilks W, et al: CD antigens 1993. *Blood* 83:879, 1994
40. Cybulsky MI, Fries JWU, Williams AJ, et al: Gene structure, chromosomal location, and basis for alternative mRNA splicing of the human VCAM1 gene. *Proc Natl Acad Sci USA* 88:7859, 1991

41. Elices MJ, Osborn L, Takada Y, et al: VCAM-1 on activated endothelium interacts with the leukocyte integrin VLA-4 at a site distinct from the VLA-4/fibronectin binding site. *Cell* 60:577, 1990
42. Bochner BS, Luscinskas FW, Gimbrone MA Jr, et al: Adhesion of human basophils, eosinophils, and neutrophils to interleukin-1-activated human vascular endothelial cells: contributions of endothelial cell adhesion molecules. *J Exp Med* 173:1553, 1991
43. Li H, Cybulsky MI, Gimbrone MA Jr, et al: An atherogenic diet rapidly induces VCAM-1, a cytokine-regulated mononuclear leukocyte adhesion molecule, in rabbit aortic endothelium. *Arteriosclerosis Thromb* 139:197, 1993
44. Witztum JL, Steinberg D: Role of oxidized low density lipoprotein in atherogenesis. *J Clin Invest* 88:1785, 1991
45. Berliner JA, Territo MC, Sevanian A, et al: Minimally modified low density lipoprotein stimulates monocyte endothelial interactions. *J Clin Invest* 85:1138, 1990
46. Kume N, Cybulsky MI, Gimbrone MA Jr: Lysophosphatidylcholine, a component of atherogenic lipoproteins, induces mononuclear leukocyte adhesion molecules in cultured arterial endothelial cells. *J Clin Invest* 90:1138, 1992
47. Bevilacqua MP, Stengelin S, Gimbrone MA Jr, et al: Endothelial-leukocyte adhesion molecule 1: an inducible receptor for neutrophils related to complement regulatory proteins and lectins. *Science* 243:1160, 1989
48. Bevilacqua MP, Nelson RM: Selectins. *J Clin Invest* 91:379, 1993
49. Spertini O, Luscinskas FW, Kansas GS, et al: Leukocyte adhesion molecule-1 (LAM-1, L-selectin) interacts with an inducible endothelial cell ligand to support leukocyte adhesion. *J Immunol* 147:2565, 1991
50. Cushing SD, Berliner JA, Valente A, et al: Minimally modified low density lipoproteins induce monocyte chemotactic protein 1 in human endothelial cells and smooth muscle cells. *Proc Natl Acad Sci USA* 87:5134, 1990
51. Clinton SK, Underwood R, Hayes L, et al: Macrophage colony-stimulating factor gene expression in vascular cells and in experimental and human atherosclerosis. *Am J Pathol* 140:301, 1992
52. Poston RN, Haskard DO, Coucher JR, et al: Expression of intercellular adhesion molecule-1 in atherosclerotic plaques. *Am J Pathol* 140:665, 1992
53. Nelken NA, Coughlin SR, Gordon D, et al: Monocyte chemoattractant protein-1 in human atheromatous plaques. *J Clin Invest* 88:1121, 1991
54. O'Brien KD, Allen MD, McDonald TO, et al: Vascular cell adhesion molecule-1 is expressed in human coronary atherosclerotic plaques: implications for the mode of progression of advanced coronary atherosclerosis. *J Clin Invest* 92:945, 1993
55. Libby P, Li H: Vascular cell adhesion molecule-1 and smooth muscle activation during atherogenesis (editorial). *J Clin Invest* 92:538, 1993

Acknowledgments

Research in the author's laboratory, in the Vascular Research Division of the Department of Pathology at the Brigham and Women's Hospital, has been supported primarily by grants from the National Heart, Lung, and Blood Institute and from the American Heart Association and its Massachusetts Affiliate. The author acknowledges the contributions of his colleagues and collaborators in the experimental studies summarized here, especially by Drs. Tucker Collins, Myron Cybulsky, Noriaki Kume, Peter Libby, William Luscinskas, Nitzan Resnick, and Masayuki Yoshida.

Figure 1 Talar Agasyan. Adapted from *Vascular Endothelium in Hemostasis and Thrombosis*, edited by M. A. Gimbrone Jr., Churchill Livingstone, 1986.

Figures 2, 3 Talar Agasyan.

Figure 4 Dimitry Schidlovsky. Adapted from "Monocyte Rolling, Arrest and Spreading on IL-4–Activated Vascular Endothelium under Flow Is Mediated via Sequential Action of L-Selectin, β_1-Integrins, and β_2-Integrins," by F. W. Luscinskas, G. S. Kansas, H. Dingi, et al, in *Journal of Cell Biology* 125:1417, 1994. Used by permission.

CHAPTER 5

Vascular Cell Growth Factors and the Arterial Wall

Michael Klagsbrun, Ph.D.

Vascular endothelial cells and smooth muscle cells (SMCs) are the predominant cells found in blood vessels, the sizes of which vary from small (capillaries) to large (veins and arteries). Capillaries are composed of a contiguous monolayer of endothelial cells that self-associate to form a lumen. Occasionally, pericytes, which are smooth muscle cell–like cells, are found on the abluminal side of capillaries. Large blood vessels are composed of three distinct layers: the intima, the media, and the adventitia. The intima is composed of a single layer of endothelial cells that remains in direct contact with the circulating blood, the subendothelial basement membrane, and the internal elastic lamina. The media is composed of multiple layers of SMCs interspersed with elastic fibers. The adventitia is composed of small capillaries and connective tissue. Differences exist between large vessel and small vessel endothelia in, for example, morphological heterogeneity, expression of surface antigens, and response to growth factors. SMCs in the vessel wall are also heterogeneous.

Proliferation of vascular cells in the adult is a rare event, except in the female reproductive system, which is characterized by the cyclic and tightly regulated proliferation of capillaries in the follicle, corpus luteum, and placenta and by the proliferation of SMCs in the uterus. Angiogenesis is also an important part of the body's response to injury and occurs in a highly regulated and temporal manner. By contrast, uncontrolled proliferation of endothelial cells and SMCs is associated with pathological processes. For example, the induction of new capillary growth is a prerequisite for the growth of solid tumors,[1] and SMC hyperplasia is associated with restenosis after angioplasty[2] and the pathogenesis of atherosclerosis [*see Chapter 2*].[3]

Numerous growth factors that regulate vascular endothelial cell and SMC proliferation, as either stimulators or inhibitors, have been identified [*see Table 1*].[1,3-7] These growth factors are mitogenic and chemotactic in cell culture and in vivo. The goal of this chapter is to describe the biochemical and biologic properties of the better-characterized polypeptide vascular cell growth factors and inhibitors; to describe how vascular cell growth factors might be useful in the stimulation of desired blood vessel proliferation, such as collateral vessels; and to describe strategies aimed at controlling pathological vascular cell growth based on knowledge of these growth factors.

Vascular Cell Growth Factors

Fibroblast Growth Factor

Acidic fibroblast growth factor (aFGF, or FGF-1) and basic FGF (bFGF, or FGF-2) are structurally homologous 18-kilodalton (kd) polypeptides that are potent mitogens for both cultured endothelial cells and SMCs.[8-9] The factors aFGF and bFGF are members of a larger family of at least nine structurally homologous proteins. In addition to aFGF and bFGF, FGF-4 and FGF-5 have been shown to be mitogenic for endothelial cells. However, the vascular activities of the other members of the FGF family have not been studied nearly as extensively as have those of aFGF and bFGF. The growth factors aFGF and bFGF have certain biologic properties that are important for our understanding of their potential role in the mediation of vascular cell growth. First, they have a strong affinity for heparin and heparan sulfate. Heparan sulfate proteoglycans, which are abundant on the surface of endothelial cells and SMCs, act as relatively low-affinity binding sites for bFGF and probably for aFGF as well. The factor bFGF needs to bind to cell surface heparan sulfate proteoglycans in order to bind to high-affinity tyrosine kinase receptors and to be mitogenic.[10] Thus, cell surface heparan sulfate proteoglycans and high-affinity FGF receptors act as a dual receptor system that modulates bFGF activity. Second, aFGF and bFGF are not secreted into conditioned medium but are found to be associated mainly with the cell and with extracellular matrix. Thus, a source of endogenous bFGF after injury could be damaged cells or extracellular matrix that has been degraded by proteinases. Third, multiple high-affinity FGF receptors exist, including at least four gene products and numerous splice variants.[11] These FGF receptor variants are partly responsible for FGF family ligand specificity.

Ample evidence exists for FGF regulation of vascular cell proliferation. The factor bFGF is mitogenic for endothelial cells and SMCs and is synthesized by these cells in vitro. However, in vivo, bFGF synthesis occurs primarily after vascular injury.[12] Balloon angioplasty of the rat carotid artery results in SMC hyperplasia and intimal thickening. Endogenous bFGF is mitogenic in this model because administration of antibodies that neutralize bFGF decreases medial SMC proliferation by 80 percent.[13] Administered in vivo, aFGF and bFGF are mitogenic for both endothelial cells and SMCs. The bFGF stimulates collateral vessel formation in myocardial infarct and ischemia models[14,15] and stimulates proliferation of vasa vasorum around in-

Table 1 Vascular Cell Growth Factors and Inhibitors

	Acronym or Abbreviation	*Endothelial Cell Proliferation**	*Angiogenesis†*	*Smooth Muscle Cell Proliferation**
Acidic fibroblast growth factor	aFGF	+	+	+
Angiogenin		0	+	0
Basic fibroblast growth factor	bFGF	+	+	+
Betacellulin	BTC	0	0	+
Cartilage-derived inhibitor	CDI	–	–	0
Fibroblast growth factor–5	FGF-5	+	+	0
Heparin		0	0	–
Heparin-binding EGF-like growth factor	HB-EGF	0	0	+
hst/Kaposi fibroblast growth factor	FGF-4	+	+	0
Insulinlike growth factor–1	IGF-1	0	0	+
Interferon gamma	IFN-γ	–	0	0
Interleukin-1	IL-1	0	0	+
Interleukin-8	IL-8	0	+	0
Leukemia inhibitory factor	LIF	–	0	0
Placental growth factor	PLGF	+	0	0
Platelet-derived growth factor	PDGF	?	?	+
Platelet-derived endothelial cell growth factor	PD-ECGF	?	+	0
Platelet factor–4	PF4	–	–	0
Pleiotropin/Heparin-binding neurotrophic factor	PLN/HBNF	0	+	0
Prolactin		0	–	0
Thrombin		0	0	+
Thrombospondin	TSP	–	–	+
Transforming growth factor–α	TGF-α	+	+	0
Transforming growth factor–β	TGF-β	–	+	–,+
Tumor necrosis factor–α	TNF-α	–	+	0
Vascular endothelial growth factor/ Vascular permeability factor	VEGF/VPF	+	+	0

*Assayed in vitro
†Assayed in vivo
(–) inhibitor, (+) stimulator, (–,+) inhibitor or stimulator depending on assay conditions, (0) no effect or unknown effect, (?) conflicting data

jured arteries.[16] It also stimulates a substantial increase in SMC proliferation in arteries, but only after carotid artery injury.[17] Direct aFGF gene transfer into uninjured porcine arteries induces intimal thickening within 21 days, as well as neocapillary formation in the expanded intima.[18] These findings taken together imply that administration of FGF in vivo could have both beneficial and adverse effects in terms of vascular cell growth. On one hand, the vascularization of granulation tissue after injury and the induction of collateral vessel formation in response to ischemia in myocardium and limbs could be highly beneficial in repair of injury, as could be the vascularization of atherosclerotic plaques. On the other hand, induction of SMC proliferation in blood vessels could be quite harmful, leading to blood vessel occlusion. Thus, the administration of FGF in vivo as a therapeutic agent needs careful consideration.

Vascular Endothelial Growth Factor/Vascular Permeability Factor

Vascular endothelial growth factor (VEGF) is a 46-kd dimeric protein that is a highly specific mitogen for endothelial cells.[19,20] It is identical to vascular permeability factor (VPF), a protein that enhances the permeability of local venules and small veins.[21] VEGF/VPF has limited structural homology (about 18 to 20 percent) to platelet-derived growth factor (PDGF). However, the mitogenic target cell specificities of VEGF/VPF, an endothelial cell mitogen and angiogenesis factor, differ considerably from those of PDGF, which is a mitogen for SMCs and fibroblasts but not for endothelial cells. An important structural feature of VEGF/VPF is that it exists in four isoforms, derived by alternative splicing, of 121, 165, 189, and 206 amino acids that are similar in activity but differ in secretion profiles. $VEGF_{121}$ is readily secreted into conditioned medium, $VEGF_{165}$ is only partly secreted, and $VEGF_{189}$ and $VEGF_{206}$ are almost totally bound to cell surface and matrix. Like bFGF, VEGF/VPF (except $VEGF_{121}$) has a strong affinity for heparin, is heparin dependent for receptor binding, and is stored in matrix in association with heparan sulfate proteoglycan. VEGF/VPF binds to high-affinity receptors that are expressed mainly by endothelial cells. To date, three structurally homologous VEGF/VPF receptors have been cloned, Flt (Fms-like tyrosine kinase), KDR/Flk-1, and Flt4. These receptor tyrosine kinases are transmembrane proteins that have an extracellular domain containing seven immunoglobulin-like loops.

A primary role for VEGF/VPF is the regulation of angiogenesis in vivo. VEGF/VPF is a highly specific mitogen for endothelial cells in culture, it induces cells to invade underlying matrix to form capillarylike tubes (angiogenesis in vitro),[22] and it stimulates angiogenesis in the chorioallantoic membrane and the cornea models. VEGF/VPF and bFGF are highly synergistic in stimulating angiogenesis in vitro.[22] Analysis of embryonic development,[23] the female reproductive cycle,[24] and tumor growth[25,26] suggests that VEGF/VPF is expressed only during periods of angiogenesis in cells adjacent to blood vessels, and that VEGF/VPF receptor expression is confined to blood vessels. Thus, VEGF/VPF appears to be a pure paracrine angiogenic factor. Hypoxia regulates VEGF/VPF expression. Glioblastoma mutiforme, the most common brain tumor in humans, is highly vascular and necrotic. VEGF/VPF messenger RNA (mRNA) expression is strongly up-regulated in high-grade glioblastoma cells, particularly in cells near necrotic foci.[25] In cultured glioblastoma cells, VEGF/VPF mRNA is strongly induced after exposure to hypoxic conditions.[26] Thus, VEGF/VPF production might be a response to conditions in which tissues are insufficiently perfused, such as hypoxia and ischemia.

Although little is known about the expression of VEGF/VPF in the vasculature, SMCs have been shown to synthesize VEGF/VPF in culture.[27] Thus, one might envision that after vascular injury, VEGF/VPF might be up-regulated in SMCs, resulting in endothelial cell proliferation. Like bFGF, added VEGF/VPF augments collateral vessel development after ischemia. $VEGF_{165}$ stimulated growth of collateral vessels when it was administered to the internal iliac artery of rabbits in which the ipsilateral femoral artery was excised to induce severe unilateral hind limb ischemia.[28] VEGF/VPF might have an advantage over FGF in the treatment of ischemic conditions because it has no complicating fibroblast or SMC mitogenic activity.

Angiogenin

Angiogenin is a 14-kd angiogenic factor that was first purified from tumor cell–conditioned medium.[29] It has a 35 percent structural homology to pancreatic ribonuclease A and has ribonucleolytic activity, which is essential for angiogenin to induce neovascularization. Placental ribonuclease inhibitor, a 50-kd protein, inhibits angiogenin activity and has antitumor activity.

Angiogenin is unusual in that it was purified using an assay that measured neovascularization in vivo. Most other angiogenic factors were first identified based on their ability to stimulate endothelial cell proliferation in culture. It is now apparent that angiogenin is not an endothelial cell mitogen. Thus, it has been postulated that angiogenin is an indirect angiogenic factor, that is, a factor that does not directly stimulate endothelial cell proliferation but acts on endothelial cells in another manner or indirectly by stimulating other cells to produce endothelial cell mitogens. Angiogenin does have many effects on endothelial cells that may be related to angiogenesis. For example, angiogenin coated onto dishes, but not angiogenin in solution, supports endothelial cell adhesion and spreading, an effect inhibitable by the peptide Arg-Gly-Asp-Ser.[30] Thus, angiogenin, which binds to extracellular matrix, may act as a matrix adhesion molecule to promote angiogenesis in vitro in a way that is similar to the activity of laminin. Angiogenin also binds to receptors on endothelial cells, although these have yet to be purified and characterized. Elucidation of the mechanism of angiogenin's action would greatly increase our understanding of how indirect angiogenesis factors might act.

Platelet-Derived Growth Factor

PDGF is a dimeric growth factor that contains two distinct homologous subunits, 17-kd PDGF A and 14-kd PDGF B.[31] The transforming product of the oncogene v-*sis* is structurally homologous to PDGF B. Three forms of PDGF exist: heterodimeric PDGF AB and homodimeric PDGF AA and PDGF BB. The PDGF receptor, a 170- to 180-kd high-affinity receptor tyrosine kinase, is made up of two subunits: an α chain (which binds PDGF A or B chains) and a β chain (which binds only PDGF B chains). As a consequence,

PDGF AA binds only to the αα receptor, PDGF AB binds to the αα or αβ receptor, and PDGF BB binds to the αα, αβ, or ββ receptor.

PDGF, particularly PDGF BB, is a potent chemotactic factor and mitogen for SMC in vitro.[32] Under similar conditions, none of the PDGF isoforms are mitogenic for endothelial cells, yet some evidence indicates that PDGF BB affects some small-vessel endothelial cells because it has been demonstrated that PDGF BB is chemotactic for rat brain capillary endothelial cells in culture and that it stimulates angiogenesis in the chick chorioallantoic membrane.[33] PDGF does stimulate SMCs in vivo, but by inducing migration rather than proliferation: in an intra-arterial balloon injury model that results in neointimal thickening, antibodies that neutralize PDGF inhibit the accumulation of neointimal SMCs but not their proliferation.[34] Administration of PDGF in this injury model results in SMC migration and intimal thickening.[35] Introduction of a eukaryotic vector plasmid that encodes recombinant PDGF B by direct gene transfer into uninjured porcine ileofemoral arteries resulted in PDGF B chain synthesis and intimal hyperplasia, although it was difficult to tell whether the PDGF effect was restricted to SMC migration.[36]

PDGF is synthesized by both endothelial cells and SMCs. Endothelial cells express predominantly PDGF B mRNA in culture, whereas SMCs express predominantly PDGF A mRNA in culture. These cells also secrete PDGF protein. The PDGF gene is induced by numerous factors that might be physiologically relevant, such as thrombin, which is involved in vascular injury[37]; angiotensin II, which stimulates SMC hypertrophy[38]; oxidized low-density lipoproteins, which are associated with atherogenesis[39]; transforming growth factor–β (TGF-β)[40]; and interleukin-1 (IL-1).[41] The mitogenic activities of α-thrombin, interleukin-1, and TGF-β for SMCs are mediated by the PDGF AA that is induced by these cytokines. PDGF is thought to be involved in atherogenesis, which is considered by some to be associated with vascular injury and inflammation.[3]

Heparin-Binding Epidermal Growth Factor–like Growth Factor

Heparin-binding epidermal growth factor–like growth factor (HB-EGF) is a 20- to 22-kd, heparin-binding glycoprotein that is structurally homologous to members of the epidermal growth factor (EGF) family.[42] It consists of a C-terminal EGF-like domain and a hydrophilic N-terminal region domain that is not found in EGF and TGF-α The bifunctional domain structure of HB-EGF plays an important role in its function as an SMC mitogen. HB-EGF is a potent mitogen and chemotactic factor for SMCs in culture and is as active as PDGF for both activities in vitro.[42,43] However, whether or not HB-EGF is predominantly a chemotactic factor for SMCs in vivo, as PDGF appears to be, is not yet known. Like PDGF, HB-EGF is not mitogenic for endothelial cells. It is about 50 times more potent than its homologues, EGF and TGF-α, despite the fact that all three EGF-like molecules appear to bind to the same EGF receptor. The enhanced SMC activity of HB-EGF is apparently related to its strong affinity for heparin and SMC surface heparan sulfate proteoglycan, a property lacking in EGF and TGF-α. This heparin affinity results from an N-terminal stretch of 21 amino acids that constitutes a heparin-binding domain.[43] The binding of HB-EGF to the EGF receptor and its bioactivity are markedly down-regulated to the level of the binding and bioactivity of EGF when SMCs are incubated with heparitinase that destroys cell surface heparan sulfate proteoglycan or when they are incubated with a 21-amino-acid synthetic peptide corresponding to the HB-EGF heparin-binding domain. The chemotatic and mitogenic activities of HB-EGF for SMCs are apparently enhanced by the interaction of HB-EGF with cell surface heparin sulfate proteoglycan, as is the case for two other vascular cell growth factors, bFGF and VEGF/VPF. Like the other SMC mitogens and chemotactic factors, such as PDGF and bFGF, HB-EGF may play a role in the regulation of SMC migration and proliferation in normal and abnormal blood vessels. HB-EGF is produced by SMCs,[44] endothelial cells,[45] macrophages,[42] and T cells,[46] cells associated with vascular injury and atherogenic lesions.[3] Like PDGF, the HB-EGF gene is inducible in these cell types by agents such as tumor necrosis factor–α, phorbol ester, lysophosphatidylcholine, and thrombin, as well as growth factors such as PDGF, bFGF, and HB-EGF itself.[44,45] HB-EGF mRNA is induced rapidly and transiently after carotid artery injury in the rat,[47] and immunoreactive HB-EGF appears to be associated with macrophages and SMCs in atherosclerotic plaques obtained from human autopsy material.[48] In addition, HB-EGF, a potent SMC mitogen, is expressed in eosinophils associated with thickened microvessels in a rat pulmonary hypertension model.[49] Whether HB-EGF in these processes is associated with SMC migration or proliferation in vivo is not known. In many ways, the function of HB-EGF is similar to that of PDGF in regard to target cell specificity, regulation of gene expression, and potential involvement in vascular disease—much more so than it is to other members of the EGF family, such as EGF, TGF-α, and amphiregulin, all of which are relatively poor mitogens for SMCs.

Transforming Growth Factor–β

TGF-β, a 25-kd homodimer, is a member of a large superfamily of multifunctional proteins that are involved in the stimulation and inhibition of SMC proliferation, matrix formation, differentiation, and morphogenesis.[50] Three TGF-β isoforms with similar but not identical biologic properties have been identified: β1, β2, and β3. TGF-β is secreted in a latent form that consists of mature TGF-β, a TGF-β latency-associated protein, and the latent TGF-β binding protein. Latent TGF-β is activated by acidification and plasmin.[51] TGF-β acts by binding to specific receptors, of which three have been identified, type I (53 kd), type II (75 kd), and type III (betaglycan, 300 kd).[52] The type I and II receptors are serine/threonine kinases and are indispensable for TGF-β signaling. The type II receptor is needed for the binding of TGF-β to the type I receptor, and the type I receptor is required for signal transduction induced by the type II receptor. The type III receptor lacks a cytoplasmic protein kinase domain and may be involved in the presentation of ligands to the type I and II receptors.

In monolayer culture, TGF-β is a potent inhibitor of endothelial cell migration and proliferation.[50] However, TGF-β is a potent inducer of capillary endothelial cell tube formation in vitro in three-dimensional collagen gels, a process referred to as angiogenesis in vitro, and of angiogenesis in vivo. This apparently paradoxical effect has not been clearly explained. One possibility is that TGF-β, a potent chemoattractant for monocytes, indirectly stimulates angiogenesis by recruiting inflammatory cells that deliver direct-acting angiogenesis factors. Alternatively, the inhibition of endothelial cell proliferation may be accompanied by the differentiation of endothelial cells, for example, into capillary endothelial cell tubes, one of the later stages of angiogenesis. The ability of TGF-β to stimulate matrix production is also compatible with the formation of differentiated capillary tubes.

TGF-β can either stimulate or inhibit SMC proliferation. Stimulation of SMC proliferation occurs at low TGF-β concentrations, but inhibition occurs at high ones. The effect of TGF-β appears to be a PDGF receptor–related phenomenon. TGF-β promotes an increase in SMC endogenous PDGF production, but at high TGF-β concentrations, expression of the PDGF receptor is down-regulated, thereby attenuating the response to PDGF.[53] The proliferative activity of TGF-β for SMCs is also dependent on cell density in that it is an inhibitor of sparse SMCs but a stimulator at confluent densities or in soft agar.[40] Infusion of TGF-β1 into the balloon-injured carotid artery induces intimal thickening, perhaps by increasing SMC number and stimulating matrix production.[54]

Endogenous TGF-β appears to regulate vascular cell growth by paracrine and autocrine mechanisms. When endothelial cells are cocultured with SMCs or with pericytes, latent TGF-β is activated and the active TGF-β that is formed inhibits endothelial cell migration and proliferation.[51,55] Activation of TGF-β requires cell-to-cell contact and is mediated by plasminogen activator/plasmin activity. It has been suggested that endothelial cells express plasminogen activator/plasmin on their cell surface and that when endothelial cells and SMCs/pericytes make contact, endothelial cell plasminogen activator/plasmin activates latent TGF-β that is solely targeted to SMCs. The growth factor bFGF, a mitogen for endothelial cells, is also a potent inducer of plasminogen activator/plasmin. Thus, bFGF may activate a negative feedback mechanism in which bFGF stimulates endothelial cell proliferation that results in plasminogen activator/plasmin secretion that in turn activates TGF-β, an endothelial cell inhibitor.

Other Modulators of Vascular Cell Proliferation

Many other vascular cell polypeptide growth factors that are not as well characterized for vascular cell mitogenic activity as the ones discussed thus far are worth mentioning. These include angiogenesis factors, such as platelet-derived endothelial cell growth factor,[56] TGF-α,[57] TNF-α,[58] and interleukin-8.[59] Other SMC mitogens include interleukin-1,[41] thrombin,[37] thrombospondin,[60] insulinlike growth factor–1,[61] and betacellulin.[62]

Inhibitors of Angiogenesis

Typically, endothelial cells are quiescent in vivo, but they proliferate in diseases such as cancer, diabetic retinopathy, and arthritis. The adverse effects of blood vessel growth in diseases have generated great interest in angiogenesis inhibitors, which typically fall into two classes, direct inhibitors of angiogenesis and antagonists of angiogenic factors, such as bFGF, angiogenin, and VEGF/VPF. Angiogenesis inhibitors usually inhibit endothelial cell proliferation, capillary tube formation (angiogenesis in vitro), and neovascularization in chorioallantoic membrane or cornea models, or both. Most of these angiogenesis inhibitors are well-characterized proteins whose antiangiogenesis activity has been realized only recently. Among these proteins are thrombospondin,[63] platelet factor–4,[64] cartilage-derived inhibitor,[65] and a truncated form of prolactin.[66]

Inhibitors of Smooth Muscle Cell Proliferation

Inhibitors of SMC proliferation are not as well characterized as are angiogenesis inhibitors; the best-characterized one is heparin.[2,67] Although SMCs, like endothelial cells, are typically quiescent, SMC hyperplasia occurs in response to injury, and thus inhibitors of SMC proliferation could be quite useful. In culture, heparinlike molecules produced by endothelial cells inhibit SMC proliferation but do not inhibit endothelial cell proliferation.[68] These results suggest a paracrine mechanism in which SMC proliferation is regulated by endothelial cells. Importantly, heparin inhibits SMC proliferation in vivo.[69] Infusion of heparin into carotid arteries denuded of endothelial cells by a balloon catheter inhibits subsequent intimal thickening by inhibiting SMC migration, SMC proliferation, and accumulation of matrix.[2,69] The cellular mechanism by which heparin inhibits these three SMC activities is not established, but several possibilities have been suggested, including the inhibition of c-*myb*,[70] the suppression of a protein kinase C–dependent second-messenger pathway for c-*fos*,[71] the down-regulation of SMC growth factor receptors,[72] and the prevention of access of SMC growth factors to cell surface heparan sulfate proteoglycan.[73]

Growth Factors and Smooth Muscle Cell Hyperplasia

Arterial Injury

Arterial injury results in SMC hyperplasia. Thirty to 50 percent of atherosclerotic arteries treated by carotid angioplasty develop restenosis within three to six months after angioplasty and endarterectomy.[3] Vascular injury has been studied extensively in rat and rabbit arterial models, both in the carotid artery and in the aorta.[2] In these animals, the principal response to vascular injury is the rapid accumulation of SMCs in the intima of the blood vessel wall. Injury to arteries with a balloon catheter destroys the intima, which contains endothelial cells, damages medial SMCs, and induces medial SMC proliferation. The magnitude of the proliferative response depends on the amount of trauma. Several days after medial SMC proliferation, SMCs migrate into intima of mostly nondividing SMCs. Once in the intima, SMCs continue to proliferate, forming an intimal lesion and narrowing the lumen. The neointima consists of a thick layer of SMCs and extracellular matrix. Within four to six weeks, SMCs stop proliferating. Eventually, endothelial cells proliferate to re-endothelialize the artery, further inhibiting SMC proliferation.

It has been suggested that growth factors, in particular bFGF, play a role in intimal thickening, because neutralizing anti-bFGF antibodies administered before injury cause substantial reduction in medial SMC proliferation within two days after injury.[13] However, anti-bFGF antibodies administered four to six days after injury have no inhibitory effect, suggesting that bFGF is not involved in the chronic proliferation of intimal SMCs. In situ hybridization using an en face technique reveals that early after injury, bFGF and FGF receptor-1 mRNA levels are increased in replicating endothelial cells, especially those close to the wound edge, and in replicating SMCs.[12] Balloon injury is also accompanied by up-regulation of functional FGF receptor.[74] Taken together, these findings indicate that endogenous bFGF released from, and/or synthesized by, damaged vascular cells stimulates both SMC hyperplasia and re-endothelialization by interaction with newly available receptors. On the other hand, PDGF may be responsible for medial SMC migration into the intima, but not proliferation, because neutralizing anti-PDGF antibodies have little effect on DNA synthesis after injury, but they inhibit neointimal SMC accumulation.[34] What causes intimal SMC replication is not clear. The response to vascular injury is obviously complex, and other endothelial cell growth factors, such as VEGF/VPF, which is produced by SMCs, and HB-EGF, which is a potent SMC mitogen produced by SMCs, may be involved.

Pathogenesis of Atherosclerosis

Atherosclerosis, a major cause of death in the United States, results from an excessive inflammatory-fibroproliferative response to injury to endothelial cells and SMCs in the arterial wall[3] [*see Chapter 2*]. Fatty streaks made up of lipid-rich macrophages and T cells form within the intima and develop into fatty lesions, which are composed of layers of macrophages and SMCs, and then develop into fibrous plaques, which project into the arterial lumen and impede blood flow. Ruptures in the fibrous cap lead to sudden death from myocardial infarcts. It has been suggested that growth factors produced by cells associated with lesions (endothelial cells, SMCs, macrophages, platelets, and T cells) are mediators of atherogenesis.[3] Figure 1 gives a schematic overview of several of the growth factors that may be involved in lesion formation (FGF, PDGF, VEGF, HB-EGF, and TGF-β), their cellular sources, and their cellular targets. Mitogenic activity for endothelial cells might be involved in development of vasa vasorum, which would bring nutrients to the lesioned artery,[16] whereas mitogenic activity for SMCs might be associated with the SMC hyperplasia and matrix production evident in lesions.

Because of the potent activity of PDGF in stimulating the migration and proliferation of SMCs, PDGF has been the growth factor most extensively analyzed in atherosclerotic lesions. PDGF B mRNA is expressed in atherosclerotic segments of human artery.[75] PDGF A mRNA is expressed in mesenchymal-appearing intimal cells, which have the appearance of SMCs, whereas endothelial cells are the major sites of PDGF B mRNA expression.[76] PDGF B protein is expressed in all stages of lesion development in both human and nonhuman primate atherosclerosis.[77] The chemotactic activity of PDGF for SMCs and monocytes/macrophages contributes to the SMC hyperplasia associated with atherosclerotic plaques. However, these relationships have yet to be established experimentally for PDGF or any other growth factor.

Therapeutic Strategies

Given the contribution of angiogenesis and SMC hyperplasia to vascular disease, strategies to block inappropriate vascular cell proliferation are needed [*see Figure 2*]. One strategy has been to generate growth factor–toxin chimeric fusion proteins (mitotoxins) that bind to endothelial cells and SMCs via growth factor receptors, thereby targeting toxins that kill the cells.[74] For example, a conjugate of bFGF and saporin, which is a plant enzyme that inactivates ribosomes, kills SMCs in culture. When applied in vivo in the rat carotid artery, the bFGF-saporin conjugate killed activated, but not quiescent, SMCs. Reduction of neointimal thickening was observed at seven to 10 days, but not at 28 days. Toxin fusion proteins have also been prepared that target the EGF receptor in SMCs. For example, an EGF-diphtheria toxin fusion protein[78] and an HB-EGF–*Pseudomonas* toxin fusion pro-

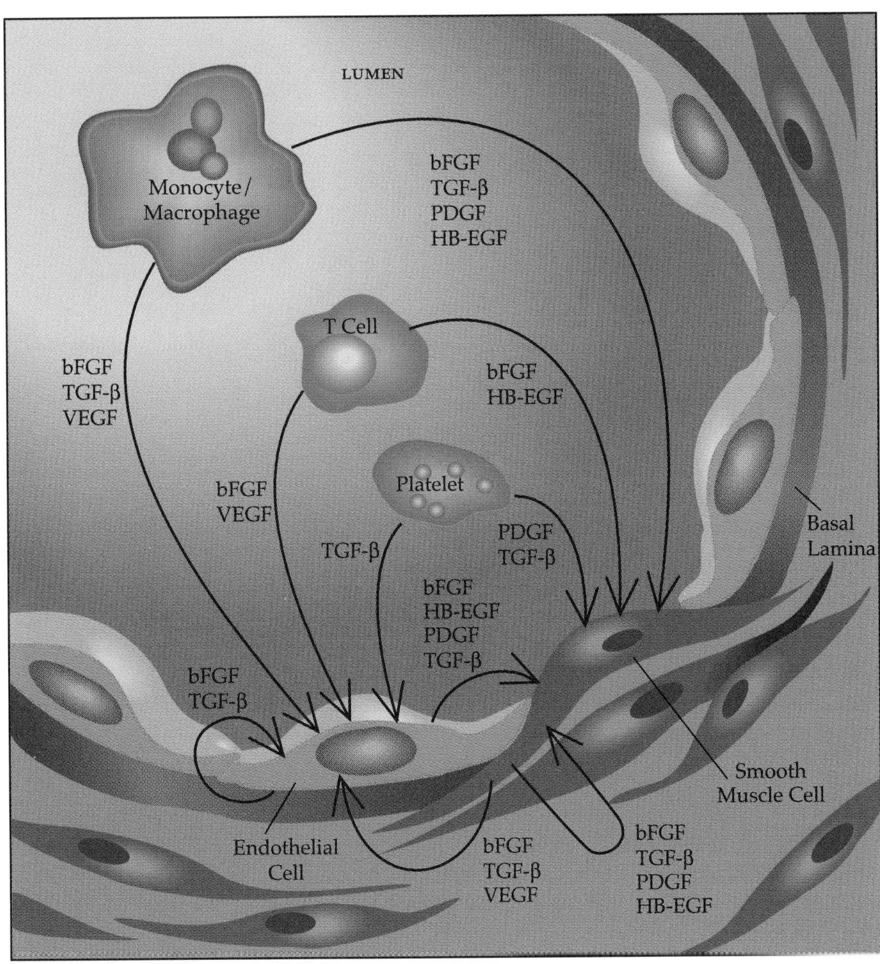

Figure 1 *A blood vessel wall is depicted showing an area denuded of endothelial cells in which smooth muscle cells have migrated toward the lumen, which contains a monocyte/macrophage, a T cell, and a platelet. Arrows indicate the possible pathways of such vascular cell growth factors as basic fibroblast growth factor (bFGF), platelet-derived growth factor (PDGF), vascular endothelial growth factor (VEGF), transforming growth factor–β (TGF-β), and heparin-binding epidermal growth factor–like growth factor (HB-EGF) from their cellular sources to their cellular targets in the blood vessel. bFGF is mitogenic for endothelial cells and smooth muscle cells, VEGF is mitogenic for endothelial cells, and PDGF and HB-EGF are mitogenic for smooth muscle cells; TGF-β is inhibitory for endothelial cells and either mitogenic or inhibitory for smooth muscle cells.*

tein[79] both killed SMCs. The use of mitotoxins is a promising approach to killing SMCs in vivo, but much more work is necessary before the toxic: therapeutic ratio of this treatment is optimized.

Because unregulated vascular cell growth factor activity might lead to SMC hyperplasia, therapeutic strategies have been developed to antagonize growth factors or their receptors, or both. Two such strategies are the use of neutralizing anti-bFGF antibodies to inhibit medial SMC proliferation and the use of anti-PDGF antibodies to block SMC migration into the intima after balloon injury.[13,34] Over the long term, however, anti-bFGF antibodies do not appreciably reduce intimal thickening. For clinical use to be made of antibodies, combinations targeted against different growth factors might be needed. Also, immune rejection of large amounts of antibody may occur with these methods.

Another approach has been to use antisense oligonucleotides to inhibit intimal arterial SMC accumulation in vivo. In a recent example of this approach, stimulation of SMC proliferation in vitro by growth factors was followed by elevated c-*myb* message levels, and this proliferation was suppressed by antisense c-*myb* oligonucleotides. In studies in vivo, application of pluronic gels containing antisense c-*myb* to rat carotid arteries subjected to balloon angioplasty resulted in minimal intimal accumulation.[80] In another study,

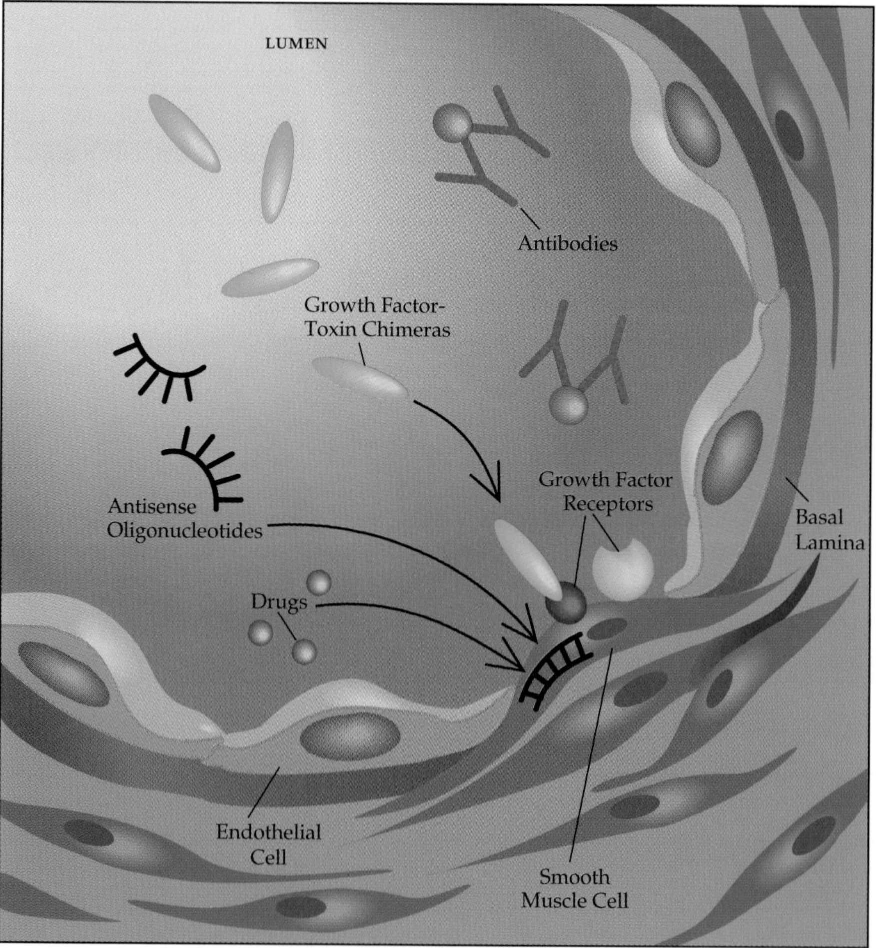

Figure 2 *Potential smooth muscle cell proliferation antagonists include growth factor–toxin chimeric fusion proteins (e.g., bFGF fused to saporin and HB-EGF fused to* Pseudomonas *exotoxin) targeted to growth factor receptors, antibodies directed against vascular cell growth factors (e.g., anti-PDGF and anti-bFGF), antisense oligonucleotides directed against oncogenes and cell cycle proteins shown to be involved in smooth muscle cell replication in vivo (e.g., c-myb, cdc2, and proliferating-cell nuclear antigen), and drugs that inhibit smooth muscle cell proliferation in vivo (e.g., heparin).*

which used inactivated hemagglutinating virus of Japan-liposome complexes as a vehicle of DNA transfer, a mixture of *cdc2* kinase antisense oligonucleotides and proliferating-cell nuclear antigen antisense oligonucleotides that were transfected into balloon-injured arteries in vivo resulted in a marked decrease in *cdc2* kinase and proliferating-cell nuclear antigen mRNA expression, inhibition of the DNA synthesis induced by balloon injury, and inhibition of neointima formation two weeks after angiopasty.[81]

Yet another strategy would be to develop drugs that directly block angiogenesis and SMC hyperplasia. Angiogenesis inhibitors and heparin have been used to inhibit SMC proliferation in vivo. Because angiotensin II induces SMC proliferation in normal and injured arterial walls, the use of angiotensin-converting enzyme inhibitors has been explored. For example, cilazapril blocks intimal thickening in balloon-injured rat carotid arteries.[2]

Future Perspectives

The rapid increase in the identification, purification, and cloning of numerous vascular cell growth factors as well as the increased knowledge of how these growth factors act holds great promise for the future modulation of vascular cell proliferation in vivo. Based on these studies, it is becoming feasible to develop therapeutic strategies aimed at either stimulating or inhibiting vascular cell proliferation in vivo. One application would be to stimulate new blood vessel growth in the heart in response to ischemia, and within atherosclerotic arteries. Potentially promising therapeutic agents for the stimulation of vessel growth are bFGF and VEGF/VPF. It is now possible to deliver recombinant growth factor or the DNA that encodes the growth factor in vivo and locally. Conversely, inhibition of vascular SMC proliferation would be desirable to control SMC hyperplasia associated with restenosis in patients who have undergone angioplasty, in those with atherosclerosis, and in those with hypertension. Detailed elucidation of vascular growth factors and their role in vascular disease would allow rational development of antagonists, such as neutralizing antibodies, antisense oligonucleotides, mitotoxins, and synthetic peptides, that mimic growth factor–receptor binding sites and act as competitive inhibitors. To be successful, these antagonists will have to be delivered to the correct location and be highly specific and nontoxic. Future studies will determine the efficacies of these approaches.

References

1. Folkman J, Klagsbrun M: Angiogenic factors. *Science* 235:442, 1987
2. Clowes AW, Reidy MA: Prevention of stenosis after vascular reconstruction: pharmacologic control of intimal hyperplasia—a review. *J Vasc Surg* 13:885, 1991
3. Ross R: The pathogenesis of atherosclerosis: a perspective for the 1990s. *Nature* 362:801, 1993
4. Klagsbrun M, Folkman J: Angiogenesis. *Peptide Growth Factors and Their Receptors. Handbook of Experimental Pharmacology*, Vol 95/II. Sporn MB, Roberts AB, Eds. Springer-Verlag, Berlin, 1990, p 549
5. Casscells W: Smooth muscle cell growth factors. *Prog Growth Factor Res* 3:177, 1991
6. Moses MA, Langer R: Inhibitors of angiogenesis. *Biotechnology* 9:630, 1991
7. Klagsbrun M, Dluz S: Smooth muscle cell and endothelial cell growth factors. *Trends Cardiovasc Med* 3:213, 1993

8. Burgess WH, Maciag T: The heparin-binding (fibroblast) growth factor family of proteins. *Annu Rev Biochem* 58:575, 1989
9. Klagsbrun M: The fibroblast growth factor family: structural properties and biological properties. *Prog Growth Factor Res* 1:207, 1989
10. Klagsbrun M, Baird A: A dual receptor system is required for basic fibroblast growth factor activity. *Cell* 67:229, 1991.
11. Partanen J, Vainikka S, Korhonen J, et al: Diverse receptors for fibroblast growth factors. *Prog Growth Factor Res* 4:69, 1992
12. Lindner V, Reidy MA: Expression of basic fibroblast growth factor and its receptor by smooth muscle cells and endothelium in injured rat arteries: an en face study. *Circ Res* 73:589, 1993
13. Lindner V, Reidy MA: Proliferation of smooth muscle cells after vascular injury is inhibited by an antibody against basic fibroblast growth factor. *Proc Natl Acad Sci USA* 88:3739, 1991
14. Yanagisawa-Miwa A, Uchida Y, Nakamura F, et al: Salvage of infected myocardium by angiogenic action of basic fibroblast growth factor. *Science* 257:1401, 1992
15. Baffour R, Berman J, Garb JL, et al: Enhanced angiogenesis and growth of collaterals by in vivo administration of recombinant basic fibroblast growth factor in a rabbit model of acute lower limb ischemia: dose-responsive effect of basic fibroblast growth factor. *J Vasc Surg* 16:181, 1992
16. Edelman ER, Nugent MA, Smith LT, et al: Basic fibroblast growth factor enhances the coupling of intimal hyperplasia and proliferation of vasa vasorum in injured rat arteries. *J Clin Invest* 89:465, 1992
17. Lindner V, Lappi DA, Baird A, et al: Role of basic fibroblast growth factor in vascular lesion formation. *Circ Res* 68:106, 1991
18. Nabel EG, Yan Z-Y, Plautz G, et al: Recombinant fibroblast growth factor-1 promotes intimal hyperplasia and angiogenesis in arteries in vivo. *Nature* 362:844, 1993
19. Ferrara N: Vascular endothelial growth factor. *Trends Cardiovasc Med* 3:244, 1993
20. Klagsbrun M, Soker S: VEGF/VPF: the angiogenesis factor found? *Curr Biol* 3:699, 1993
21. Connolly DT: Vascular permeability factor: a unique regulator of blood vessel function. *J Cell Biochem* 47:219, 1991
22. Pepper MS, Ferrara N, Orci L, et al: Potent synergism between vascular endothelial growth factor and basic fibroblast growth factor in the induction of angiogenesis in vitro. *Biochem Biophys Res Commun* 189:824, 1992
23. Millauer B, Wizigmann-Voos S, Schnürch H, et al: High affinity VEGF binding and developmental expression suggest Flk-1 as a major regulator of vasculogenesis and angiogenesis. *Cell* 72:835, 1993
24. Shweiki D, Itin A, Neufeld G, et al: Patterns of expression of vascular endothelial growth factor (VEGF) and VEGF receptors in mice suggest a role in hormonally regulated angiogenesis. *J Clin Invest* 91:2235, 1993
25. Plate KH, Breier G, Weich HA, et al: Vascular endothelial growth factor is a potential tumour angiogenesis factor in human gliomas in vivo. *Nature* 359:845, 1992
26. Shweiki D, Itin A, Soffer D, et al: Vascular endothelial growth factor induced by hypoxia may mediate hypoxia-initiated angiogenesis. *Nature* 359:843, 1992
27. Tischer E, Mitchell R, Hartman T, et al: The human gene for vascular endothelial growth factor. *J Biol Chem* 266:11947, 1991
28. Takeshita S, Zheng LP, Brogi E, at al: Therapeutic angiogenesis: a single intraarterial bolus of vascular endothelial growth factor augments revascularization in a rabbit ischemic hind limb model. *J Clin Invest* 93:662, 1994
29. Riordan JF, Vallee BL: Human angiogenin, an organogenic protein. *Br J Cancer* 57:587, 1988
30. Soncin F: Angiogenin supports endothelial and fibroblast cell adhesion. *Proc Natl Acad Sci USA* 89:2232, 1992
31. Raines EW, Bowen-Pope DF, Ross R: Platelet-derived growth factor. *Peptide Growth factors and Their Receptors. Handbook of Experimental Pharmacology*, Vol 95/I. Sporn MB, Roberts AB, Eds. Springer-Verlag, Berlin, 1990, p 173
32. D'Amore PA, Smith SR: Growth factor effects on cells of the vascular wall: a survey. *Growth Factors* 8:61, 1993
33. Risau W, Drexler H, Mironov V, et al: Platelet-derived growth factor is angiogenic in vivo. *Growth Factors* 7:261, 1992
34. Ferns GAA, Raines EW, Sprugel KH, et al: Inhibition of neointimal smooth muscle accumulation after angioplasty by an antibody to PDGF. *Science* 253:1129, 1991

35. Jawein AD, Bowen-Pope D, Lindner V, et al: Platelet-derived growth factor promotes smooth muscle cell migration and intimal thickening in a rat model of balloon angioplasty. *J Clin Invest* 89:507, 1992
36. Nabel EG, Yang Z, Liptay S, et al: Recombinant platelet-derived growth factor B gene expression in porcine arteries induces intimal hyperplasia in vivo. *J Clin Invest* 91:1822, 1993
37. Okazaki H, Majesky MW, Harker LA, et al: Regulation of platelet-derived growth factor ligand and receptor gene expression by α-thrombin in vascular smooth muscle cells. *Circ Res* 71:1285, 1992
38. Naftilan, AJ, Pratt RE, Dzau VJ: Induction of platelet-derived growth factor A-chain and c-*myc* gene expressions by angiotensin II in cultured rat vascular smooth muscle cells. *J Clin Invest* 83:1419, 1989
39. Zwijsen RM, Japenga SC, Heijen AM: Induction of platelet-derived growth factor chain A gene expression in human smooth muscle cells by oxidized low density lipoproteins. *Biochem Biophys Res Commun* 186:1410, 1992
40. Majack RA, Majesky MW, Goodman LV: Role of PDGF-A expression in the control of vascular smooth muscle cell growth by transforming growth factor-β. *J Cell Biol* 111:239, 1990
41. Raines EW, Dower SK, Ross R: Interleukin-1 mitogenic activity for fibroblasts and smooth muscle cells is due to PDGF-AA. *Science* 243:393, 1989
42. Higashiyama S, Abraham JA, Miller J, et al: A heparin-binding growth factor secreted by macrophage-like cells that is related to EGF. *Science* 251:936, 1991
43. Higashiyama S, Abraham JA, Klagsbrun M: Heparin-binding EGF-like growth factor stimulation of smooth muscle cell migration: dependence on interactions with cell surface heparan sulfate. *J Cell Biol* 122:933, 1993
44. Dluz SM, Higashiyama S, Damm D, et al: Heparin-binding EGF-like growth factor expression in cultured fetal human vascular smooth muscle cells: induction of mRNA levels and secretion of active mitogen. *J Biol Chem* 268:18330, 1993
45. Yoshizumi M, Kourembanas S, Temizer DH, et al: Tumor necrosis factor increases transcription of the heparin-binding epidermal growth factor-like growth factor gene in vascular endothelial cells. *J Biol Chem* 267:9467, 1992
46. Blotnick M, Peoples G, Freeman M, et al: T lymphocytes synthesize and export heparin-binding epidermal growth factor-like growth factor and basic fibroblast growth factor, mitogens for vascular cells and fibroblasts: differential production and release by $CD4^+$ and $CD8^+$ cells. *Proc Natl Acad Sci USA* 91:2890, 1994
47. Reidy M: (Unpublished data)
48. Miyagawa J, Higashiyama S, Kawata S, et al: Localization of heparin-binding EGF-like growth factor in the smooth muscle cells and macrophages of human atherosclerotic plaques. *J Clin Invest* 95:404, 1995
49. Powell P, Klagsbrun M, Jones R: Eosinophils expressing heparin-binding EGF-like growth factor localize around microvessels in pulmonary hypertension. *Am J Pathol* 193:1, 1993
50. Roberts AB, Sporn MB: The transforming growth factor-βs. *Peptide Growth Factors and Their Receptors, Handbook of Experimental Pharmacology*, Vol 95/I. Sporn MB, Roberts AB, Eds. Springer-Verlag, Berlin, 1990, p 491
51. Sato Y, Okada F, Abe M, et al: The mechanism for the activation of latent TGF-β during co-culture of endothelial cells and smooth muscle cells: cell type specific targeting of latent TGF-β to smooth muscle cells. *J Cell Biol* 123:1249, 1993
52. Lin HY, Lodish HF: Receptors for the TGF-β superfamily: multiple polypeptides and serine/threonine kinases. *Trends Cell Biol* 3:14, 1993
53. Battegay EJ, Raines EW, Seifert RA, et al: TGF-β induces bimodal proliferation of connective tissue cells via complex control of an autocrine PDGF loop. *Cell* 63:515, 1990
54. Majesky M, Lindner V, Twardzik DR et al: Production of transforming growth factor-β 1 during repair of arterial injury. *J Clin Invest* 88:904, 1991
55. Antoneli-Orlidge AA, Saunders KB, Smith SR, et al: An activated form of transforming growth factor beta is produced by co-cultures of endothelial cells and pericytes. *Proc Natl Acad Sci USA* 86:4544, 1989
56. Miyazono K, Okabe T, Urabe A, et al: Purification and properties of an endothelial cell growth factor from human platelets. *J Biol Chem* 262:4098, 1987
57. Schreiber AB, Winkler ME, Derynck R: Transforming growth factor-alpha: a more potent angiogenic mediator than epidermal growth factor. *Science* 232:1250, 1986
58. Leibovich SJ, Polverini SJ, Shepard HM, et al: Macrophage-induced angiogenesis is mediated by tumor necrosis factor-α. *Nature* 329:630, 1987
59. Koch AE, Polverini PJ, Kunkel SL, et al: Interleukin-8 as a macrophage-derived mediator of angiogenesis. *Science* 258:1798, 1992

60. Bagavandoss P, Wilks JW: Specific inhibition of endothelial cell proliferation by thrombospondin. *Biochem Biophys Res Commum* 170:867, 1990
61. Khorsandi MJ, Fagin JA, Gianella-Neto D, et al: Regulation of insulin-like growth factor-1 and its receptor in rat aorta after balloon denudation. *J Clin Invest* 90:1926, 1992
62. Shing Y, Christofori G, Hanahan D, et al: Betacellulin: a mitogen from pancreatic B cell tumors. *Science* 259:1604, 1993
63. Good DJ, Polverini PJ, Rastinejad F, et al: A tumor suppressor-dependent inhibitor of angiogenesis is immunologically and functionally indistinguishable from a fragment of thrombospondin. *Proc Natl Acad Sci USA* 87:6624, 1990
64. Maione TE, Gray GS, Petro J, et al: Inhibition of anigogenesis by recombinant human platelet factor-4 and related peptides. *Science* 247:77, 1990
65. Moses MA, Sudhalter J, Langer R. Identification of an inhibitor of neovascularization from cartilage. *Science* 248:1408, 1990
66. Clapp C, Martial JA, Guzman RC, et al: The 16-kilodalton N-terminal fragment of human prolactin is a potent inhibitor of angiogenesis. *Endocrinology* 133:1292, 1993
67. Jackson RL, Busch SJ, Cardin AD: Glycosaminoglycan: molecular properties, protein interactions, and role in physiological processes. *Physiol Rev* 71:481, 1991
68. Castellot JJ, Addonizio ML, Rosenberg R, et al: Cultured endothelial cells produce a heparin-like inhibitor of smooth muscle cell growth. *J Cell Biol* 90:372, 1981
69. Clowes AW, Karnovsky MJ: Suppression by heparin of smooth muscle cell proliferation in injured arteries. *Nature* 265:625, 1977
70. Reilly CF, Kindy MS, Brown KE, et al: Heparin prevents vascular smooth muscle cell progression through the G_1 phase of the cell cycle. *J Biol Chem* 264:6990, 1989
71. Pukac LA, Ottlinger ME, Karnovsky MJ: Heparin suppresses specific second messenger pathways for protooncogene expression in rat vascular smooth muscle cells. *J Biol Chem* 268:19173, 1993
72. Reilly CF, Fritze LMS, Rosenberg RD: Heparin-like molecules regulate the number of epidermal growth factor receptors on vascular smooth muscle cells. *J Cell Physiol* 136:23, 1988
73. Nugent MA, Karnovsky MJ, Edelman ER: Vascular cell-derived heparan sulfate shows coupled inhibition of basic fibroblast growth factor binding and mitogenesis in vascular smooth muscle cells. *Circ Res* 73:1051, 1993
74. Casscells W, Lappi DA, Baird A: Molecular atherectomy for restenosis. *Trends Cardiovasc Med* 3:235, 1993
75. Barrett TB, Benditt EP: Platelet-derived growth factor gene expression in human atherosclerotic plaques and normal artery wall. *Proc Natl Acad Sci USA* 85:2810, 1988
76. Wilcox JN, Smith KM, Williams LT, et al: Platelet-derived growth factor mRNA detection in human atherosclerotic plaques by in situ hybridization. *J Clin Invest* 82:1134, 1988
77. Ross R, Masuda J, Raines EW, et al: Localization of PDGF-B protein in macrophages in all phases of atherogenesis. *Science* 248:1009, 1990
78. Pickering JG, Bacha PA, Weir L, et al: Prevention of smooth muscle cell outgrowth from human atherosclerotic plaque by a recombinant cytotoxin specific for the epidermal growth factor receptor. *J Clin Invest* 91:724, 1993
79. Mesri EA, Ono M, Kreitman RJ, et al: The heparin-binding domain of the heparin-binding EGF-like growth factor can target *Pseudomonas* exotoxin to kill cells exclusively through heparan sulfate proteoglycans. *J Cell Sci 107*: 2559, 1994
80. Simons M, Edelman ER, DeKeyser J-L, et al: Antisense c-*myb* oligonucleotides inhibit intimal arterial smooth muscle cell accumulation in vivo. *Nature* 359:67, 1992
81. Morishita R, Gibbons GH, Ellison KE, et al: Single intraluminal delivery of antisense *cdc2* kinase and proliferating-cell nuclear antigen oligonucleotides results in chronic inhibition of neointimal hyperplasia. *Proc Natl Acad Sci USA* 90:8474, 1993

Acknowledgments

The writing of this chapter was supported by NIH grants CA37392 and CA45548.

Figures 1, 2 Dana Burns-Pizer.

CHAPTER 6

Gene Therapy for Cardiovascular Disease

Elizabeth G. Nabel, M.D., Gary J. Nabel, M.D., Ph.D.

The goal of gene therapy is to alter the genetic program of cells to prevent or treat a congenital or acquired illness. This technique introduces genes that have been altered in the laboratory, called recombinant genes, into target cells whose biologic function requires modification. The therapeutic goal may be to provide missing genetic material, to correct defective genes, or to augment the function of genes already present to enhance their therapeutic or immunologic effects.

Principles of Gene Transfer

Any application of gene therapy first requires that the gene of interest be identified, cloned, and sequenced. The gene can then be introduced into a host cell, where the product encoded by the gene may have a therapeutic effect.[1] To begin the transfection process, the coding region of the recombinant gene (in the form of complementary DNA [cDNA]) is ligated into a vector [*see Figure 1*]. This cDNA is transcribed to messenger RNA (mRNA), which in turn is translated into the corresponding protein. Generally, vectors must be used to transfer genes into cells because most cells are resistant to the uptake of foreign DNA. The vectors penetrate the wall of the target cell with varying efficiency, depending on the cell type. The recombinant gene usually enters the target cell cytoplasm by receptor-mediated endocytosis or after membrane fusion of a carrier molecule. In the cytoplasm, the DNA is released from endosomes and translocates to the nucleus by unknown mechanisms. The recombinant gene may replicate in the host by integration into the host genome or through extrachromosomal replication.

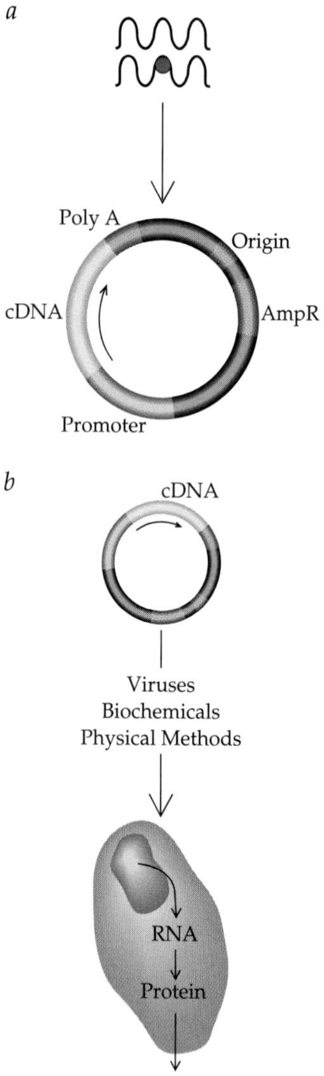

The new gene undergoes transcription into mRNA and is translated into protein by host enzymes, culminating in expression of the recombinant gene products. The period of gene expression, which may be stable or transient, can be used to study various cellular functions and to provide gene products that have therapeutic value.

Recombinant genes can be transferred to the host in two ways. Ex vivo, or cell-mediated, gene transfer consists of removing autologous cells from the intended host and growing them in cell culture in the laboratory. The recombinant genes used to change or transfect the cultured cells are introduced in vitro by various methods. Studies of transfection in vitro have usually employed electroporation, diethylaminoethyl-dextran incubation, calcium phosphate coprecipitation, or different viral carriers to transfect the harvested cells. After a period of incubation, the transfected cells are reintroduced into the host by injection or infusion. Ex vivo gene transfer allows both the introduction of recombinant genetic material into a specific cell type and analysis of its effects in vitro before the material is reintroduced into the host. In addition, cells transfected in vitro can be stored for limited periods of time before use. Ex vivo gene transfer has been successfully achieved in numerous circumstances. However, the method is both time consuming and costly, and cell lines required for in vitro transfection cannot be grown from some tissues or animals.

In vivo gene transfer employs direct injection or catheter-based infusion of recombinant genes, either carried by vectors or alone, to introduce the genetic material directly into the host. This method is attractive because of its relative simplicity and speed. However, gene expression cannot yet be precisely regulated in vivo. In addition, transfection cannot yet be targeted to specific cells. The development of promoters active only in a specific type of cell may alleviate the latter difficulty.

The efficacy of various vectors and recombinant genes is usually studied in vitro. Cell-mediated and direct gene transfer may be used to study the effects of the recombinant genes in various animal models. Because some vectors, such as retroviruses and adenoviruses, may have deleterious effects on the host, their toxicity, pattern of replication, and specificity must be carefully analyzed. Only after these studies are successfully completed can the recombinant gene of interest be used in clinical trials.

a

Poly A
Origin
cDNA
AmpR
Promoter

b

cDNA
Viruses
Biochemicals
Physical Methods
RNA
Protein

Figure 1 *Principles of gene transfer. The complementary DNA (cDNA) is ligated into a plasmid expression vector (a) and transfected into target cells (b). Expression of the recombinant cDNA within the target cell may have autocrine, paracrine, or systemic effects.*

Cardiovascular Applications of Gene Therapy

Because of its intimate and extensive communication with many other structures in the human body, the cardiovascular system is a target of great interest for gene therapy studies. The vascular system may be employed to deliver recombinant genes to other organs, such as the liver and kidneys. Because of its anatomically localized nature, cardiovascular disease has less stringent requirements for gene therapy than does correction of an inherited genetic defect. Recombinant genes can be directly transferred to the affected site, and transient rather than lifelong expression of the recombinant gene may be acceptable and is frequently desirable.

Currently, cardiovascular applications of gene transfer involve gene augmentation to restore, enhance, or inhibit normal genetic function without removing the genes already present. Both ex vivo and in vivo gene transfer techniques have been used in preclinical studies and clinical trials of gene transfer into the cardiovascular system.

Studies of the effects of recombinant genes on the cardiovascular system that involve cell-mediated gene transfer have used autologous endothelial or smooth muscle cells grown and transfected in the laboratory before reimplantion via catheter into the host blood vessel.[2-4] Genetically modified canine endothelial cells have been successfully seeded onto Dacron grafts and reimplanted into the host carotid arteries,[5] and vascular stents have been seeded with genetically modified endothelial cells in vitro.[6] The demonstration that genetically modified endothelial cells could populate arteries or vascular prostheses has raised the possibility that genes can be introduced into these cells to optimize the function of arteries, vascular grafts, or stents. Another use of ex vivo transfection can be found in a human gene therapy trial for familial hypercholesterolemia that used autologous hepatocytes transfected in culture with a retroviral vector containing a human low-density lipoprotein receptor gene and then reinstilled via infusion catheter into a patient's vena cava.[7] This trial is discussed in greater detail in Chapter 7.

Studies of in vivo gene transfer to the cardiovascular system have used catheters or direct injection to deliver vectors carrying modified genes directly into target cells or tissues [*see Figure 2*].[8] Research using a double-balloon catheter to deliver recombinant genes directly into the vasculature includes studies of the arterial effects of recombinant fibroblast growth factor–1[9]; recombinant platelet-derived growth factor B[10]; transforming growth factor–β1[11]; a human class I major histocompatibility complex gene, HLA-B7[12]; the marker gene luciferase[13-15]; and others.[16] A porous balloon catheter with perfusion capabilities has been used to deliver liposome vectors carrying a marker gene to intact canine femoral arteries.[14] DNA has been applied onto a hydrogel angioplasty balloon to deliver genes directly to arteries,[17] and genes have been injected into subcutaneous tumor nodules in a human gene therapy trial of immunotherapy for patients with metastatic melanoma.[18,19]

One impediment to direct gene transfer into the vascular system is the slow replication of vascular endothelial cells in the resting state. This quality limits the efficacy of some vectors, such as the retrovirus, that require cell proliferation for expression of the recombinant gene.[20] Other vectors, such as cationic liposomes and recombinant adenoviral vectors, have been developed to attempt to overcome this problem.

Vectors

Transfection in vivo is generally accomplished with the assistance of vectors, which facilitate the delivery and entry into the host cells of the recombinant genetic material. To be effective, vectors must be able to overcome the cell's natural resistance to foreign DNA. Viral vectors include the retrovirus, adenovirus, and adenoviral conjugates. Nonviral vectors include liposomes, biolistics (from biological ballistic), and physical injection.[21]

Viral Vectors

Because of the efficiency with which viruses can infect mammalian cells, viral vectors were among the first to be studied. Viral entry into cells requires the presence of the appropriate viral receptor on the target cell. Once in the cell, the virus uses host cell biosynthetic pathways to produce viral DNA, RNA, and protein. The viral vectors employed in preclinical gene transfer studies include retroviruses, adenoviruses, adeno-associated viruses, and herpesviruses. Retroviruses and adenoviruses are the viral vectors primarily used in studies of gene transfer to cardiovascular tissue.

Retrovirus

Retroviruses are RNA viruses that, unlike many viruses, do not destroy the cell they infect. In the natural life cycle of retroviruses, they enter cells via a retroviral receptor. Once in the cell, viral RNA in the cytoplasm is copied by reverse transcriptase into DNA. After integration into the host cell nucleus, viral RNA and proteins are synthesized in the host cytoplasm and assembled, and new viral particles bud through the cell membrane.

Retroviruses are valuable as vectors for recombinant genes because they have the ability to stably infect many mammalian cells.[22] Retroviral vectors are engineered to incorporate the new gene and are replication defective in the host cell. Because of their ability to become part of the infected cell, the effects of retroviral vectors can be dangerous to the host if reproduction of the viral part of the vector is not controlled. To prevent the reproduction of wild-type retrovirus, retroviral vectors are engineered to be replication incompetent by removing the viral structural genes necessary for replication while leaving the packaging signal intact.[23] The altered retroviral DNA is transfected into a packaging cell line, which contains plasmids that encode all of the retrovirus structural genes that are under control of the regulatory sequences of the viral promoter but lack the packaging signal.[24] The vector transcripts are recognized by the packaging mechanism, and a replication-deficient virion is produced. A further precaution against generation of wild-type virus is the introduction of multiple modifications of the helper provirus so that more than one recombination event is required to generate wild-type virus.

Retroviruses provide stable expression of recombinant genes with relative ease in mammalian cells. The efficiency of gene transfer into vascular cells via retroviral vectors is relatively low; approximately 5 to 10 percent of vascular endothelial cells have been transfected in vitro, and fewer than 0.1 to 1 percent of vascular endothelial cells have been transfected in vivo.[15,25] Studies have shown that retroviral vectors are probably effective only in replicating cells,[20] thus limiting the utility of this vector.

Despite the careful construction of replication-defective retroviral vectors, the safety of their use for long-term gene transfer in vivo is not yet known. Generation of wild-type virus that produced lymphomas was reported in one study that introduced retroviral vectors into hematopoietic stem cells via bone marrow transplantation in primates.[26] In contrast, five-month studies of serum and peripheral blood lymphocytes revealed no wild-type retroviral recombination after direct transfer into porcine arteries.[8] Direct transfection employing retroviral injection has recently received approval for use in human studies by the Recombinant DNA Advisory Committee of the National Institutes of Health.

Other deficiencies of retroviral vectors include relative lability of the viral particles, so that in primates and humans, the virus may be inactivated in vivo by a complement-mediated process. In addition, the size of cDNA insert that can be accommodated by the vector is relatively small, generally less than 5 kilobases.

In summary, retroviruses are versatile vectors that readily infect mammalian cells, express the recombinant gene product without killing the host cell, and have the ability to integrate into the genome of the host cell. The requirement for host cell replication to produce the recombinant gene product, the size constraint on the DNA insert that can be incorporated into the vector, and the possibility that deleterious wild-type virus can be produced through uncontrolled combinations or mutagenesis are all drawbacks that have stimulated the search for other viral and nonviral vectors.

Adenovirus

The adenovirus is a nonenveloped, double-stranded DNA virus that is regarded as a useful vector for in vivo gene delivery for many reasons. Adenoviruses attach to an adenoviral lipoprotein receptor on a broad range of mammalian cells. Adenoviruses integrate into the host genome at low frequency and are maintained in the nucleus transiently, primarily as an episome. They do not require cell replication for transfer and expression of recombinant genes. This characteristic overcomes the impediment to gene transfer presented by the slow replication of cardiovascular endothelial cells. Adenoviral vectors can be produced in very high titer, often greater than 10^9 plaque-forming units per milliliter, which is several logs higher than can be generated with retroviral vectors.[27] In addition, these vectors are relatively stable and are amenable to purification and concentration. They can accommodate large cDNA inserts. Adenoviruses have not been associated with human malignancies or chronic infections.

Adenoviral vectors can be made replication defective by deletion of viral replication genes and replacement with a new gene of interest. The cell line used to construct the replication-defective adenoviral vector is the human embryonic kidney cell line 293, which contains a copy of an important adenoviral replication gene, *E1a*. Transfection of plasmids that contain a relevant cDNA in a partial adenoviral genome together with another fragment of adenoviral DNA into the 293 packaging cells generates the replication-defective adenovirus.

At the present time, limitations of these first-generation adenoviral vectors exist for in vivo studies. At least one of the adenoviral gene products, a viral protein expressed late in replication, is specifically toxic to cells. In addition, a number of viral proteins normally expressed by the adenovirus may induce immune responses directed against the host cells, or they may induce shutoff of host protein synthesis, or both of these actions may occur. Research is ongoing to characterize the immune response against viral capsid proteins and to construct second-generation vectors that lack late replication genes.

Expression of adenoviral gene products is transient, generally lasting less than one month. The stability and duration of gene expression in target tissues require further study. Reporter genes delivered by intravenous injection of adenovirus into neonatal mice have been expressed for up to 12 months in murine muscle; however, expression in adult murine muscle was lost by four weeks,[28] and low-density lipoprotein receptor expression in murine liver persisted for only several weeks.[29]

Finally, the safety and potential toxicity of adenoviral infection for human therapy are still unknown. In animal models, endobronchial delivery of adenovirus is associated with peribronchial inflammation and alveolar edema,[30] and intravenous infusion of virus has been associated with lymphocytic infiltration of murine livers.[29]

Despite these drawbacks, adenoviral vectors have successfully achieved gene transfer to many organs in various models, including cardiac[31] and skeletal muscle,[28] arteries,[31-34] brain,[35] lung epithelium,[36-38] and liver.[29, 39] The ability of adenoviruses to transfer genetic material efficiently into lung epithelial cells has stimulated interest in the use of this vector to provide gene therapy for patients with cystic fibrosis.[40, 41]

In summary, advantages of adenoviral vectors include their growth to high titer, their efficient infection of various mammalian cells, and their expression in nondividing cells in vivo. They are relatively stable, can be purified and concentrated, and can accommodate large cDNA inserts. The high efficiency of gene transfer via adenoviral vectors suggests the possible therapeutic value of this regimen in diseases in which short-term gene expression may be required, such as restenosis. Finally, the extrachromosomal replication of adenovirus makes it less likely that adenovirus will cause mutation by random integration and dysregulation of important host cellular genes.

Adenovirus-Augmented, Receptor-Mediated Gene Delivery

Another adenoviral delivery system uses specific ligands, such as transferrin, conjugated to DNA through a cationic polymer, polylysine.[42-45] The complex enters cells by receptor-mediated endocytosis through binding of the transferrin ligand to the transferrin receptor. A second component of the vector is a photochemically inactivated, replication-defective adenovirus that is linked directly to the DNA. After the DNA complex binds to the transferrin receptor, the complex is internalized into lysosomes. The virus lowers pH in the lysosomes, triggering a conformational change that disrupts the endosome, releasing DNA into the cytoplasm for transport to the nucleus.

Advantages of adenovirus-augmented, receptor-mediated gene delivery include a moderately efficient transfer of DNA via ligand receptor binding and receptor-mediated endocytosis. Because the DNA and virus are separate structures, alterations can be made in either the gene or the virus. This system also permits the use of other synthetic or natural ligands (i.e., a ligand to the asialoglycoprotein receptor, antibodies to cell surface receptors) and other viruses.[46] However, the stability and duration of gene expression after receptor-mediated gene delivery depend on the specific ligand and viral components. The safety of these vectors for clinical use has yet to be determined, and the effect of these vectors in vascular cells and myocytes has not been defined.

Nonviral Vectors

Interest in avoiding the infectious complications of the viral vector systems has stimulated the study of other methods of gene delivery, including the use of nonviral vectors, such as cationic liposomes, biolistics, and physical injection.

Cationic Liposomes

Negatively charged DNA can be incorporated into cationic liposomes, which are attracted to lipid molecules because they are positively charged. Initially, the efficiency of DNA encapsulation into conventional uncharged or anionic liposomes was low because the internal volume of liposomes is usually smaller than the foreign gene. In addition, transfection efficiency was low because conventional liposomes did not efficiently bypass lysosomal degradation. Cationic liposomes were developed in the late 1980s to overcome these deficiencies.[47] These liposomes interact with the negatively charged DNA and deliver the nucleic acid to the cell through mechanisms that are not fully defined. To some extent, this process allows a portion of the polynucleotide to bypass lysosomal degradation. Some of the introduced DNA translocates to the cell nucleus, where it is maintained largely in an extrachromosomal form.

DNA-liposome complexes form rapidly in aqueous solution via an electrostatic interaction that is always dependent on the molar ratio between the DNA and the liposomes.[48] Although gene expression is not always permanent, it lasts weeks to months. Safety and toxicity studies of DNA liposome delivery by catheter or by intravenous or intratumoral injection in mice, rabbits, and pigs have detected transfection at the site of delivery,[8] with minimal risk of mutagenesis and toxicity in vivo.[16, 49, 50]

Cells receiving liposome-mediated gene transfer in vivo include vascular endothelial cells,[8-15] lung epithelial cells,[51] and tumor cells.[52] This vector has also been used in a human gene therapy protocol for malignant melanoma treatment and for catheter-based gene delivery in humans.[18, 19]

The prototypic cationic lipid is DOTMA (*N*[1-(2,3-dioleyloxy)propyl]-*N,N,N*-trimethylammonium chloride).[47] When mixed with an equimolar amount of DOPE (dioleoylphosphatidylethanolamine), DOTMA forms a cationic liposome, commercially available as Lipofectin (Bethesda Research Laboratories, Gaithersburg, MD). Another cationic liposome, composed of DC-cholesterol (3b[*N*-(*N'N'*-dimethylaminoethane)-carbamoyl] cholesterol) and DOPE, has proved to be nontoxic to cells over a wide range of concentrations in vitro and is metabolized in vivo.[53] This vector has provided efficient gene transfer into vascular cells and into malignant tumors in vivo.[16,52] Recently, new formulations of cationic liposomes have been developed to improve transfection efficiency, including DMRIE/DOPE (1,2-dimyristyloxypropyl-3-dimethylhydroxyethyl ammonium bromide/dioleoylphosphatidylethanolamine)[50] and DOSPA/DOPE (Lipofectamine, or

2,3-dioleyloxy-*N*-[2(sperminecarboxamido)ethyl]-*N,N*-dimethyl-1-propanaminiumtrifluoroacetate/dioleolyphosphatidylethanolamine).

As is the case with all transfection methods, the expression levels and stability obtained with cationic liposomes depend on the plasmid expression vector, cell line, and host cell. For example, differences in the type of target cell, plasmid, and mixture of DOTMA with DOPE require individual adjustments. Unlike anionic liposomes, which are primarily cleared by the reticuloendothelial system, cationic liposomes are often inactivated by polyvalent, negatively charged serum components. Because of this, serum-free conditions at the transfection site, such as those provided by the double-balloon catheter, are important.

Cationic liposomes are safe vectors for direct gene transfer because they contain no viral sequences and transfection is limited primarily to the site of transfection.[8,16] Cationic liposomes can accept large amounts of DNA, they are strongly attracted to the target cell, and they are minimally degraded in endosomes. Further modifications of these vectors will improve their efficiency and the duration of gene expression.

Particle-Mediated (Biolistic) Gene Transfer

Particle-mediated gene delivery can also be employed to deliver recombinant DNA in vitro and in vivo. Plasmid DNA is precipitated onto the surface of microscopic metal beads (~1 μm in diameter). The microprojectiles, which are accelerated with a wave of expanding helium gas or water vapor, can then be used to transduce cells in vitro or to penetrate tissues to a depth of several cell layers to deliver foreign DNA to the skin or internal organs of anesthetized animals. Expression of the gene is high for several days and then falls off but is detectable for several weeks.[54] This approach may be useful for situations in which transient expression is required within a localized region of tissue, such as genetic immunization of mice against foreign antigens.[55] Particle-mediated gene transfer could be adapted to transduce unstimulated cells and possibly to deliver recombinant genes and other nondividing cells, such as T cells or hematopoietic progenitor cells. Preliminary studies using this technique have achieved 0.1 to 10 percent recombinant gene expression in $CD4^+$ T cells in vitro,[56] and this method is being tested in a clinical protocol against acquired immunodeficiency syndrome.[56]

Physical Injection

The introduction of foreign genes into cardiac and skeletal muscle by direct injection has been an exciting recent development in myocyte transfection. In skeletal muscle, no gene delivery vector was necessary to achieve significant levels of transgene expression.[57] Further studies suggest that in the fully differentiated skeletal myocytes, gene sequences are maintained as nuclear episomes but are not integrated into the nucleus.[58] Physical injection has been employed to transfer genes to cardiac muscle,[59] to introduce transduced myoblasts into skeletal muscle,[60] and to introduce cationic liposome vectors carrying HLA-B7 immunogenic plasmids into melanoma tumors.[19]

Naked DNA

Another approach to the introduction of DNA into arteries is to coat DNA vectors onto balloon catheters using polymer gels. During balloon inflation, DNA is directly introduced throughout the full thickness of the arterial wall with minimal tissue damage. In vivo studies on rabbit arteries showed that gene transfer could be successfully accomplished by use of the hydrogel-coated catheter.[17] Another DNA delivery system is a pluronic gel, which has been used successfully to deliver antisense oligonucleotides to the adventitial surfaces of arteries.[61]

Gene Transfer into the Vasculature

Early preclinical work in vascular gene transfer used reporter genes to study the effectiveness of viral and nonviral vectors to introduce genes into the vasculature. Although these studies are continuing, more recent work is focusing on the introduction of new DNA or gene sequences into target somatic cells as a means of providing therapy for cardiovascular disorders. The therapeutic goal of gene therapy can be (1) to provide or augment the in vivo synthesis of a missing or defective gene product or (2) to suppress the synthesis of a deleterious gene product. Innovative techniques of gene transfer include seeding of recombinant genes onto arteries or vascular prostheses,[2, 5, 62] direct transferring of genes into coronary and peripheral arteries,[8-15] and injection of recombinant genes into cardiac muscle.[59,63] Other preclinical studies focus on understanding the pathophysiology of cardiovascular disease. Examples of techniques used in these studies include direct gene transfer of growth factors into arteries to study their role in the stimulation of smooth muscle cell proliferation, as occurs in restenosis,[9-11] and to develop gene therapies for cardiovascular disease, such as the use of antisense oligonucleotides to inhibit smooth muscle cell proliferation.[61, 64, 65]

Within the vascular system, two cells involved in the production of vascular disease, endothelial cells and smooth muscle cells, are specific targets for genetic intervention. The endothelium forms a monolayer of approximately 10^5 cells/cm^2 on the luminal surface of all blood vessels. Endothelial cells regulate hemostasis, vascular contractility, cellular proliferation, and inflammatory mechanisms in the vessel wall. Thus, because of their important anatomic and pathogenic roles, endothelial cells are potential carriers, either locally or systemically, of therapeutic agents, including anticoagulant, vasodilatory, angiogenic, or growth inhibitory factors. The role of the endothelium in vascular biology is discussed in Chapter 4.

Vascular smooth muscle cells compose the media of arteries and exert the contractile force that provides arterial tone. In vascular disease states, these cells proliferate in the intima in response to vessel injury, contributing to the development of intimal hyperplasia.[66] Because of their central role in the development of stenotic vascular lesions, smooth muscle cells are important targets for gene transfer. In addition, their multilayered configuration provides a larger reservoir than does the single layer of endothelial cells for the synthesis of recombinant gene products.

These two cell types are important targets for the application of gene therapy to vascular and other diseases. Because of their continuity with the bloodstream, endothelial cells could deliver therapeutic gene products with anticoagulant, anti-inflammatory, vasodilatory, or antiproliferative effects, thereby providing treatment for systemic or inherited disease in another organ system. Recombinant genes secreted from endothelial and vascular smooth muscle cells might have autocrine and paracrine effects on adjacent vascular cells and could alter local cellular growth, thereby providing treatment for vascular injury or disease.

Cell-Mediated Gene Transfer

Ex vivo transfection of endothelial and smooth muscle cells has been demonstrated in several animal models. Transfected endothelial cells were seeded onto denuded porcine iliofemoral arteries via a double-balloon catheter [*see Figure 2*].[2] Genetically modified vascular smooth muscle cells were also seeded onto denuded porcine iliofemoral arteries. These cells were observed subsequently in the intima and media of seeded arteries.[3, 4] Seeding of autologous transduced endothelial cells onto rat skeletal muscle capillaries was also shown to be feasible.[67]

Vascular ex vivo gene transfer may have an important role to play in device technology as a means of effecting fibrinolysis on the surface of vascular devices that are highly predisposed to thrombosis. Genetically modified canine endothelial cells seeded onto prosthetic grafts and reimplanted in vivo into canine coronary arteries produced reporter gene expression for at least five weeks,[5] and stents were seeded in vitro with genetically modified sheep endothelial cells.[6] Seeding of genetically modified smooth muscle cells was achieved both in denuded pig arteries[3] and denuded rat arteries.[4,62] Other studies addressing this issue have improved the conditions for increasing protein expression from retrovirally transduced endothelial cells and for increasing the number and longevity of seeded cells.[68, 69]

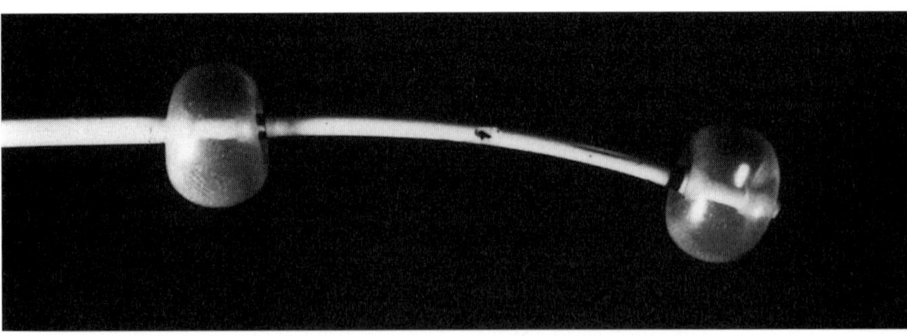

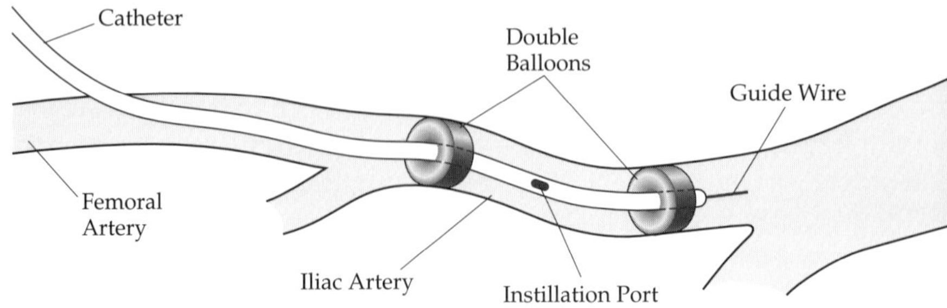

Figure 2 *Double-balloon catheter used for in vivo gene transfer into the vasculature. Inflation of the proximal and distal balloons creates a protected arterial space into which vectors carrying DNA particles can be infused through a central port.*

Direct Gene Transfer

Recombinant DNA has been delivered directly to normal and injured peripheral and coronary arteries of many species by catheters or by local injection. The transfer of genes in vivo into various components of the cardiovascular system depends on several variables, including animal species, type of artery (muscular, elastic), vector, concentration of vector, and delivery system.

Expression of a reporter gene in iliofemoral arteries of pigs after direct gene transfer with retrovirus or cationic liposome vectors demonstrated the feasibility of in vivo transfer of recombinant genes into the vasculature.[8] In this study, reporter gene expression was observed for at least five months after retroviral infection and was limited to the site of arterial infusion. The failure to observe gene expression in other arteries or organs, including the kidney, the lung, the liver, and the spleen, suggested the relative safety of this gene transfer model; retroviral replication was not observed in the sera or lymphocytes of the experimental animals. Subsequent studies employed surgical or percutaneous approaches to the transfer of marker genes to coronary or peripheral arteries of dogs.[13, 14] Percutaneous gene transfer has also been shown to be possible in normal and balloon-dilated atherosclerotic arteries of rabbits.[15]

These studies of retrovirus- or liposome-mediated gene transfection into specific sites in arteries have demonstrated gene expression in endothelial and smooth muscle cells. Expression of recombinant proteins from these cells can exert local autocrine and paracrine effects. For example, direct transduction of the human class I major histocompatibility complex gene HLA-B7 into porcine arteries demonstrated focal inflammation at the transduction sites.[12] Gene transfer using liposomes complexed with a heat-inactivated virus, hemagglutinating virus of Japan, to examine the effect of angiotensin-converting enzyme on renin gene expression in rat vascular smooth muscle cells revealed an increase in angiotensin II and smooth muscle cell proliferation after transfection.[70]

Direct gene transfer has been used as a somatic transgenic model to define gene expression and function in the arterial wall. Our laboratory has examined the biology of three recombinant growth factor genes, platelet-derived growth factor B (PDGF B),[10] fibroblast growth factor (FGF-1, or acidic FGF),[9] and transforming growth factor–β1 (TGF-β1).[11] Although data from human atherosclerosis specimens suggest an important role for these growth factors in human vascular disease, their direct effects within arteries in vivo are poorly understood. The advantage of gene transfer is that a recombinant gene can be transfected into a focal artery segment, where its expression and effects on arterial function can be evaluated.

To address the role of the *PDGF B* gene in vivo, we transfected a plasmid expression vector encoding a human *PDGF B* gene into porcine arteries. Transfer of plasmid DNA was documented by polymerase chain reaction, and expression of recombinant mRNA was confirmed by reverse transcriptase polymerase chain reaction. Recombinant PDGF BB protein was detected in transduced arteries by immunohistochemistry using a monoclonal antibody against human PDGF BB. Arteries transfected with a *PDGF B* gene demonstrated severe intimal thickening, characterized by increased cellularity and smooth muscle cell proliferation in contrast to control arteries transduced with a reporter gene [*see Figure 3*]. Quantitative morphometric studies confirmed a significant difference in intimal-to-medial ratio between arteries transfected with PDGF B and control arteries.

We have also examined the role of FGF-1 in vascular pathology. Intimal thickening was also observed in FGF-1–transduced arteries. Interestingly, in FGF-1–transduced vessels with expanded intima, intimal angiogenesis was present. This intimal angiogenesis was not evident in vessels transduced with other growth factor genes, including *PDGF* and *TGF-β1*. These studies support a role for FGF-1 in the stimulation of vascular angiogenesis in vivo. Further studies from our laboratory examined the expression of a secreted active form of TGF-β1 in porcine arteries; *TGF-β1* gene–transduced arteries were associated with increased synthesis of procollagen and extracellular matrix proteins, including proteoglycans and reticulin. In summary, the results of our studies examining recombinant growth factor gene expression in vivo suggest that intimal hyperplasia is not uniform. Growth factors have overlapping, but distinct, effects on the development of intimal hyperplasia. The implications of these studies are that for a complex biologic process like restenosis, interfering with a single growth factor gene product is probably insufficient to inhibit intimal hyperplasia when multiple redundant pathways are involved. Rather, strategies that target factors or pathways common to these growth factors may be more beneficial.

Recent studies employing adenoviral vectors have shown high-level transfer of reporter genes into the peripheral and coronary arteries and the myocardium in mice,[28] rabbits,[31] sheep,[32] rats,[33] and pigs.[34] Direct in vivo transfection of sheep carotid arteries and veins with replication-incompetent adenoviral vectors containing a bacterial reporter gene and a human cystic fibrosis transmembrane regulator gene resulted in expression of the reporter gene up to 14 days after infection.[32] Barr and associates have shown that genes can be expressed in the myocardium after percutaneous transluminal administration of an adenoviral vector encoding the *lac*-Z gene into rabbit coronary arteries.[31] In addition, recombinant gene expression has been demonstrated in porcine pulmonary arteries by a percutaneous approach.[34] In general, after adenoviral infection of arteries in multiple species, gene expression is transient, with peak expression occurring within the first week and diminishing by one month. Loss of transgene expression may be secondary to loss of viral genome, promoter extinction, or immune response against viral proteins. Adenoviral vectors are being modified to improve the duration of gene expression and to minimize immune responses. These vectors hold promise for gene transfer studies in the vasculature because of their high efficiency.

In summary, gene transfer has been performed in vascular tissue using ex vivo and direct approaches, in which viral and nonviral vectors were used in several animal species. Studies have used reporter genes to quantify levels of gene expression and to determine cell types that have been transfected. In addition, investigations of the pathophysiology of vascular disease have been conducted, and new therapeutic approaches to treating vascular disease have been explored. Major challenges include the optimization and regulation of gene expression.

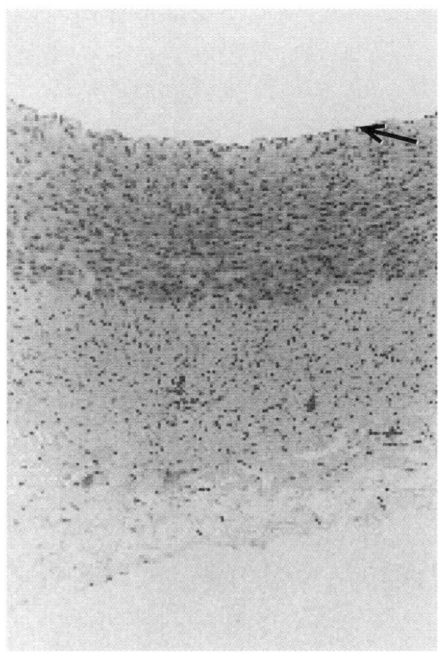

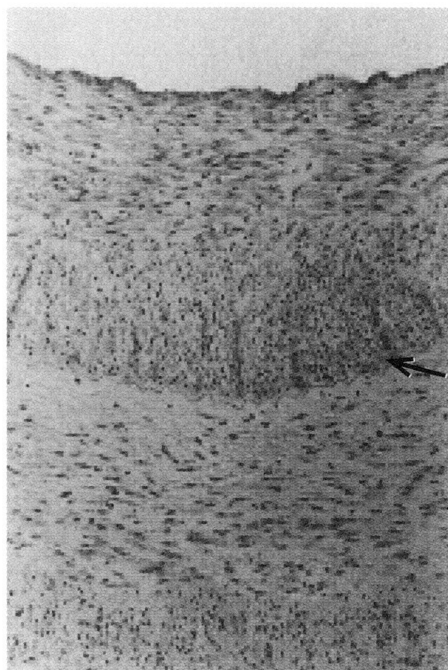

Figure 3 *Light microscopy of porcine iliofemoral arteries 21 days after in vivo infusion of liposome vectors carrying the* E. coli *β-galactosidase reporter gene (left) or a recombinant* PDGF B *gene (right). Intimal thickening is evident in the arteries transfected by the* PDGF *gene (right), compared with no intimal proliferation in arteries transfected by the reporter gene (left). The arrows denote the internal elastic lamina (hematoxylin-eosin × 100).*

Antisense Oligonucleotides

Antisense oligonucleotides are single-stranded DNA molecules synthesized with a base-pair sequence that is complementary to the mRNA sequence of a cellular gene.[71] They enter cells by simple diffusion and are not targeted to specific cell types. Binding of the antisense RNA to the native RNA creates a double-stranded RNA hybrid that inhibits translation of the mRNA. Oligonucleotides may be equally effective in replicating and nonreplicating cells and do not contain viral sequences. However, they are relatively unstable compounds and may be rapidly degraded within cells. To suppress cellular mRNA, therefore, antisense oligonucleotides must reach most vascular cells for a prolonged contact time. Antisense oligonucleotides directed against c-*myb*,[72] c-*myc*,[73] nonmuscle myosin,[72] and proliferating-cell nuclear antigen[73] have been used in vitro to suppress smooth muscle cell replication. Recent reports of antisense oligonucleotides targeted to c-*myb*,[61] *cdc*2 kinase, proliferating-cell nuclear antigen,[64] and *cdk*2 kinase[65] have suggested that this approach may limit intimal hyperplasia in an injured rat carotid artery model. However, differences in the effectiveness of antisense oligonucleotides in injured arteries have been reported, and these differences in vivo may be a function of variability in animal species, type of artery, oligonucleotide length and chemistry, concentration of oligonucleotide, and delivery method. Although the results of these studies suggest the potential of this approach, some technical features require refinement.

Gene Transfer into Muscle Cells

Injection of genetically modified myoblasts has potential as a gene transfer system for the delivery of recombinant proteins into the circulation. Injection of transduced myoblasts into skeletal muscle may produce therapeutic proteins, which can be secreted into the circulation at physiologic levels.[60,74] Transplantation of cardiac myocytes has been limited, however, by the difficulty of growing and manipulating these cells in culture and by their fully differentiated nature. Recombinant genes have been expressed in rat hearts for several months after direct plasmid DNA injection.[59,63] Murine C2C12 myoblasts transfected with human growth hormone via retroviral vectors expressed physiologic levels of human growth hormone into the serum for three weeks[60] and three months[74] after injection into the hind limbs of mice. In another study, injected myoblasts that were transfected with human factor IX via retroviral vectors secreted factor IX into the circulation for up to one month.[75]

Infusion of replication-defective adenoviruses into coronary arteries of rabbits produced a high percentage (60 to 80 percent) of cardiac myocyte transfection.[31] This percentage was 50 to 100 times higher than that observed after direct DNA injections into the heart.[59] Although expression was transient, this model of myocyte transfection appears promising.

Clinical Trials

In the United States, gene therapy clinical protocols are subject to approval and regulation by the National Institutes of Health Recombinant DNA Advisory Committee and the Food and Drug Administration. More than 80 clinical trials of gene transfer/therapy have been approved thus far; several are applicable to the cardiopulmonary field and include an ex vivo trial for familial hypercholesterolemia[7] and several trials to treat cystic fibrosis.[40, 41] A recently completed trial of direct DNA–liposome-mediated transfection for immunotherapy against melanoma has established the feasibility and safety of direct DNA introduction into humans by both direct injection and catheter-based infusion into the vasculature[19] [*see Figure 4*].

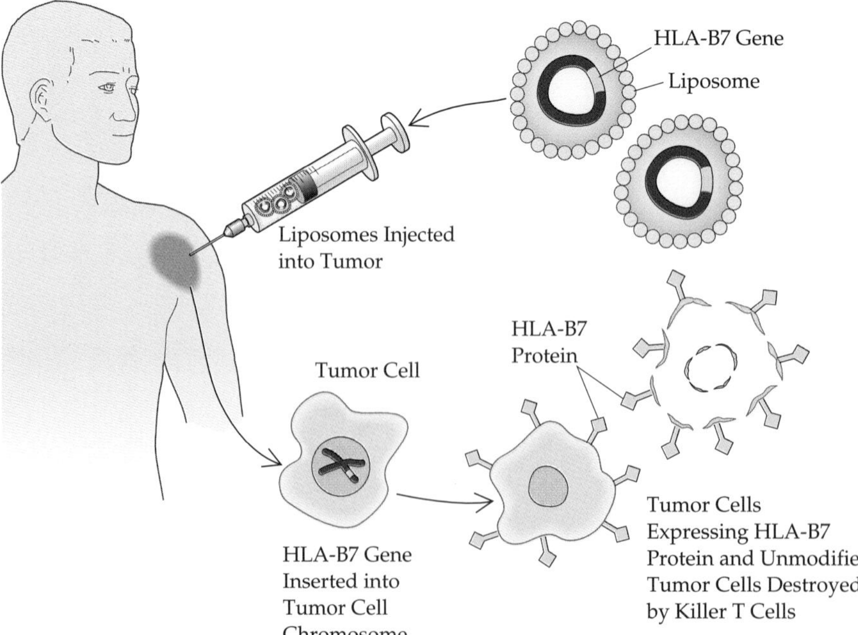

Figure 4 *Trial of direct gene transfer achieved by injection of cationic liposomes carrying the immunogenic HLA-B7 gene. Cells expressing the transfected HLA-B7 gene are recognized as foreign by the patient's immune system, and killer T cells destroy not only these tumor cells but also, by an unknown mechanism, some unmodified tumor cells.*

Conclusion

Many scientific challenges must be met before human gene therapy can be used to its full potential to treat cardiovascular disorders. The identification of target genes and an understanding of disease pathophysiology are important goals, as is an understanding of the regulation of gene expression. Modifications in vectors to improve transfection efficiency and duration of gene expression, to minimize toxicity, and to target genes to particular organs will facilitate these efforts.

Despite these hurdles, gene therapy has much to offer in the treatment of cardiovascular disorders. The pathology in many acquired cardiovascular diseases is anatomically localized. Although atherosclerosis is a systemic disorder, the critical lesions in most instances are located at specific sites in the circulation. Thus, focal arterial disease is a major target for gene therapy of the vascular system. During angioplasty procedures, recombinant DNA may be introduced into the coronary artery at the angioplasty site to modify cellular proliferation. Other genetic interventions, including thrombolytic, angiogenic, or growth factor genes, could be introduced at the time of intervention for the treatment of myocardial or tissue ischemia.

In the past decade, rapid growth has occurred in our understanding of the molecular and cellular biology of the cardiovascular system. Gene transfer is a new approach to the investigation of the pathophysiology of cardiovascular diseases, and genetic interventions for the treatment of these disorders are likely to be implemented in the future.

References

1. Watson JD, Gilman M, Witkowski J, et al: *Recombinant DNA*, 2nd ed. Scientific American Books, New York, 1992
2. Nabel EG, Plautz G, Boyce FM, et al: Recombinant gene expression in vivo within endothelial cells of the arterial wall. *Science* 244:1342, 1989
3. Plautz G, Nabel EG, Nabel GJ: Introduction of vascular smooth muscle cells expressing recombinant genes in vivo. *Circulation* 83:578, 1991
4. Lynch CM, Clowes MM, Osborne WR, et al: Long-term expression of human adenosine deaminase in vascular smooth muscle cells of rats: a model for gene therapy. *Proc Natl Acad Sci USA* 89:1138, 1992
5. Wilson JM, Birinyi LK, Salomon RN, et al: Implantation of vascular grafts lined with genetically modified endothelial cells. *Science* 244:1344, 1989
6. Dichek DA, Neville RF, Zweibel JA, et al: Seeding of intravascular stents with genetically engineered endothelial cells. *Circulation* 80:1347, 1989
7. Grossman M, Raper SE, Kozarsky K, et al: Successful ex vivo gene therapy directed to liver in a patient with familial hypercholesterolemia. *Nature Genetics* 6:335, 1994
8. Nabel EG, Plautz G, Nabel GJ: Site-specific gene expression in vivo by direct gene transfer into the arterial wall. *Science* 249:1285, 1990
9. Nabel EG, Yang Z-Y, Plautz D, et al: Recombinant fibroblast growth factor-1 promotes intimal hyperplasia and angiogenesis in arteries in vivo. *Nature* 362:844, 1993
10. Nabel EG, Yang A, Liptay S, et al: Recombinant platelet-derived growth factor B gene expression in porcine arteries induces intimal hyperplasia in vivo. *J Clin Invest* 91:1822, 1993
11. Nabel EG, Shum L, Pompili VJ, et al: Direct gene transfer of transforming growth factor β1 into arteries stimulates fibrocellular hyperplasia. *Proc Natl Acad Sci USA* 90:10759, 1993
12. Nabel EG, Plautz G, Nabel GJ: Transduction of a foreign histocompatibility gene into the arterial wall induces vasculitis. *Proc Natl Acad Sci USA* 89:5157, 1992
13. Lim CS, Chapman GD, Gammon RS, et al: Direct in vivo gene transfer into the coronary and peripheral vasculatures of the intact dog. *Circulation* 83:2007, 1991

14. Chapman GD, Lim CS, Gammon RS, et al: Gene transfer into coronary arteries of intact animals with a percutaneous balloon catheter. *Circ Res* 71:27, 1992
15. Leclerc G, Gal D, Takeshita S, et al: Percutaneous arterial gene transfer in a rabbit model: efficiency in normal and balloon-dilated atherosclerotic arteries. *J Clin Invest* 90:936, 1992
16. Nabel EG, Gordon D, Yang Z-Y, et al: Gene transfer in vivo with DNA-liposome complexes: lack of autoimmunity and gonadal localization. *Hum Gene Ther* 3:649, 1992
17. Riessen R, Rahimizadeh H, Blessing E, et al: Arterial gene transfer using pure DNA applied directly to a hydrogel-coated angioplasty balloon. *Hum Gene Ther* 4:749, 1993
18. Nabel GJ, Chang A, Nabel EG, et al: Clinical protocol: immunotherapy of malignancy by in vivo gene transfer into tumors. *Hum Gene Ther* 3:399, 705, 1992
19. Nabel GJ, Nabel EG, Yang Z-Y, et al: Direct gene transfer with DNA liposome complexes in melanoma: expression, biologic activity, and lack of toxicity in humans. *Proc Natl Acad Sci USA* 90:11307, 1993
20. Miller DO, Adam MA, Miller AD: Gene transfer by retrovirus vectors occurs only in cells that are actively replicating at the time of infection. *Mol Cell Biol* 10:4239, 1990
21. Mulligan RC: The basic science of gene therapy. *Science* 260:926, 1993
22. Varmus H: Retroviruses. *Science* 240:1427, 1988
23. Danos O, Mulligan RC: Safe and efficient generation of recombinant retroviruses with amphotropic and ecotropic host ranges. *Proc Natl Acad Sci USA* 85:6460, 1988
24. Cone RD, Mulligan RC: High-efficiency gene transfer into mammalian cells: generation of helper-free recombinant retrovirus with broad mammalian host range. *Proc Natl Acad Sci USA* 81:6349, 1984
25. Flugelman MY, Jaklitsch MT, Newman KD, et al: Low level in vivo gene transfer into the arterial wall through a perforated balloon catheter. *Circulation* 3:1110, 1992
26. National Institutes of Health Recombinant DNA Advisory Committee, Bethesda, MD. *National Institutes of Health* 6:1, 1993
27. Gerard RD, Meidell RS: Adenovirus-mediated gene transfer. *Trends Cardiovasc Med* 3:171, 1993
28. Stratford-Perricaudet LK, Makeh I, Perricaudet M, et al: Widespread long-term gene transfer to mouse skeletal muscles and heart. *J Clin Invest* 90:626, 1992
29. Herz J, Gerard RD: Adenovirus-mediated transfer of low density lipoprotein receptor gene acutely accelerates cholesterol clearance in normal mice. *Proc Natl Acad Sci USA* 90:2812, 1993
30. Simon RH, Engelhardt JF, Yang Y, et al: Adenovirus-mediated transfer of the CFTR gene to lung of nonhuman primates: toxicity study. *Hum Gene Ther* 4:771, 1993
31. Barr E, Carroll J, Kalynych AM, et al: Percutaneous transluminal gene transfer into the heart using replication-defective recombinant adenovirus. *Gene Ther* 1:51, 1994
32. Lemarchand P, Jones M, Yamada I, et al: In vivo gene transfer and expression in normal uninjured blood vessels using replication-deficient recombinant adenovirus vectors. *Circ Res* 72:1132, 1993
33. Guzman RJ, Lemarchand P, Crystal RG, et al: Efficient and selective adenovirus-mediated gene transfer into vascular neointima. *Circulation* 88:2838, 1993
34. Muller DWM, Gordon D, San H, et al: Percutaneous pulmonary vascular gene transfer and expression. *Circ Res* 75:1039, 1994
35. Davidson BL, Allen ED, Kozarsky KF, et al: A model system for in vivo gene transfer into the central nervous system using an adenoviral vector. *Nature Genetics* 3:219, 1993
36. Rosenfeld MA, Siegfried W, Yoshimura K, et al: Adenovirus-mediated transfer of a recombinant α1-antitrypsin gene to the lung epithelium in vivo. *Science* 252:431, 1991
37. Rosenfeld MA, Yoshimura K, Trapnell BC, et al: In vivo transfer of the human cystic fibrosis transmembrane conductance regulator gene to the airway epithelium. *Cell* 68:143, 1992
38. Engelhardt JF, Yang Y, Stratford-Perricaudet LD, et al: Direct gene transfer of human CFTR into human bronchial epithelia of xenografts with E1-deleted adenoviruses. *Nature Genetics* 4:27, 1993
39. Ishibashi S, Brown MS, Goldstein JL, et al: Hypercholesterolemia in low density lipoprotein receptor knockout mice and its reversal by adenovirus-mediated gene delivery. *J Clin Invest* 92:883, 1993
40. Zabner J, Couture LA, Gregory RJ, et al: Adenovirus-mediated gene transfer transiently corrects the chloride transport defect in nasal epithelia of patients with cystic fibrosis. *Cell* 75:207, 1993

41. Crystal RG, McElvaney NG, Rosenfeld MA, et al: Administration of an adenovirus containing the human CFTR cDNA to the respiratory tract of individuals with cystic fibrosis. *Nature Genetics* 8:92, 1994

42. Cotten M, Wagner E, Zatloukal K, et al: High-efficiency receptor-mediated delivery of small and large (48 kilobase) gene constructs using the endosome-disruption activity of defective or chemically inactivated adenovirus particles. *Proc Natl Acad Sci USA* 89:6094, 1992

43. Wagner E, Zatloukal K, Cotten M, et al: Coupling of adenovirus to transferrin-polylysine/DNA complexes greatly enhances receptor-mediated gene delivery and expression of transfected genes. *Proc Natl Acad Sci USA* 89:6099, 1992

44. Wagner E, Zenke M, Cotten M, et al: Transferrin-polycation conjugates as carriers for DNA uptake into cells. *Proc Natl Acad Sci USA* 87:3410, 1990

45. Curiel DT, Agarwal S, Wagner E, et al: Adenovirus enhancement of transferrin-polylysine-mediated gene delivery. *Proc Natl Acad Sci USA* 88:8850, 1991

46. Wu GY, Wilson JM, Shalaby F, et al: Receptor-mediated gene delivery in vivo: partial correction of genetic analbuminemia in Nagase rats. *J Biol Chem* 266:14338, 1991

47. Felgner PL, Ringold GM: Cationic liposome-mediated transfection. *Nature* 337:387, 1989

48. Felgner PL: Particulate systems and polymers for in vitro and in vivo delivery of polynucleotides. *Adv Drug Deliv* 5:163, 1990

49. Stewart MJ, Plautz GE, Del Buono L, et al: Gene transfer in vivo with DNA-liposome complexes: safety and acute toxicity in mice. *Hum Gene Ther* 3:267, 1992

50. San H, Yang Z-Y, Pompili VJ, et al: Safety and toxicity of a novel cationic lipid formulation for human gene therapy. *Hum Gene Ther* 4:781, 1993

51. Coutelle C, Caplen N, Hart S, et al: Gene therapy for cystic fibrosis. *Arch Dis Child* 68:437, 1993

52. Plautz GE, Yang ZY, Gao X, et al: Immunotherapy of malignancy by in vivo gene transfer into tumors. *Proc Natl Acad Sci USA* 90:4645, 1993

53. Gao X, Huang L: A novel cationic liposome reagent for efficient transfection of mammalian cells. *Biochem Biophys Res Commun* 179:280, 1991

54. Williams RS, Johnston SA, Riedy M, et al: Introduction of foreign genes into tissues of living mice by DNA-coated microprojectiles. *Proc Natl Acad Sci USA* 88:2726, 1991

55. Tang D, DeVit M, Johnston SA: Genetic immunization is a simple method for eliciting an immune response. *Nature* 356:152, 1992

56. Nabel GJ, Fox BA, Post L, et al: A molecular genetic intervention for AIDS—effects of a transdominant negative form of Rev. *Hum Gene Ther* 5:79, 1994

57. Wolff JA, Malone RW, Williams P, et al: Direct gene transfer into mouse muscle in vitro. *Science* 247:1465, 1990

58. Wolff JA, Williams P, Acsadi G, et al: Conditions affecting direct gene transfer into rodent muscle in vivo. *Biotechnology* 11:474, 1991

59. Lin H, Parmacek MS, Morle G, et al: Expression of recombinant genes in myocardium in vivo after direct injection of DNA. *Circulation* 82:2217, 1990

60. Barr E, Leiden JM: Systemic delivery of recombinant proteins by genetically modified myoblasts. *Science* 254:1507, 1991

61. Simons M, Edelman ER, DeKeyser JL, et al: Antisense c-*myb* oligonucleotides inhibit intimal arterial smooth muscle cell accumulation in vivo. *Nature* 359:67, 1992

62. Clowes MM, Lynch CM, Miller AD, et al: Long-term biological response of injured rat carotid artery seeded with smooth muscle cells expressing retrovirally introduced human genes. *J Clin Invest* 93:644, 1994

63. Buttrick PM, Kass A, Kitsis RN, et al: Behavior of genes directly injected into the rat heart in vivo. *Circ Res* 70:193, 1992

64. Morishita R, Gibbons GH, Ellison KE, et al: Single intraluminal delivery of antisense *cdc2* kinase and proliferating-cell nuclear antigen oligonucleotides results in chronic inhibition of neointimal hyperplasia. *Proc Natl Acad Sci USA* 90:8474, 1993

65. Morishita R, Gibbons GH, Ellison KE, et al: Intimal hyperplasia after vascular injury is inhibited by antisense *cdk2* kinase oligonucleotides. *J Clin Invest* 93:1458, 1994

66. Ross R: The pathogenesis of atherosclerosis: a perspective for the 1990s. *Nature* 362:801, 1993

67. Messina LM, Podrazik RM, Whitehill TA, et al: Adhesion and incorporation of *lac-Z*-transduced endothelial cells into the intact capillary wall in the rat. *Proc Natl Acad Sci USA* 89:12018, 1992

68. Podrazik RM, Whitehill TA, Ekhterae D, et al: High-level expression of recombinant human tPA in cultivated canine endothelial cells under varying conditions of retroviral gene transfer. *Ann Surg* 216:233, 1992

69. Kahn ML, Lee SW, Dichek DA: Optimization of retroviral vector-mediated gene transfer into endothelial cells in vitro. *Circ Res* 71:1508, 1992

70. Morishita R, Gibbons GH, Kaneda Y, et al: Novel and effective gene transfer technique for study of vascular renin angiotensin system. *J Clin Invest* 91:2580, 1993

71. Weintraub HM: Antisense RNA and DNA. *Sci Am* 262:40, 1990

72. Simons M, Rosenberg RD: Antisense nonmuscle myosin heavy chain and c-*myb* oligonucleotides suppress smooth muscle cell proliferation in vitro. *Circ Res* 70:835, 1992

73. Biro S, Fu Y-M, Yu Z-X, et al: Inhibitory effects of antisense oligodeoxynucleotides targeting c-*myc* mRNA on smooth muscle cell proliferation and migration. *Proc Natl Acad Sci USA* 90:654, 1993

74. Dhawan J, Pan LC, Pavlath GK, et al: Systemic delivery of human growth hormone by injection of genetically engineered myoblasts. *Science* 254:1509, 1991

75. Yao SM, Kurachi K: Expression of human factor IX in mice after injection of genetically modified myoblasts. *Proc Natl Acad Sci USA* 89:3357, 1992

Acknowledgments

Figure 1 Talar Agasyan. Adapted from "Gene Transfer and Vascular Disease," by Nabel EG, Pompili VJ, Plautz GE, et al, in *Cardiovascular Research* 28:445, 1994, and *Molecular Cell Biology,* 2nd ed., by J. Darnell, H. Lodish, and D. Baltimore, Scientific American Books, New York, 1990.

Figure 2 Tom Moore. Adapted from "Recombinant Gene Expression in vivo within Endothelial Cells of the Arterial Wall," by Nabel EG, Plautz G, Boyce FM, et al, in *Science* 244:1342, 1989.

Figure 3 From "Recombinant Platelet-Derived Growth Factor B Gene Expression in Porcine Arteries Induces Intimal Hyperplasia in vivo," by Nabel EG, Yang A, Liptay S, et al, in *Journal of Clinical Investigation* 91:1822, 1993.

Figure 4 Tom Moore. Adapted from "Clinical Trials Put Gene Therapy to the Test," by Contie VL, in *National Center for Research Resources Reporter* 16:1, 1992.

CHAPTER 7

Gene Therapy for Lipid Disorders

Daniel J. Rader, M.D., James M. Wilson, M.D., Ph.D.

Lipoproteins are macromolecular complexes that transport lipids within the circulation. In addition to lipids (unesterified and esterified cholesterol, triglycerides, and phospholipids), lipoproteins also contain proteins termed *apolipoproteins*. Apolipoproteins serve various physiologic functions in lipoprotein metabolism, acting as cofactors for enzymes, ligands for cell-surface receptors, and structural proteins for lipoprotein biosynthesis [*see Table 1*]. Quantitation of certain apolipoproteins has an increasingly important role in the clinical risk assessment for atherosclerotic cardiovascular disease.[1]

Lipoproteins and Atherosclerosis

Lipoprotein Metabolism

The major classes of lipoprotein particles are chylomicrons, very low density lipoproteins (VLDL), intermediate-density lipoproteins (IDL), low-density lipoproteins (LDL), and high-density lipoproteins (HDL) [*see Figure 1*]. In the metabolism of these lipoproteins, dietary fat is absorbed and packaged into chylomicrons, which contain as their major protein a form of apolipoprotein (apo) B called apoB-48. The triglycerides in chylomicrons are hydrolyzed in the capillaries of peripheral tissues by the endothelial enzyme lipoprotein lipase, which requires apoC-II as a cofactor. The resulting chylomicron remnants are then removed from the circulation by the liver via a process that involves the binding of apoE to a putative remnant (or apoE) receptor in the liver. The liver repackages the lipid and secretes triglyceride-rich

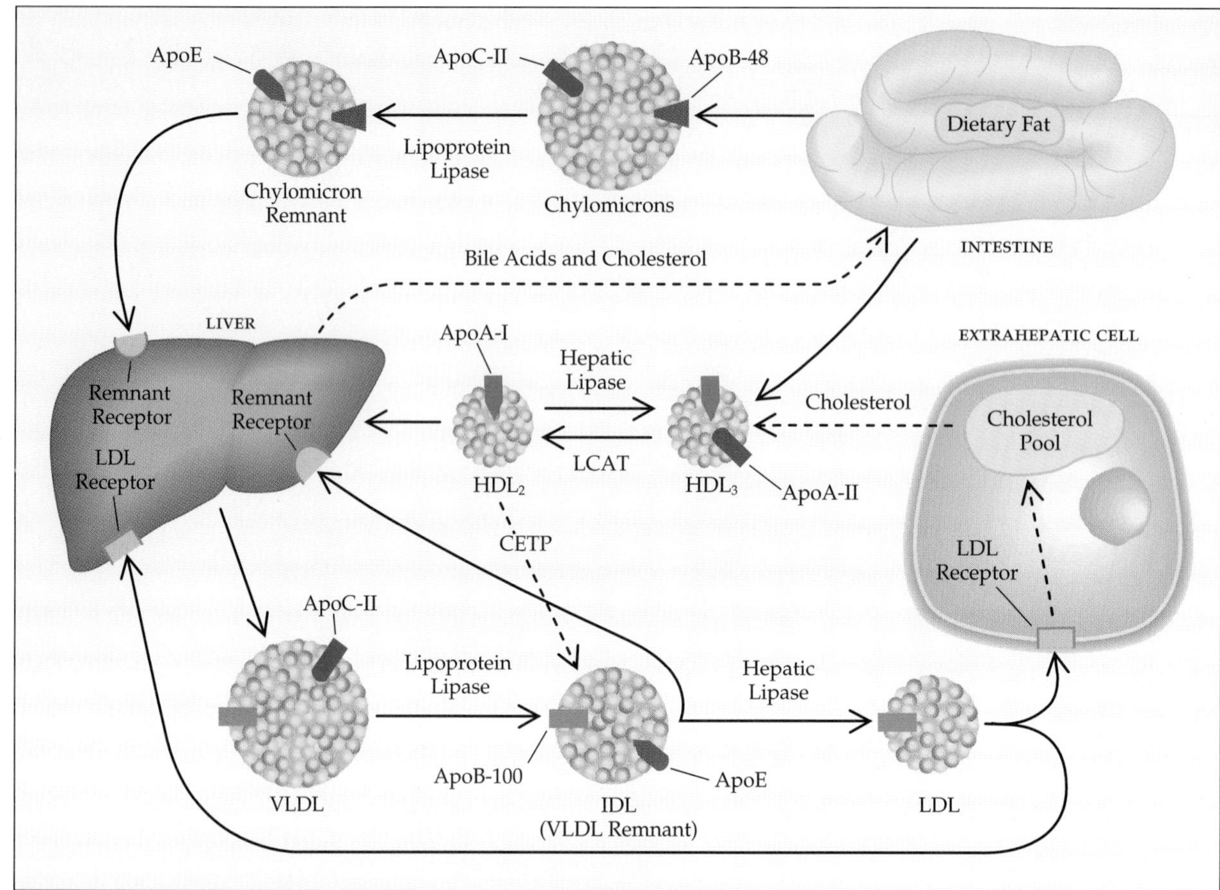

Figure 1 *The schematic diagram shows the metabolism of the major lipoproteins within the plasma. The intestine absorbs dietary fat into chylomicrons that contain apoB-48. Lipoprotein lipase and its cofactor, apoC-II, hydrolyze chylomicrons to remnants that are taken up by the liver by the binding of apoE. The liver secretes lipids as VLDL with apoB-100. VLDL is hydrolyzed to IDL, some of which is taken up by the liver. IDL is further hydrolyzed by hepatic lipase to become LDL. Hepatic and extrahepatic cells remove LDL from the circulation when apoB-100 binds to the LDL receptor. HDL is thought to remove excess cholesterol from cells and target it to the liver for excretion in the bile. The metabolism of lipoproteins is shown by solid arrows, and the transport of cholesterol, when not contained within lipoproteins, is indicated by broken arrows.*

lipoproteins known as VLDL, which contain as their major protein a form of apoB called apoB-100. After hydrolysis, some VLDL remnants (also known as IDL) are removed from the circulation by the liver, probably also by binding of apoE to the remnant (or apoE) receptor. However, other VLDL remnants are further processed by hepatic lipase with eventual conversion to LDL. LDL transports cholesteryl ester and vitamin E to peripheral tissues, but a significant amount of plasma LDL is eventually removed from the circulation by the liver via the binding of apoB-100 to the hepatic LDL receptor.[2]

The metabolism of HDL involves several different enzymes and transfer proteins but is not completely understood.[3] The major apolipoproteins of HDL are apoA-I and apoA-II. The liver and intestine are the major sources of newly synthesized HDL particles, which are thought to interact with peripheral cells to remove excess cholesterol [*see Figure 1*]. Unesterified cholesterol in nascent HDL is a substrate for the plasma enzyme lecithin:cholesterol acyltransferase, resulting in the formation of cholesteryl ester and enlargement of the HDL particle. HDL cholesteryl ester can be transferred to apoB-containing lipoproteins (such as LDL) by the cholesteryl ester transfer protein and be returned to the liver via the LDL receptor [*see Figure 1*]. HDL may also deliver some cholesterol directly to the liver. The removal of excess cholesterol from peripheral cells and delivery to the liver for excretion in the bile is a process that has been termed *reverse cholesterol transport.*

Lipoproteins therefore can be either atherogenic or antiatherogenic depending on their composition and physical properties. Therapeutic modulation of lipoprotein metabolism requires a thorough understanding of the different lipoproteins and their effects on atherosclerosis. The next sections review the current state of knowledge regarding specific atherogenic and antiatherogenic lipoproteins.

Atherogenic Lipoproteins

LDL and Oxidized LDL

The epidemiological and clinical evidence indicating a causal association between plasma levels of LDL cholesterol and risk of atherosclerotic disease is abundant. Interventions designed to decrease plasma LDL concentrations have proved effective in the primary and secondary prevention of coronary heart disease, further supporting the hypothesis that LDL is causally related to the atherosclerotic process.[4] It is currently believed that the atherogenic properties of LDL may be largely mediated by the formation of oxidatively modified LDL in vivo.[5] Therefore, in addition to decreasing the levels of LDL, interventions targeted to the prevention of LDL oxidation may be effective in preventing atherosclerosis.

Table 1 The Major Apolipoproteins and Associated Lipoproteins

Apoliprotein	*Lipoprotein*	*Function*
ApoA-I	HDL	Structural protein for HDL Activator of LCAT
ApoA-II	HDL	Structural protein for HDL
ApoA-IV	HDL, chylomicrons	Activator of LPL and LCAT
ApoB-100	VLDL, IDL, LDL	Structural protein for VLDL and LDL Ligand for binding to LDL receptor
ApoB-48	Chylomicrons, remnants	Structural protein for chylomicrons
ApoC-II	Chylomicrons, VLDL	Essential cofactor for LPL
ApoC-III	Chylomicrons, VLDL, HDL	Inhibitor of lipoprotein binding to receptors
ApoE	Remnants, VLDL, LDL, HDL	Ligand for binding to LDL receptor Ligand for binding to remant (apoE) receptor
Apo(a)	Lp(a)	Structural protein for Lp(a) Inhibitor of plasminogen activation

HDL—high-density lipoproteins; IDL—intermediate-density lipoproteins; LDL—low-density lipoproteins; VLDL—very low density lipoproteins; LPL—lipoprotein lipase; LCAT—lecithin:cholesterol acyltransferase.

Remnant Lipoproteins

Triglyceride-rich lipoproteins (chylomicrons, VLDL) undergo lipolysis by lipoprotein lipase [*see Figure 1*]. The residual remnant lipoproteins are enriched in cholesterol relative to triglyceride and therefore are potentially more atherogenic. (In this chapter, *remnants* is used as a term for both partially delipidated chylomicrons and VLDL.) ApoB-48–containing chylomicron remnants are cleared from the circulation primarily by the liver via a receptor-mediated process involving the binding of apoE. ApoB-100–containing VLDL remnants can be either catabolized via a similar apoE-mediated mechanism or converted to LDL in a process that involves hepatic lipase. The factors that determine the fraction of VLDL remnants that are taken up directly by the liver instead of being converted to LDL are not completely understood.

The evidence that remnant lipoprotein particles are atherogenic is derived from various sources. Remnant lipoproteins are capable of producing foam cell formation in vitro. Several animal models of atherosclerosis are characterized by increased plasma levels of remnant lipoproteins. Human conditions that result in elevated levels of remnant lipoproteins are associated with an increased risk of atherosclerosis.[6] In contrast, conditions involving elevated plasma levels of triglyceride-rich lipoproteins (familial chylomicronemia, familial hypertriglyceridemia) but not lipoprotein remnants are not associated with premature atherosclerosis.

Lipoprotein(a)

Lp(a) is an LDL-like lipoprotein that contains an additional protein known as apo(a).[7] The *apo(a)* gene is highly homologous to that of plasminogen,[8] and experimental data implicate Lp(a) as an inhibitor of plasminogen activation.[9] Many cross-sectional studies and some prospective studies have demonstrated that the risk of myocardial infarction and stroke is correlated with plasma Lp(a) concentrations.[1] It has been suggested that Lp(a) levels may account for much of the familial predisposition to premature coronary heart disease that cannot be accounted for by other known heritable factors.

Evidence indicates that Lp(a) plays a direct role in atherogenesis. Atherosclerotic plaque from human aortas, coronary bypass vein grafts resected at reoperation, and atherosclerotic coronary artery plaque from monkeys all contain substantial amounts of Lp(a). Transgenic mice expressing apo(a) develop more atherosclerosis on a high-fat diet than do control mice.[10] Lp(a) may be proatherogenic at least partly because of its interference with the fibrinolytic system,[9] but more studies are required to determine the mechanisms by which Lp(a) predisposes to atherosclerosis.

Plasma levels of Lp(a) are under strong genetic control. The *apo(a)* gene itself accounts for greater than 90 percent of the variation in plasma Lp(a) concentrations.[11] The apo(a) protein exhibits a highly variable size polymorphism that is related to the number of plasminogenlike kringle-4 repeats present in the *apo(a)* gene. There is an inverse correlation between the size of the apo(a) isoform and the Lp(a) concentration: the largest isoforms are associated with the lowest levels of Lp(a), and the smallest isoforms with the highest levels. Variation in the size of apo(a), as assessed by apo(a) genotyping, has been estimated to account for about 70 percent of the variation in plasma Lp(a) concentrations.[11] The effect of apo(a) size on plasma Lp(a) levels is not due to an effect on the catabolism of Lp(a) but to an effect on the production rate of Lp(a).[12] Lp(a) concentrations also vary substantially within each apo(a) isoform class. Kinetic studies indicate that variation in the production rate of Lp(a) is the major determinant of variation in plasma Lp(a) levels among individuals with the same apo(a) phenotype but different Lp(a) levels.[13] The pathways of intravascular Lp(a) metabolism and the mechanism by which Lp(a) is taken up and degraded are not well understood.

Antiatherogenic Lipoproteins

High-Density Lipoproteins

Epidemiological studies have consistently demonstrated a strong inverse correlation between plasma concentrations of HDL cholesterol and the incidence of coronary heart disease.[14] Plasma concentrations of apoA-I are highly correlated with HDL levels and are also inversely associated with coronary risk. Patients with a genetic deficiency of apoA-I develop premature coronary heart disease in the third to fifth decade of life.[3] The epidemiological and clinical data suggest that HDL and apoA-I may be antiatherogenic, or directly protective against the development of coronary heart disease. Animal studies support this concept. One potential mechanism by which HDL could be antiatherogenic is that of reverse cholesterol transport, by which HDL are thought to promote cholesterol efflux from peripheral tissues and deliver it to the liver for excretion in the bile [*see Figure 1*]. Other potential antiatherogenic effects of HDL and apoA-I include the protection of LDL from oxidation, the protection of endothelial cells from the cytotoxic effect of LDL, and the stimulation and stabilization of the vasodilator prostacyclin.[3]

Despite the strong epidemiological association of HDL and coronary heart disease, not all individuals with low levels of HDL and apoA-I appear to be at increased risk for premature coronary heart disease.[15] This observation has given rise to the concept that specific subclasses of HDL exist that may be more directly protective than others. Despite an extensive literature concerning the relative predictive value of the major density subfractions of HDL, HDL_2 and HDL_3, the overall body of data indicate that neither HDL subfraction (HDL_2 or HDL_3) is substantially more predictive of coronary heart disease risk.[16] Instead, it has been proposed that a subclassification based on apolipoprotein composition may provide greater insight into the ability to predict coronary risk.[17] Although all HDL particles contain apoA-I, only about one half to two thirds also contain apoA-II. This difference gives rise to two major subclasses of HDL particles: those that contain both apoA-I and apoA-II (called LpA-I:A-II) and those that contain apoA-I but not apoA-II (called LpA-I). Epidemiological, cell culture, and animal studies have suggested that LpA-I may be more specifically antiatherogenic than LpA-I:A-II. However, more studies are required to establish whether the plasma concentration of LpA-I is a more specific predictor of coronary heart disease risk than plasma HDL or total apoA-I concentrations.

Lipid Disorders Associated with Premature Atherosclerosis

Conditions Associated with Elevated LDL

Familial Hypercholesterolemia

Plasma concentrations of LDL are strongly influenced by heritable factors. On the basis of multiple epidemiological studies, the genetic heritability of LDL levels has been estimated to be approximately 50 percent. Some specific monogenetic factors that cause elevated plasma LDL levels are known. Genetic defects in the LDL receptor are among the most common familial cause of elevated LDL and result in a condition known as familial hypercholesterolemia.[2] Familial hypercholesterolemia is an autosomal codominant condition: the heterozygous form is associated with LDL levels in the 250- to 500-mg/dl range, whereas the homozygous form of the disease causes LDL cholesterol levels in the 500- to 1,000-mg/dl range. Heterozygous familial hypercholesterolemia has a population frequency of approximately one in 500 and results in tendon xanthomas and premature coronary heart disease in the fourth to sixth decades. Homozygous disease, which occurs in about one in a million individuals, is a clinical syndrome characterized by generalized tendon and planar xanthomas and markedly premature coronary heart disease in childhood or adolescence. Patients with heterozygous disease can often be treated with medication to lower the LDL to acceptable levels, whereas homozygotes can only be managed by plasma exchange or LDL apheresis, a form of LDL dialysis in which the LDL is physically removed from the blood.[18] Even if treated with LDL apheresis, however, homozygous patients remain at high risk for atherosclerotic vascular disease.

Familial Defective ApoB

A mutation in apoB-100 has been described that causes decreased ability of LDL to bind to the LDL receptor and produces a phenotype similar to familial hypercholesterolemia. This genetic syndrome has been termed familial defective apoB-100.[19] Clinically, these patients are similar to patients with familial hypercholesterolemia in that they are hypercholesterolemic, can have tendon xanthomas, and are at increased risk for premature coronary heart disease. The cause of familial defective apoB-100 is a single amino acid change in the region of apoB that binds to the LDL receptor. Heterozygosity for this mutation, an arginine to glutamine substitution at residue 3500 of the apoB protein, is relatively common in some populations. For example, in white populations in Europe and North America, this mutant allele is present in approximately one in 500 people, making it as common as heterozygous familial hypercholesterolemia and one of the most common familial causes of hypercholesterolemia. Patients generally respond to treatment with drugs that up-regulate the LDL receptor, such as 3-hydroxy-3-methylglutaryl coenzyme A (HMG-CoA) reductase inhibitors and bile acid sequestrants. This response suggests that intervention to increase LDL receptor expression could be one strategy to treat this disorder.

Familial Combined Hyperlipidemia

Another genetic condition that is associated with elevated LDL levels and premature coronary heart disease is *familial combined hyperlipidemia*.[20] Familial combined hyperlipidemia is an important cause of premature coronary heart disease, with estimates that approximately 10 percent of myocardial infarction survivors under age 60 have this condition. In this autosomal dominant disorder, multiple lipoprotein phenotypes (elevated triglycerides, cholesterol, or both) can occur in the same family and even in a single individual over time; many patients also have low HDL cholesterol levels. Familial combined hyperlipidemia is characterized by the presence of increased amounts of small, dense LDL in the plasma. One metabolic basis of this disorder appears to be overproduction of apoB-containing lipoproteins by the liver, but not all patients with the disease phenotype have been found to have increased hepatic apoB production. The molecular basis of familial combined hyperlipidemia is not known and is likely to be heterogeneous. One report suggested linkage with the apoA-I/C-III/A-IV gene cluster on chromosome 11q, but this has not been confirmed.[21] Some kindreds may be heterozygous for a defect in lipoprotein lipase.[22] Regardless of etiology, many patients with familial combined hyperlipidemia respond to HMG-CoA reductase inhibitors, suggesting that upregulation of LDL receptor activity may contribute to lowering of LDL levels in this condition as well.

Conditions Associated with Elevated Remnant Lipoproteins

Familial Dysbetalipoproteinemia

ApoE is synthesized by many tissues, but the apoE in plasma is derived largely from the liver. ApoE exists in three common genetically determined isoforms in humans, known as apoE2, E3, and E4.[23] The most common form is apoE3, but the E2 allele exists in 7 percent and the E4 allele in 14 percent of the general population. The apoE4 allele is associated with elevated LDL levels and is independently associated with coronary heart disease risk.[1] Homozygosity for the apoE2 allele is associated with familial dysbetalipoproteinemia, also known as type III hyperlipoproteinemia.[6] Not all individuals homozygous for apoE2 (approximately 0.5 percent of the population) have familial dysbetalipoproteinemia, suggesting that another factor is required for expression of the hyperlipidemia.[6] ApoE2 contains an amino acid substitution near the receptor-binding region of apoE that results in poor binding to the LDL receptor and remnant receptor and therefore results in reduced clearance of remnant lipoproteins from the plasma. Patients with familial dysbetalipoproteinemia have an increased risk of premature atherosclerosis, despite plasma LDL cholesterol levels that are usually lower than normal and HDL levels that are generally within the normal range. Genetic deficiency of apoE also results in substantially elevated levels of lipoprotein remnants and is associated with an increased risk of premature atherosclerotic disease.[24] Deficiency of hepatic lipase is also associated with increased plasma levels of remnant lipoproteins and premature atherosclerosis.[25] Intervention to increase plasma levels of apoE3 would likely result in accelerated removal of remnant lipoproteins in these disorders.

Postprandial Hyperlipoproteinemia

Postprandial lipoproteins are a form of remnant lipoprotein.[26] It has been suggested that postprandial lipoproteins may be atherogenic.[27] Two studies in individuals with angiographically proven premature coronary heart disease and normal fasting lipid levels demonstrated significantly greater postprandial lipemia than in matched controls.[28] These data support the concept that postprandial remnant lipoproteins are atherogenic and suggest that methods to decrease postprandial lipemia in susceptible individuals could impact favorably on atherosclerosis progression.

Secondary Hyperlipoproteinemias

Elevation of plasma remnant lipoprotein concentrations is common secondary to metabolic disorders such as nephrotic syndrome, chronic renal failure, and diabetes mellitus. These disorders have also been associated with increased Lp(a) levels.[7] The increased risk of premature atherosclerosis associated with these disorders may be in part because of elevated remnant lipoproteins. Intervention to decrease remnant particles in patients with these disorders could retard the progression of atherosclerotic disease.

Conditions Associated with Decreased HDL

Plasma concentrations of HDL cholesterol are highly influenced by genetic factors, with the genetic heritability of HDL cholesterol levels estimated to be approximately 50 percent. Genetic factors affecting HDL levels are incompletely understood, and only a few monogenic disorders resulting in low HDL levels have been identified. Patients with deletions of or nonsense mutations in the *apoA-I* gene have the inability to synthesize apoA-I, have virtually absent HDL, and develop premature coronary heart disease in the third to fifth decade.[29] Other missense or nonsense mutations in *apoA-I* can result in low HDL levels, but these have not been clearly identified to have an increased risk of premature coronary heart disease. Mutations in the lecithin:cholesterol acyltransferase gene can result in very low levels of HDL, diffuse corneal opacities, and, in some cases, anemia and progressive renal disease. These patients also do not have evidence of an increased risk of premature coronary heart disease, possibly because they have a selective decrease in LpA-I:A-II and relatively normal levels of LpA-I,[30] the subfraction of HDL thought to be specifically protective against coronary disease.

In contrast, most patients with low HDL do not have evidence of mutations in either the *apoA-I* or the lecithin:cholesterol acyltransferase gene and do appear to have an increased risk of premature coronary heart disease. Low HDL levels are often associated with other lipid abnormalities, such as hypertriglyceridemia or familial combined hyperlipidemia. However, the syndrome of primary hypoalphalipoproteinemia (low HDL) is defined by the presence of isolated low HDL with otherwise normal lipids. In many, but not all, kindreds it is associated with premature coronary heart disease. It has been ascribed to a major dominant gene, the nature of which has not been established. Intervention to raise HDL levels in individuals with low HDL levels could theoretically protect them from the development or progression of coronary heart disease.

Lipoprotein Metabolism and the Liver

The liver plays a central role in lipoprotein metabolism and the maintenance of cholesterol homeostasis. It produces the majority of the plasma apolipoproteins; synthesizes substantial amounts of new cholesterol; removes chylomicron remnants, LDL, and HDL cholesterol from the circulation via specific cell surface receptors; and converts cholesterol to bile acids [*see Figure 2*].

A large number of gene products influence cholesterol and lipoprotein metabolism and therefore may play a role in the development of atherosclerosis. In addition to the apolipoproteins, these include plasma enzymes and transfer proteins, cell surface receptors and binding proteins, and intracellular enzymes and transfer proteins [*see Table 2*].

Gene therapy directed toward modulation of lipids to prevent or treat atherosclerosis must either decrease levels of atherogenic lipoproteins or increase levels of antiatherogenic lipoproteins. Because the liver is the critical

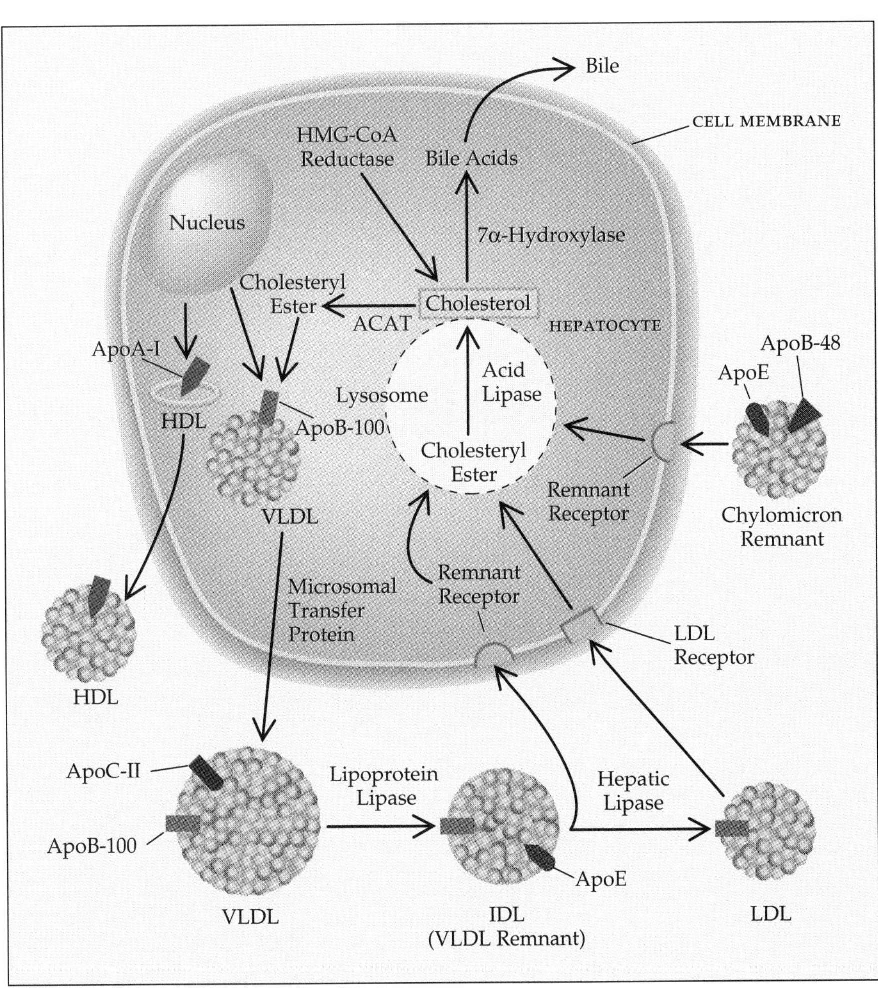

Figure 2 *The schematic diagram shows the metabolism of cholesterol and lipoproteins by the hepatocyte. Intracellular cholesterol is derived from new synthesis via HMG-CoA reductase or from hydrolysis by acid lipase of cholesteryl esters derived from uptake of lipoprotein. Cholesterol can be converted to bile acids, excreted directly into the bile, or esterified to cholesteryl ester by ACAT for secretion in VLDL.*

Table 2 Gene Products Other than Apolipoproteins That May Influence Lipoprotein Metabolism

Plasma enzymes and transfer proteins	Lipoprotein lipase (LPL) Hepatic lipase (HL) Lecithin:cholesterol acyltransferase (LCAT) Cholesteryl ester transfer protein (CETP)
Cell surface receptors and cellular binding proteins	LDL receptor LDL receptor–related protein (LRP) VLDL receptor Scavenger receptor HDL-binding protein (HBP)
Intracellular biosynthetic enzymes, hydrolytic enzymes, and transfer proteins	HMG-CoA reductase 7α-Hydroxylase Lysosomal acid lipase (AL) Microsomal transfer protein (MTP) Acyl coenzyme A:cholesterol acyltransferase (ACAT)

organ for lipoprotein metabolism, there is a major focus on liver-directed somatic gene transfer to modulate lipoproteins and prevent atherosclerotic vascular disease. Therefore, the principles of liver-directed gene transfer are reviewed in the following section.

Principles of Liver-Directed Somatic Gene Transfer

Ex Vivo Liver-Directed Gene Transfer

Retroviruses

Retroviruses are RNA viruses that are attractive vehicles for therapeutic gene transfer because they have the capability to integrate stably into the host genome and result in persistent expression of the transgene.[31] Once the retrovirus infects a cell, viral RNA is converted to double-stranded DNA, which is then integrated into the host genome. To integrate, however, retroviruses require active host cell replication. Because hepatocytes are not actively dividing under normal circumstances, retroviruses cannot be easily used for in vivo liver-targeted gene transfer. However, primary hepatocytes in culture undergo cell division for a brief period. If the hepatocytes are infected with a recombinant retrovirus during this time, stable integration can occur. This principle has been used to develop methods for ex vivo liver-directed gene transfer using recombinant retroviruses.[32] In this approach, a portion of the liver is removed, the primary hepatocytes are placed in culture and infected with a recombinant retrovirus containing the gene of interest, and then the transduced cells are reintroduced into the host liver.[33] This approach was first used for a therapeutic transgene in a rabbit model of LDL receptor deficiency[34] and led to the development of the first human clinical trial of liver-directed gene therapy.

In Vivo Liver-Directed Gene Transfer

ADENOVIRUSES

Adenoviruses are double-stranded DNA viruses that are tropic for respiratory epithelium in humans and have been used to direct gene transfer to multiple tissue types in animals.[35] After host cell infection, adenoviral DNA migrates to the nucleus, where it remains episomal rather than integrating into the host genome. Interest in the use of recombinant adenoviruses for liver-directed gene transfer was sparked by the demonstration that when injected intravenously, adenoviruses efficiently infect the liver and result in a high level of hepatic transgene expression.[36] Replication-defective adenoviruses have been developed that have a deletion of an entire region (the *E1a* gene and part of the *E1b* gene) required for replication.[35] As a result, these viruses can infect cells and result in transgene expression, but they cannot actively replicate. Recombinant adenoviruses have been used successfully to achieve in vivo liver-directed gene transfer and expression of several different genes in mice,[36-39] rats,[40] and rabbits.[41]

Despite their attractiveness for in vivo liver-directed gene transfer, use of adenoviruses has some drawbacks. Current adenoviral vectors do not result in persistent hepatic expression of the transgene beyond a few weeks in animal models. In mice, recombinant adenoviruses stimulate a cellular immune response, leading to hepatic inflammation and destruction of the genetically modified hepatocytes. This probably occurs because of adenoviral protein expression despite the deletion that renders the virus replication-defective.[42] Further inactivation of another essential gene (*E2a*) results in less inflammation and substantially longer recombinant gene expression in mouse liver.[43] In rabbits, the second administration of a recombinant adenovirus failed to result in further transgene expression, probably because of the development of neutralizing antibodies to the first dose.[41] Efforts are ongoing to engineer recombinant adenoviruses to achieve less immunogenicity of the virus and greater persistence of transgene expression.

DNA-PROTEIN COMPLEXES

The liver expresses cell surface receptors that are specific for certain plasma proteins such as the asialoglycoprotein receptor and the transferrin receptor. This principle has been used to target DNA to the liver in vivo by coupling the DNA with a specific protein ligand to form DNA-protein complexes. Injection of these complexes would be expected to result in specific targeting to the liver in vivo. This approach has been used successfully in rats using asialo-orosomucoid to target genes to the liver.[44,45] It was also used to target the delivery of the LDL receptor gene to the livers of rabbits deficient in the LDL receptor.[46] Examination of livers harvested up to 11 weeks after injection demonstrated transgene DNA that was episomal and not integrated into the host genome.[47]

Despite these promising initial results, DNA-protein complexes result in relatively low levels of expression of transgenes in the liver, at least in part because they are targeted to the lysosome and degraded.[45] One approach to overcome this problem has been the use of a replication-incompetent adenovirus as an endosomal lysis agent. When adenovirus is cointernalized with the DNA-protein complexes, either separately[48] or directly coupled to the complexes,[49,50] gene expression is considerably enhanced. Investigation is ongoing to modify DNA-protein complexes further to escape lysosomal degradation and achieve higher levels of persistent expression in liver.

Liposomes

Liposomes are large spherical or discoidal structures composed primarily of phospholipids that orient themselves so that the polar head groups interact with the aqueous outer environment and the fatty acyl chains point in toward a hydrophobic core. They are nontoxic, nonimmunogenic, and stable in plasma, making them attractive vehicles for delivery of substances to cells. DNA can be placed within the liposome core and protected from degradation in the plasma. Liposomes have been used for in vivo gene transfer to rat liver.[51] However, the lack of tissue specificity and the low levels of gene expression have limited the applicability of liposomes to liver-directed gene transfer.

Liver-Directed Gene Transfer to Decrease LDL: The LDL Receptor

Liver-Directed LDL-Receptor Gene Transfer in Animals

Familial hypercholesterolemia has been a valuable paradigm for the investigation of liver-directed gene transfer. A natural animal model of homozygous familial hypercholesterolemia is the Watanabe heritable hyperlipidemic (WHHL) rabbit. These rabbits are homozygous for a mutation in the LDL receptor that results in impaired receptor activity and severe hypercholesterolemia and atherosclerosis similar to that in the human disease. Ex vivo retrovirally mediated gene transfer of the LDL-receptor gene was successfully achieved in WHHL rabbits, resulting in temporary[34] and ultimately long-term[52] improvement in hypercholesterolemia. A similar ex vivo protocol was used to express the human LDL-receptor gene in dog[53] and baboon[54] hepatocytes. These studies led to the development and implementation of a clinical protocol for ex vivo gene therapy for homozygous familial hypercholesterolemia in humans.

Recombinant adenoviral vectors have been used in animals to achieve liver-directed LDL-receptor gene transfer and expression in vivo. Injection of normal mice with a recombinant adenovirus containing the human LDL-receptor complementary DNA resulted in a high level of transient human LDL-receptor expression in the liver and enhanced the catabolism of labeled LDL.[37] Injection of a recombinant adenovirus containing the LDL-receptor gene into LDL-receptor gene knockout mice successfully (but transiently) reduced cholesterol levels to the normal range.[38] Recombinant adenovirus has also been used successfully to transfer the LDL-receptor gene to WHHL rabbit liver in vivo, resulting in substantial lowering of cholesterol.[41] Livers harvested three days after adenovirus infusion were analyzed by immunohistochemical methods with an antibody to the human LDL receptor and found to have 50 percent of hepatocytes positive for binding to the antibody. Western blot analysis of membrane fractions with the same antibody revealed the recombinant-derived human LDL receptor. Serum cholesterol levels in all five animals receiving the recombinant virus fell significantly to a nadir at seven days. In three of five rabbits, cholesterol returned to baseline within two weeks, but cholesterol levels in two animals remained at a lower level for the entire three-week experiment. WHHL rabbits injected with a control virus had no change in their cholesterol levels. The decreased cholesterol levels in the treated rabbits were demonstrated to be caused by increased LDL catabolism by the performance of ^{125}I-LDL turnover studies.

Liver-Directed LDL-Receptor Gene Transfer in Humans

A clinical protocol for ex vivo liver-directed gene therapy for homozygous familial hypercholesterolemia was initiated in 1992.[55] To be considered for this protocol, a patient with homozygous familial hypercholesterolemia must have documented coronary artery disease. Serial baseline lipid tests are performed in the months before gene therapy. The patient undergoes a surgical resection of the left lateral segment of the liver and has a Hickman catheter placed in the inferior mesenteric vein. Primary hepatocytes are isolated and, after two days, are infected with a recombinant murine retrovirus containing the human LDL-receptor gene. Hepatocytes are harvested the next day and reinfused into the patient via the Hickman catheter. Blood is drawn serially after therapy and assayed for cholesterol and other lipids in a blinded fashion. The first patient to be treated on this protocol had a decrease of approximately 20 percent in her LDL cholesterol levels, which has persisted for over 18 months since therapy.[56]

Efforts to develop in vivo methods for targeting the LDL receptor to human liver are ongoing. One step toward this goal was the demonstration that a recombinant adenovirus successfully transferred the LDL receptor complementary DNA into human familial hypercholesterolemia hepatocytes in vitro.[57] New and more effective protocols for liver-directed gene therapy of homozygous familial hypercholesterolemia will be developed over the next several years. Ultimately, liver-directed LDL-receptor gene transfer may prove to be of therapeutic benefit in many patients with substantially elevated LDL levels, regardless of primary etiology.

Liver-Directed Gene Transfer to Decrease Remnant Lipoproteins: Apolipoprotein E

Animal Studies of ApoE Infusion and Overexpression

ApoE is a critical ligand for the clearance of chylomicron and VLDL remnant lipoproteins. ApoE knockout mice develop extremely high levels of remnants and severe atherosclerosis on a chow diet.[58,59] To date, no apoE gene transfer studies in animals have been reported. However, existing animal data indicate that intervention to increase plasma apoE results in a decrease in remnants as well as LDL. WHHL rabbits have elevated levels of remnants and LDL; when purified apoE was infused, the serum cholesterol levels fell significantly because of reductions in both remnants and LDL.[60] Transgenic mice that overexpress apoE are resistant to diet-induced hypercholesterolemia[61] and exhibit much faster catabolism of VLDL and LDL.[62] Transgenic mice expressing apoC-III develop hypertriglyceridemia but, if crossed with apoE transgenic mice, normalize their lipid values.[63] Therefore, the animal data strongly indicate that apoE is required for remnant lipoprotein clearance and that increasing plasma apoE levels by infusion or transgenesis results in accelerated catabolism of remnants and LDL and lowering of serum cholesterol.

Prospects for Therapeutic ApoE *Gene Transfer in Humans*

The epidemiological, clinical, and animal data suggest that specific intervention to increase apoE levels would lower remnant lipoprotein levels in humans. However, no controlled data in humans exist to indicate that intervention to lower lipoprotein remnant levels would impact favorably on atherosclerosis. One trial of the effect of lipid lowering in the primary prevention of coronary heart disease enrolled patients with elevated non-HDL cholesterol, and statistical analysis of the results suggested that the subgroup who benefited most from treatment was that with elevated triglycerides, suggestive of increased remnant particles.[64] However, clinical trials have not yet been carried out specifically to evaluate the effect of selectively decreasing remnant particles in the primary or secondary prevention of coronary heart disease.

Enhancing the hepatic expression of apoE is an attractive potential mechanism to lower plasma remnant levels, as apoE is the primary ligand that mediates the uptake and degradation of these lipoprotein particles from the plasma. Expression of apoE3 in patients with familial dysbetalipoproteinemia would be expected to substantially lower plasma levels of remnant particles. Even other causes of elevated remnants, such as postprandial hyperlipidemia and some secondary hyperlipidemias, may be effectively treated by increasing plasma apoE levels. Furthermore, because VLDL remnants that remain in the plasma are converted to LDL, increased expression of apoE would be expected to lower LDL levels as well. Therefore, hepatic apoE expression could be used as a mechanism to lower plasma levels of atherogenic lipoproteins (remnants and LDL) regardless of the underlying cause of the hyperlipidemia.

Liver-Directed Gene Transfer to Increase HDL: Apolipoprotein A-I

Animal Studies: ApoA-I Infusion and Overexpression

ApoA-I is required for the normal formation of HDL. ApoA-I knockout mice have extremely low levels of HDL cholesterol.[65] Animal studies have provided substantial evidence that apoA-I is directly protective against atherosclerosis and that intervention to raise HDL or apoA-I levels could be beneficial. Intravenous infusion of HDL in cholesterol-fed rabbits resulted in regression of atherosclerotic lesions.[66] Overexpression of human apoA-I in transgenic mice raised HDL levels and inhibited atherogenesis.[67] ApoA-I transgenic rabbits have recently been successfully generated,[68] and studies in these rabbits will elucidate the protective effect of apoA-I overexpression.

Prospects for Therapeutic ApoA-I *Gene Transfer in Humans*

Epidemiological and animal data suggest that specific intervention to raise HDL levels could be beneficial in humans. Further supporting this concept is the observation that genetic syndromes of high HDL, termed familial hyperalphalipoproteinemia, are associated with longevity and decreased incidence of coronary heart disease.[69] One known genetic cause of elevated HDL levels is deficiency of the cholesteryl ester transfer protein (CETP), which results in markedly elevated HDL and apoA-I levels and may be associated with decreased risk of coronary heart disease.[70] Other kindreds with high HDL levels who do not have CETP deficiency have also been described. One individual with familial hyperalphalipoproteinemia was found to have increased production of apoA-I associated with longevity in her extended pedigree.[71] This suggests that therapy to increase endogenous apoA-I production could raise HDL levels and may protect against the development or progression of coronary heart disease.

Currently, no direct data exist in humans to indicate that interventions to raise HDL levels would reduce the development of coronary heart disease. One primary prevention drug trial enrolled patients with elevated non-HDL cholesterol, but statistical analysis of the results suggested an independent benefit of raising HDL cholesterol levels.[64] However, clinical trials have not yet been carried out specifically to evaluate the effect of selectively raising HDL levels on the development or progression of atherosclerosis. One difficulty with designing such a trial is that drugs that raise HDL levels generally also lower LDL and remnant lipoprotein levels. Therefore, the first true clinical trial of the specific effect of raising HDL on development or progression of atherosclerosis in humans may require the use of specific *apoA-I* gene transfer rather than a pharmacological agent.

Conclusion

In attempts to prevent or treat atherosclerosis, the plasma lipoproteins are an attractive target for modulation because a wealth of data indicate that some lipoproteins are highly atherogenic and some are strongly antiatherogenic. However, the ability to specifically modulate levels of these lipoproteins with traditional pharmacological therapy is limited. Extensive animal data indicate that liver-directed gene expression has the ability to lower levels of specific atherogenic lipoproteins or raise levels of antiatherogenic lipoproteins and thereby potentially to reduce atherosclerosis progression. These data suggest that liver-directed gene transfer in humans directed toward modulation of lipoproteins could be a highly effective method to prevent the progression or even cause regression of atherosclerosis. The testing of these hypotheses in clinical trials awaits the further development of technology for more effective methods of somatic liver-directed gene transfer in humans.

References

1. Rader DJ, Hoeg JM, Brewer HB Jr: Quantitation of plasma apolipoproteins in the primary and secondary prevention of coronary artery disease. *Ann Intern Med* 120:1012, 1994
2. Brown MS, Goldstein JL: A receptor-mediated pathway for cholesterol homeostasis. *Science* 232:34, 1986
3. Tall AR, Plasma high density lipoproteins: metabolism and relationship to atherogenesis. *J Clin Invest* 86:379, 1990
4. Summary of the second report of the National Cholesterol Education Program (NCEP) Expert Panel on Detection, Evaluation, and Treatment of High Blood Cholesterol in Adults (Adult Treatment Panel II). *JAMA* 269:3015, 1993
5. Steinberg D, Parthasarathy S, Carew TE, et al: Beyond cholesterol: modifications of low-density lipoprotein that increase its atherogenicity. *N Engl J Med* 230:915, 1989
6. Brewer HB Jr, Zech LA, Gregg RE, et al: Type III hyperlipoproteinemia: diagnosis, molecular defects, pathology, and treatment. *Ann Intern Med* 98:623, 1983
7. Rader DJ, Brewer HB Jr: Lipoprotein(a): clinical approach to a unique atherogenic lipoprotein. *JAMA* 267:1109, 1992
8. McLean JW, Tomlinson JE, Kuang WJ, et al: cDNA sequence of human apolipoprotein(a) is homologous to plasminogen. *Nature* 330:132, 1987
9. Miles LA, Plow EF: Lp(a): an interloper in the fibrinolytic system. *Thromb Haemost* 63:331, 1990
10. Lawn RM, Wade DP, Hammer RE, et al: Atherogenesis in transgenic mice expressing human apolipoprotein(a). *Nature* 360:670, 1992
11. Boerwinkle E, Leffert CC, Lin J, et al: Apolipoprotein(a) gene accounts for greater than 90% of the variation in plasma lipoprotein(a) concentrations. *J Clin Invest* 90:52, 1992
12. Rader DJ, Cain W, Ikewaki K, et al: The inverse association of plasma lipoprotein(a) concentrations with apolipoprotein(a) isoform size is not due to differences in Lp(a) catabolism but to differences in production rate. *J Clin Invest* 93:2758, 1994
13. Rader DJ, Cain W, Zech LA, et al: Variation in Lp(a) concentration among individuals with the same apo(a) isoform is determined by the rate of Lp(a) production. *J Clin Invest* 91:443, 1993
14. Gordon DJ, Rifkind BM: High-density lipoprotein—the clinical implications of recent studies. *N Engl J Med* 321:1311, 1989
15. Rader DJ, Ikewaki K, Duverger N, et al: Markedly decreased plasma high density lipoprotein levels without premature coronary atherosclerosis caused by rapid catabolism of apolipoproteins A-I and A-II. *Lancet* 342:1455, 1993
16. Miller NE: Associations of high-density lipoprotein subclasses and apolipoproteins with ischemic heart disease and coronary atherosclerosis. *Am Heart J* 113:589, 1987
17. Fruchart JC, Ailhaud G: Apolipoprotein A-containing lipoprotein particles: physiological role, quantification, and clinical significance. *Clin Chem* 38:793, 1992
18. Gordon BR, Kelsey SF, Bilheimer DW, et al: Treatment of refractory familial hypercholesterolemia by low-density lipoprotein apheresis using an automated dextran sulfate cellulose adsorption system. *Am J Cardiol* 70:1010, 1992
19. Tybjærg-Hansen A, Humphries S: Familial defective apolipoprotein B-100: a single mutation that causes hypercholesterolemia and premature coronary artery disease. *Atherosclerosis* 96:91, 1992
20. Kwiterovich PO Jr: Genetics and molecular biology of familial combined hyperlipidemia. *Curr Opin Lipidol* 4:133, 1993
21. Wojciechowski AP, Farrall M, Cullen P, et al: Familial combined hyperlipidemia linked to the apolipoprotein AI-CIII-AIV gene cluster on chromosome 11q23-q24. *Nature* 349:161, 1991
22. Babirak SP, Brown BG, Brunzell JD: Familial combined hyperlipidemia and abnormal lipoprotein lipase. *Arteriosclerosis Thromb* 12:1176, 1992
23. Davignon J, Gregg RE, Sing CF: Apolipoprotein E polymorphism and atherosclerosis. *Arteriosclerosis* 8:1, 1988
24. Schaefer EJ, Gregg RE, Ghiselli G, et al: Familial apolipoprotein E deficiency. *J Clin Invest* 78:1206, 1986
25. Connelly PW, Maguire GF, Lee M, et al: Plasma lipoproteins in familial hepatic lipase deficiency. *Arteriosclerosis* 10:40, 1990

26. Schneeman BO, Kotite L, Todd K, et al: Relationships between the responses of triglyceride-rich lipoproteins in blood plasma containing apolipoproteins B-48 and B-100 to a fat-containing meal in normolipidemic humans. *Proc Natl Acad Sci USA* 90:2069, 1993
27. Zilversmit DB: Atherogenesis: a postprandial phenomenon. *Circulation* 60:473, 1979
28. Miesenbock G, Patsch JR: Postprandial hyperlipidemia: the search for the atherogenic lipoprotein. *Curr Opin Lipidol* 3:196, 1992
29. Norum RA, Lakier JB, Goldstein S, et al: Familial deficiency of apolipoproteins A-I and C-III and precocious coronary-artery disease. *N Engl J Med* 306:1513, 1982
30. Rader DJ, Ikewaki K, Duverger N, et al: Rapid catabolism of apolipoprotein A-II and high density lipoproteins containing apoA-II in classic LCAT deficiency and fish-eye disease. *J Clin Invest* 93:321, 1994
31. Salmons B, Günzburg WH: Targeting of retroviral vectors for gene therapy. *Hum Gene Ther* 4:129, 1993
32. Friedmann T: Progress toward human gene therapy. *Science* 244:1275, 1989
33. Raper SE, Wilson JM: Cell transplantation in liver-directed gene therapy. *Cell Transplant* 2:381, 1993
34. Wilson JM, Chowdhury NR, Grossman M, et al: Temporary amelioration of hyperlipidemia in low density lipoprotein receptor–deficient rabbits transplanted with genetically modified hepatocytes. *Proc Natl Acad Sci USA* 87:8437, 1987
35. Kozarsky K, Wilson JM: Gene therapy: adenovirus vectors. *Curr Opin Genet Dev* 3:499, 1993
36. Stratford-Perricaudet L, Levero M, Chasse JF, et al: Evaluation of the transfer and expression in mice of an enzyme-encoding gene using a human adenovirus vector. *Hum Gene Ther* 1:241, 1990
37. Herz J, Gerard RD: Adenovirus-mediated transfer of the low density lipoprotein receptor gene acutely accelerates clearance in normal mice. *Proc Natl Acad Sci USA* 90:2812, 1993
38. Ishibashi S, Brown M, Goldstein J, et al: Hypercholesterolemia in low density lipoprotein receptor knockout mice and its reversal by adenovirus-mediated gene delivery. *J Clin Invest* 92:883, 1993
39. Smith T, Mehaffey M, Kayda D, et al: Adenovirus mediated expression of therapeutic plasma levels of human factor IX in mice. *Nature Genet* 5:397, 1993
40. Jaffe H, Danel C, Longenecker G, et al: Adenovirus-mediated in vivo gene transfer and expression in normal rat liver. *Nature Genet* 1:372, 1992
41. Kozarsky KF, McKinley DR, Austin LL, et al: In vivo correction of LDL receptor deficiency in the Watanabe heritable hyperlipidemic rabbit with recombinant adenoviruses. *J Biol Chem* 269:13695, 1994
42. Yang Y, Nunes F, Berencs K, et al: Cellular immunity to viral antigens limits E1-deleted adenoviruses for gene therapy. *Proc Natl Acad Sci USA* 91:4407, 1994
43. Engelhardt JF, Ye X, Doranz B, et al: Ablation of E2a in recombinant adenoviruses improves transgene persistence and decreases imflammatory response in mouse liver. *Proc Natl Acad Sci USA* 91:6196, 1994
44. Wu CH, Wilson JM, Wu GY: Targeting gene delivery and persistent expression of a foreign gene driven by mammalian regulatory elements in vivo. *J Biol Chem* 264:16985, 1989
45. Wu GY, Wilson JM, Shalaby F, et al: Receptor-mediated gene delivery in vivo. *J Biol Chem* 266:14338, 1991
46. Wilson JM, Grossman M, Wu CH, et al: Hepatocyte-directed gene transfer in vivo leads to transient improvement of hypercholesterolemia in low density lipoprotein receptor-deficient rabbits. *J Biol Chem* 267:963, 1992
47. Wilson JM, Grossman M, Wu CH, et al: A novel mechanism for achieving transgene persistence in vivo after somatic gene transfer into hepatocytes. *J Biol Chem* 267:11483, 1992
48. Cristiano RJ, Smith LC, Woo S: Hepatic gene therapy: adenovirus enhancement of receptor-mediated gene delivery and expression in primary hepatocytes. *Proc Natl Acad Sci USA* 90:2122, 1993
49. Michael S, Huang C, Romer M, et al: Binding-incompetent adenovirus facilitates molecular conjugate-mediated gene transfer by the receptor-mediated endocytosis pathway. *J Biol Chem* 268:6866, 1993
50. Cristiano RJ, Smith LC, Kay MA, et al: Hepatic gene therapy: efficient gene delivery and expression in primary hepatocytes utilizing a conjugated adenovirus-DNA complex. *Proc Natl Acad Sci USA* 90:11548, 1993
51. Kaneda Y, Iwai K, Uchida T: Increased expression of DNA cointroduced with nuclear protein in adult rat liver. *Science* 243:375, 1989

52. Chowdhury JR, Grossman M, Gupta S, et al: Long-term improvement of hypercholesterolemia after ex vivo gene therapy in LDLR-deficient rabbits. *Science* 254:1802, 1991
53. Grossman M, Wilson JM, Raper S: A novel approach for introducing hepatocytes into the portal circulation. *J Lab Clin Med* 121:472, 1993
54. Grossman M, Raper S, Wilson JM: Transplantation of genetically modified autologous hepatocytes into nonhuman primates: feasibility and short-term toxicity. *Hum Gene Ther* 3:501, 1992
55. Wilson JM, Grossman M, Raper SE, et al: Clinical protocol: ex vivo gene therapy of familial hypercholesterolemia. *Hum Gene Ther* 3:179, 1992
56. Grossman M, Raper S, Kozarsky K, et al: Successful ex vivo gene therapy directed to the liver in a patient with familial hypercholesterolemia. *Nature Genet* 6:335, 1994
57. Kozarsky K, Grossman M, Wilson JM: Adenovirus-mediated correction of the genetic defect in hepatocytes from patients with familial hypercholesterolemia. *Somat Cell Mol Genet* 19:449, 1993
58. Plump A, Smith J, Hayek T, et al: Severe hypercholesterolemia and atherosclerosis in apolipoprotein E-deficient mice created by homologous recombination in ES cells. *Cell* 71:343, 1992
59. Zhang S, Reddick R, Piedrahita J, et al: Spontaneous hypercholesterolemia and arterial lesions in mice lacking apolipoprotein E. *Science* 258:468, 1992
60. Yamada N, Shimano H, Mokuno H, et al: Increased clearance of plasma cholesterol after injection of apolipoprotein E into Watanabe heritable hyperlipidemic rabbits. *Proc Natl Acad Sci USA* 86:665, 1989
61. Shimano H, Yamada N, Katsuki M, et al: Overexpression of apolipoprotein E in transgenic mice: marked reduction in plasma lipoproteins except high density lipoprotein and resistance against diet-induced hypercholesterolemia. *Proc Natl Acad Sci USA* 89:1750, 1992
62. Shimano H, Yamada N, Katsuki M, et al: Plasma lipoprotein metabolism in transgenic mice overexpressing apolipoprotein E: accelerated clearance of lipoproteins containing apolipoprotein B. *J Clin Invest* 90:2084, 1992
63. De Silva H, Lauer S, Wang J, et al: Overexpression of human apolipoprotein C-III in transgenic mice results in an accumulation of apolipoprotein B48 remnants that is corrected by excess apolipoprotein E. *J Biol Chem* 269:2324, 1994
64. Frick MH, Elo O, Haapa K, et al: Helsinki Heart Study: primary-prevention trial with gemfibrozil in middle-aged men with dyslipidemia: safety of treatment, changes in risk factors, and incidence of coronary heart disease. *N Engl J Med* 317:1237, 1987
65. Williamson R, Lee D, Hagaman J, et al: Marked reduction of high density lipoprotein cholesterol in mice genetically modified to lack apolipoprotein A-I. *Proc Natl Acad Sci USA* 89:7134, 1992
66. Badimon JJ, Badimon L, Fuster V: Regression of atherosclerotic lesions by high density lipoprotein plasma fraction in the cholesterol-fed rabbit: New York 10029. *J Clin Invest* 85:1234, 1990
67. Rubin EM, Krauss RM, Spangler EA, et al: Inhibition of early atherogenesis in transgenic mice by human apolipoprotein AI. *Nature* 353:265, 1991
68. Hoeg JM, Vaisman BL, Demosky SJ, et al: Development of transgenic Watanabe heritable hyperlipidemic rabbits expressing human apolipoprotein A-I [abstract]. *Circulation* 88:I-2, 1993
69. Glueck CJ, Fallat RW, Millett F, et al: Familial hyper-alpha-lipoproteinemia: studies in eighteen kindreds. *Metabolism* 24:1243, 1975
70. Inazu A, Brown ML, Hesler CB, et al: Increased high-density lipoprotein levels caused by a common cholesteryl-ester transfer protein gene mutation. *N Engl J Med* 323:1234, 1990
71. Rader DJ, Schaefer JR, Lohse P, et al: Increased production of apolipoprotein A-I associated with elevated plasma levels of high density lipoproteins, apoA-I, and LpA-I in a patient with familial hyperalphalipoproteinemia. *Metabolism* 42:1429, 1993

Acknowledgments

Figures 1, 2 Dimitry Schidlovsky.

CHAPTER 8

Thrombosis

Robert D. Rosenberg, M.D., Ph.D., William C. Aird, M.D.

Advances in biochemical, molecular genetic, and clinical investigative techniques have provided us with a detailed understanding of the structures of the coagulation system's plasma proteins and receptors, as well as a more sophisticated appreciation of the function of the coagulation mechanism in humans. This knowledge has improved our understanding of the role of the hypercoagulable state in acute coronary syndromes and has also led to the development of new anticoagulants for the treatment of coronary artery thrombosis.

The Blood Coagulation Mechanism

The prototype transformations of the coagulation mechanism involve an enzyme precursor, or zymogen, that is normally present in the blood. This substance is transformed into a trypsinlike protease (serine protease) either by a conformational alteration or by a converting enzyme that cleaves peptide bonds. The rate of this reaction may be accelerated by nonenzymatic cofactors that are able to either alter zymogen conformation or bind the converting enzyme and the zymogen close together on an appropriate surface. Once the serine protease is generated, it is free to act as an enzyme on its natural substrates and transform them into biologically potent species or ultimately produce fibrin. However, the serine protease may also encounter plasma components that neutralize its activity or prevent its generation. These inhibitory substances contain peptide sequences similar to those within the protease's natural substrates. The interaction of the serine protease with these unique regions triggers conformational events that prevent

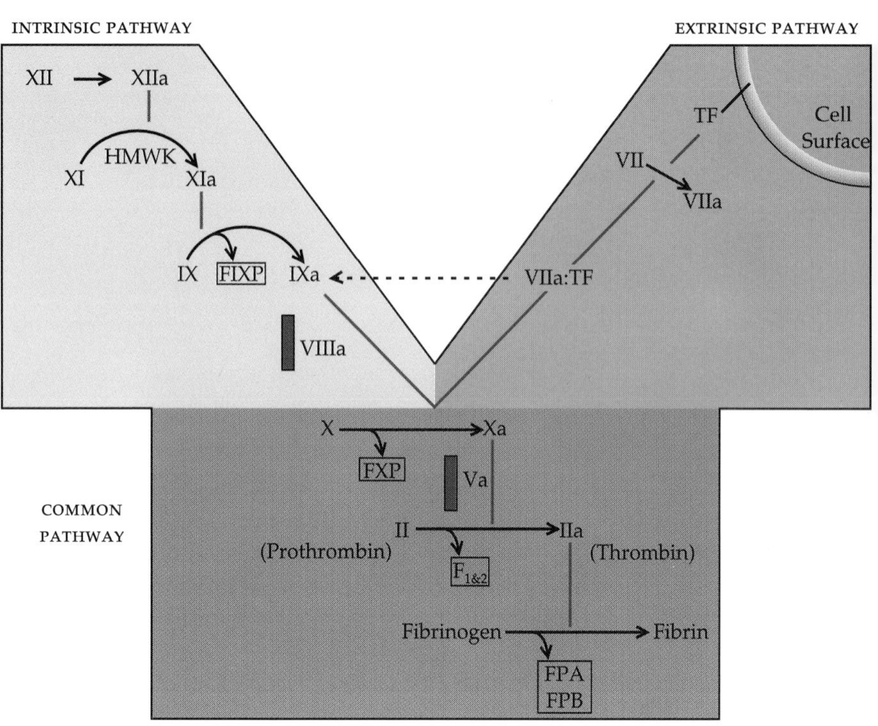

Figure 1 *The blood coagulation mechanism. The intrinsic and extrinsic pathways generate factor Xa of the common pathway, which ultimately leads to the formation of fibrin clot. "Cross talk" between the extrinsic and intrinsic cascades occurs through the activation of factor IX by the factor VIIa–tissue factor (VIIa:TF) complex (dashed arrow). Activation peptides FIXP, FXP,* F_{1+2}*, FPA, and FPB are indicated in blue boxes. HMWK, high-molecular-weight kininogen; FPA, fibrinopeptide A; FPB, fibrinopeptide B. Filled rectangles, cell surface.*

bond hydrolysis and generates stable inactive enzyme–enzyme inhibitor complexes.

During evolution, homologous sets of zymogens, converting enzymes, cofactors, and inhibitors arise as a result of gene duplication and mutation. This situation has led to the development of a linked series of reactions in which a zymogen is converted into a serine protease that then catalyzes the subsequent precursor to protease transition. This multistage system permits both amplification and modulation of the initial stimulus that sets the coagulation mechanism into action [*see Figure 1*].

The activation of the intrinsic pathway is initiated by the exposure of collagen, basement membrane, or microfibrillar substance to the blood. Factor XII, a zymogen with a single polypeptide chain (molecular weight, 80 kilodaltons [kd]), binds to these subendothelial structures and is converted via conformational and proteolytic events to an active serine protease, XIIa.[1] The generation of factor XIIa is enhanced by an autocatalytic circuit that involves the zymogens prekallikrein and plasminogen as well as the cofactor high-molecular-weight kininogen. With the aid of the cofactor high-molecular-weight kininogen, factor XIIa is then able to rapidly cleave factor XI, a zymogen with two identical polypeptide chains that are connected by disulfide bonds (molecular weight, 80 kd × 2). Factor XIa generated by this process is then able to interact with factor IX, a zymogen with a single polypeptide chain whose molecular weight is 57 kd.[2] The conversion of factor IX to factor IXa requires two peptide bond scissions that result in the release of an activation peptide, factor IX activation peptide (FIXP). Factor IXa then cleaves factor X zymogen at a single site to produce the serine protease factor Xa in conjunction with the release of an activation peptide, factor X activation peptide (FXP). Factor X is a zymogen that circulates as a two-chain species whose structure is quite homologous to that of factor IX (molecular weight, 55 kd). In vivo, the conversion of factor X to factor Xa is dramatically enhanced by a cofactor termed factor VIIIa in conjunction with Ca^{2+} ions and an activated platelet surface. The structure of factor VIII (molecular weight, 300 kd) has been defined by molecular cloning.[3,4]

The activation of the extrinsic pathway is initiated by exposure to the blood of a membrane-bound glycoprotein termed tissue factor. The structure of this component was determined by molecular cloning. Tissue factor has a short cytoplasmic domain, a hydrophobic membrane-spanning sequence, and an extracellular binding region.[5-8] Tissue factor is able to form a stable complex with a plasma protein termed factor VII/VIIa. This component is quite homologous in structure to prothrombin, factor IX, and factor X, and it is present in the blood at very low levels. It is unclear whether factor VII is activated by a conformational change induced by its interaction with tissue factor or whether factor VIIa is produced by an active enzyme before factor VIIa binds to tissue factor. Subsequently, factor X interacts with the factor VII/VIIa–tissue factor complex and is rapidly converted to factor Xa via proteolytic cleavages that are identical to those occurring during the intrinsic activation of the zymogen.

Prothrombin is a single-chain zymogen (molecular weight, 69 kd) that is composed of a C-terminal half that will ultimately constitute thrombin and an N-terminal half termed prothrombin fragment 1+2 (F_{1+2}). Prothrombin fragment possesses multiple γ-carboxyglutamic acid and triple-looped subdomains that are involved in binding to phospholipid and factor Va. Once the extrinsic and intrinsic pathways have generated sufficient factor Xa, this enzyme can convert prothrombin to thrombin. This event is accomplished by multiple scissions of the zymogen, which liberate the N-terminal F_{1+2}, a small 13-amino-acid polypeptide, and the two-chain disulfide-linked enzyme IIa.[9] In vitro, this sequence of events proceeds slowly, and many hours are needed for thrombin generation. In vivo, the process is dramatically accelerated by the action of a cofactor termed factor V/Va in conjunction with calcium ions and the activated platelet surface.[10] Factor V consists of a minimally active single polypeptide chain (molecular weight, 286 kd) that contains several types of internal repeats or domains that are homologous to those of factor VIII, as well as a unique connecting region of 31 tandem repeats. The minimally active factor V is converted to the extremely potent factor Va by the action of thrombin or factor Xa or both. The conversion process involves multiple scissions that remove the central connecting region and allow the C-terminal heavy chain and the N-terminal light chain to function. The light chain interacts with the activated platelet surface and binds factor Xa, whereas the heavy chain complexes with prothrombin. The net effect of these actions is to bring the serine protease and the zymogen into proximity and thereby accelerate the production of thrombin about 300,000-fold.

Fibrinogen is a plasma protein (molecular weight, 340 kd) that is composed of three pairs of polypeptide chains.[11,12] The six chains are held together by numerous disulfide bridges, with the N-terminal regions of all polypeptide chains maintained in a rigid symmetric configuration within a central E nodule. These chains emerge from this region to form two lateral bundles, each containing a single set of three chains that intertwine to form two nodular structures, termed D domains, that contain the C-terminal segments of two of these chains. Thus, fibrinogen is a dumbbell-shaped molecule with two smaller lateral D domains and a larger central E domain [*see Chapter 11, Figure 5*]. Once thrombin evolves, it cleaves two sets of polypeptides within the central E nodule to liberate a 16-amino-acid and a 14-amino-acid polypeptide termed fibrinopeptide A and fibrinopeptide B, respectively. The release of these polypeptides unmasks a specific set of sites within the E nodule that allows this region to interact with areas in the D nodules of other fibrin molecules. The staggered array of E nodule–D nodule interactions permits the generation of large polymers, which create the fibrin meshwork.

The Natural Anticoagulation Mechanisms That Regulate the Generation of Thrombin

The tissue factor pathway inhibitor (TFPI) is a lipoprotein-associated plasma protein (molecular weight, 35 kd) that controls factor VII/VIIa–tissue factor complex activity [*see Figure 2*]. TFPI possesses three tandem, repeated serine protease inhibitor domains whose functions are similar to those of antithrombin.[13-16] The suppression of extrinsic pathway activity is accomplished by rapid formation of an interaction product between TFPI, factor VIIa–tissue factor, and factor Xa. The inhibition of factor VIIa–tissue factor is wholly dependent upon the presence of factor Xa, whereas factor Xa can be inhibited in the absence of factor VIIa–tissue factor. The first inhibitor domain of TFPI is involved in its binding to factor VIIa–tissue factor, whereas the second inhibitor domain of TFPI simultaneously complexes with factor Xa. The function of the third inhibitory domain remains enigmatic.

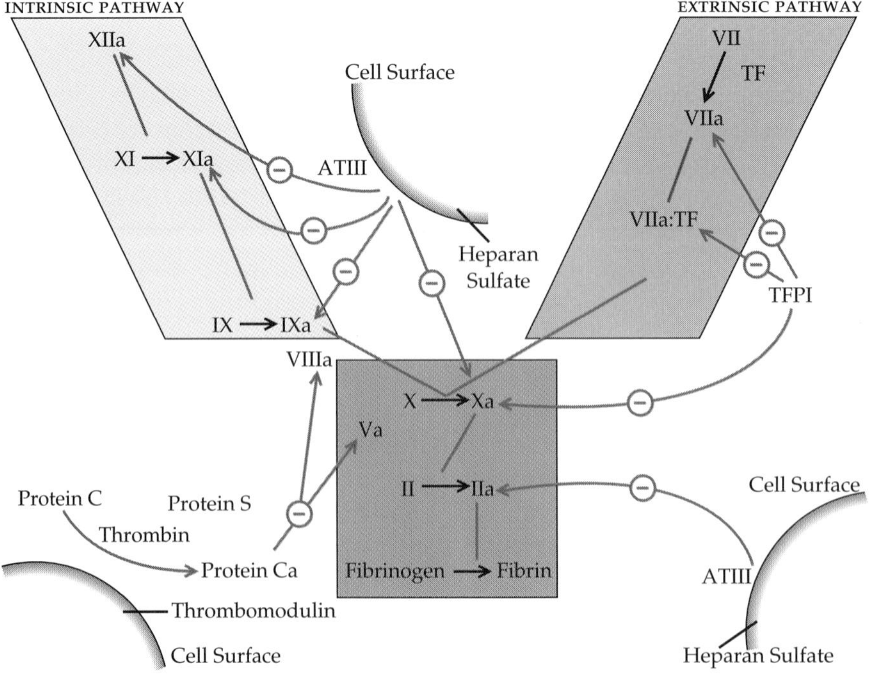

Figure 2 The natural anticoagulant mechanisms. Tissue factor pathway inhibitor (TFPI) suppresses extrinsic pathway activity through the formation of a complex with factor VIIa–tissue factor (VIIa:TF) and Xa. The protein C–thrombomodulin mechanism, consisting of thrombomodulin, thrombin, protein C, and protein S, inactivates factors Va and VIIIa. Antithrombin III (ATIII) inhibits thrombin and factors IXa, Xa, XIa, and XIIa. This reaction is enhanced several orders of magnitude by the presence of anticoagulantly active heparin or heparan sulfate synthesized by the blood vessel wall.

Thus, multifunctional TFPI is designed to allow formation of the factor VII/VIIa–tissue factor complex but then to suppress extrinsic pathway activity by simultaneously binding the two serine proteases within the interaction product.[17] This novel multicomponent interaction allows basal function of the factor VII–tissue factor complex pathway and subsequent suppression of the system after extensive generation of factors VIIa and Xa.

The protein C–thrombomodulin mechanism modulates the activity of the cofactors of the coagulation mechanism. Protein C is a zymogen (molecular weight, 41 kd) that consists of a heavy and a light chain joined by a disulfide bridge.[18,19] Thrombomodulin is an endothelial cell receptor (molecular weight, 100 kd) whose structure contains a highly charged N-terminal domain, six homologous epidermal growth factor repeats similar to those of the low-density lipoprotein receptor, a highly glycosylated region that is rich in serine and threonine, a membrane-spanning sequence, and a short cytoplasmic tail.[20,21] Thrombin and protein C assemble on the three epidermal growth factor type B repeats closest to the membrane and allow thrombomodulin to rapidly cleave a single peptide bond in protein C. This cleavage generates protein Ca and a 14-amino-acid activation peptide. Once evolved, protein Ca is able to cleave the heavy chains of factors Va and VIIIa, thereby inactivating these cofactors by preventing subsequent interactions with prothrombin or factor X.[22-24] Protein S and another, as yet unidentified, protein appear to be required as cofactors in this process. Thus, the generation of thrombin initiates a complex series of events that destroy activated cofactors and ultimately suppress the production of this enzyme.

The antithrombin III–heparan sulfate mechanism regulates the activity of most of the serine proteases of the coagulation mechanism other than factor VIIa and protein Ca. Antithrombin III is a plasma protein (molecular weight, 56 kd) that contains a C-terminal arginine-serine reactive site, which interacts with serine proteases, as well as an N-terminal set of positive residues, which bind heparin and heparan sulfate.[25] The drug heparin, which is isolated from pig mucosa or beef lung, as well as heparan sulfate, which is synthesized by endothelial cells of the blood vessel wall, contains a specific sequence of monosaccharide residues that bind tightly to antithrombin III. In the absence of the polysaccharide, antithrombin III slowly neutralizes the proteolytic enzymes of the coagulation mechanism, including thrombin, factor Xa, factor IXa, factor XIa, and factor XIIa, via a serine active site–arginine reactive site interaction. The addition of small amounts of anticoagulantly active heparin or heparan sulfate allows the polysaccharide to bind to positive sites on antithrombin III and thereby enhance several thousand–fold the rate of enzyme–protease inhibitor complex formation.[25] The acceleration of protease inhibitor action mainly results from a polysaccharide-induced conformational change in the inhibitor, but it also occurs because binding of the polysaccharide brings the enzyme and the protease inhibitor into proximity. After the enzyme-inhibitor complex is formed, the polysaccharide is displaced from the interaction product, binds to free antithrombin III, and thereby catalyzes multiple rounds of enzyme-inhibitor complex formation. Considerable data have shown that in vivo, the blood vessel wall synthesizes anticoagulantly active heparan sulfate proteoglycans, which bind antithrombin III and permit the protease inhibitor to be selectively activated at blood–vessel wall interfaces where enzymes of the coagulation cascade are generated.[26-29] Thus, antithrombin III is critically placed to neutralize these enzymes and thereby protect natural surfaces against thrombus formation.

The Hypercoagulable State and Coronary Heart Disease

For many years, clinicians have sought to develop blood tests that can be used to predict coronary artery thrombotic events in high-risk patients. Recent advances in our knowledge of the biochemistry of the blood clotting mechanism have led to the design of specific immunoassays that detect in vivo generation of coagulation system enzymes.

Coagulation system zymogens are transformed into serine proteases by converting enzymes and cofactors. Previous attempts to monitor these processes have been directed at measuring the levels of zymogens (factor VII, prothrombin, protein C), inhibitors (antithrombin, TFPI), or substrates (fibrinogen). These components are present in large excess within the blood, and only a small percentage of them are converted into active enzymes, enzyme-inhibitor complexes, or altered substrates. Thus, attempts to monitor hypercoagulable states by measuring the ambient levels of zymogens, inhibitors, or substrates, or by determining their catabolic rates in the circulation, have generally been of limited utility. Direct measurement of the blood levels of coagulation enzymes has been impossible in most cases because these serine proteases are rapidly neutralized by the natural anticoagulant mechanisms shown in Figure 2.

Faced with these obstacles, most investigators have resorted to developing immunoassays for peptides liberated from zymogens during their conversion to serine proteases (activation peptides), for enzyme-inhibitor complexes, or for peptides that are released from fibrinogen by thrombin. These assays have been developed through two general approaches. First, specific antibody populations have been generated that recognize new antigenic sites (neoepitopes) on the activation peptides or enzyme-inhibitor complexes that are completely hidden in the parent zymogen or inhibitor. Second, sample processing procedures have been developed that efficiently remove zymogens or substrates from plasma before it is assayed and thereby reduce the need for antibodies that can completely distinguish between the peptide or enzyme inhibitor complex and the cross-reacting parent species. Most assays were initially developed in academic laboratories, but methods for determining plasma levels of F_{1+2} and fibrinopeptide A are now available in kit form from several manufacturers. F_{1+2} is the 31-kd polypeptide released from the amino terminal end of prothrombin during its conversion to thrombin and is therefore a marker for factor Xa activity. Fibrinopeptide A is a 16-amino-acid peptide that is cleared from the α chain of fibrinogen during its transition to fibrin and is therefore a marker for thrombin action.

These assays have been used to establish the in vivo pathways responsible for the activation of the coagulation system under basal conditions (i.e., in the absence of thrombosis or provocative stimuli). The studies have been carried out in patients with inherited coagulation factor deficiencies and in primates infused with anti–tissue factor antibody. Patients with factor VII deficiency, but not factor XI deficiency, have reduced levels of FIXP,[30-31] FXP, and prothrombin activation peptide, whereas, patients with deficiencies of factor VIII or factor IX have normal levels of FXP and F_{1+2}.[32] These data suggest that in the basal state, the extrinsic (factor VII–tissue factor) pathway, not the intrinsic pathway, is mainly responsible for the activation of factor X and prothrombin. The importance of the factor VII–tissue factor pathway was confirmed by a study in which relatively small doses of recombinant factor VIIa were infused into factor VII–deficient patients.[33] The results showed a substantial elevation in plasma concentrations of FIXP, FXP, and F_{1+2} and imply that factor VIIa interacts with preexisting tissue factor sites on monocytes or the blood vessel wall and then activates factor X. Previous investigators have expressed doubts about whether or not tissue factor is normally in contact with the blood. This issue has been addressed by a study in which factor VIIa was infused into normal chimpanzees, resulting in significant increases in the levels of FIXP, FXP, and F_{1+2}.[34] Metabolic turnover studies with radiolabeled FIXP, FXP, and F_{1+2} indicated that the elevated levels of activation peptides result from accelerated conversion of factor IX, factor X, and prothrombin into their respective serine proteases. The administration of a potent monoclonal antibody to tissue factor, which suppresses the in vitro activity of the factor VIIa–tissue factor complex, abolished the elevated concentrations of FXP and F_{1+2} mediated by the recombinant protein and, to a lesser extent, also suppressed the basal levels of FIXP and FXP. Thus, the factor VII–tissue factor pathway is constitutively active and is largely responsible for the activation of factor IX, factor X, and prothrombin in the basal state.

The basal function of the intrinsic cascade has also been examined by a study in which purified factor IX concentrate was administered to individuals with hemophilia B, who have a congenital deficiency of this factor.[33] Infusions of the zymogen significantly increased the concentrations of FIXP, which were initially greatly decreased, but did not raise the levels of FXP or F_{1+2}. Furthermore, the infusions of highly purified factor VIII concentrates in patients with hemophilia A produced no significant change in the concentrations of FXP or F_{1+2}.[33] These observations strongly suggest that generation of the factor IXa–factor VIIIa cell surface complex is insufficient to activate factor X under basal conditions. It has been hypothesized that in response to vascular injury or thrombotic stimuli, the factor VII–tissue factor pathway produces sufficient free thrombin or factor Xa to generate factor VIIIa or to create a natural surface (e.g., an activated platelet) on which the factor IXa–factor VIIIa cell surface complex can be assembled [*see Figure 3*]. The subsequent accelerated production of factor Xa would then induce a burst of thrombin activity that would overwhelm normal inhibitory mechanisms and lead to thrombus formation.

These conclusions have important implications for the detection of hyperactive hemostatic mechanisms. The hypercoagulable state can be defined as the presence of increased factor Xa generation (as judged by higher concentrations of F_{1+2}) with little or no elevation in the level of free thrombin (as judged by normal or minimally elevated levels of fibrinopeptide

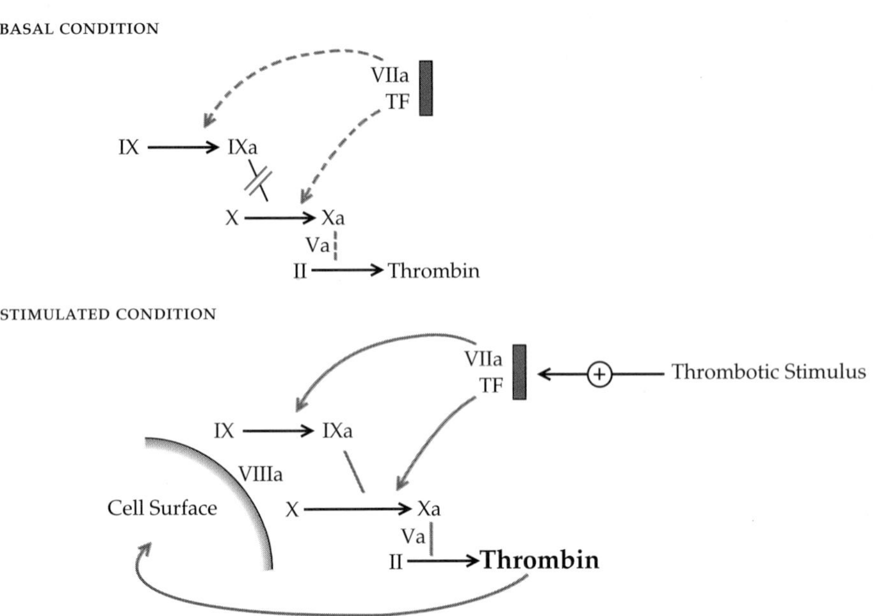

Figure 3 *In vivo pathways of coagulation. Under basal conditions, generation of factor IXa–factor VIIIa cell surface complex is insufficient to activate factor X. Stimulation of the extrinsic cascade may produce sufficient free thrombin to generate anticoagulantly active factor IXa–factor VIIIa platelet surface complex, resulting in a burst of Xa activity and, ultimately, clot formation. Filled rectangles, cell surface.*

A).[35] Patients with these biochemical abnormalities would be poised to generate sufficient factor Xa or thrombin to activate the dormant intrinsic cascade. This activation could produce a burst of thrombin that would overwhelm normal inhibitory mechanisms and thereby induce arterial or venous thrombosis. This definition of the hypercoagulable state has been partially validated by studying patients with congenital hypercoagulable states that resulted from protein C and protein S deficiencies as well as normal persons as they age.[30,36,37]

These assays have allowed investigators to determine whether or not activation of the coagulation mechanism plays a role in the development of unstable angina and myocardial infarction. Several investigations initially demonstrated that the hemostatic mechanism is activated during the onset of these disorders.[38-41] Plasma levels of fibrinopeptide A, platelet-release proteins, and fibrinogen/fibrin degradation products are elevated in the acute phases of unstable angina and myocardial infarction, indicating production and lysis of intracoronary fibrin-platelet thrombi.[40,42-44] However, levels of these markers rapidly return to normal, suggesting that activation of the coagulation mechanisms may only coincide with an acute thrombotic episode.

To further examine the utility of determining the extent of coagulation system activity, Merlini and associates[45] compared F_{1+2} and fibrinopeptide A plasma levels in a population with unstable angina or acute myocardial infarction with those in a control population (healthy individuals or those with stable angina) that was matched for age and sex. The study population consisted of 112 consecutive individuals (admitted to a single medical center) experiencing the initial onset of unstable angina or acute myocardial infarction. Patients with comorbid conditions that are known to augment or suppress coagulation system activity or to alter the metabolic behavior of F_{1+2} or fibrinopeptide A, or those who were ingesting drugs known to affect hemostasis,[46] were prospectively excluded. The patients with acute coronary syndromes were followed up for six months after discharge, a regimen that allowed the patients to be characterized as exhibiting an uneventful clinical course or as experiencing additional cardiac events. The patients with an uneventful clinical course were reinvestigated to ascertain whether patients with a single episode of an acute coronary syndrome but no further evidence of active vascular disease exhibit a persistent hypercoagulable state.

At the patients' admission, plasma concentrations of F_{1+2} and fibrinopeptide A were significantly elevated in those with unstable angina or acute myocardial infarction, compared with concentrations in the control population; these elevations reflect the presence of ongoing intracoronary thrombosis. Previous investigations had documented elevated plasma levels of fibrinopeptide A in 60 to 80 percent of patients during the acute phase of these disorders, but no data are available for F_{1+2}.[40,42,43] The normal plasma concentrations of F_{1+2} and fibrinopeptide A in a minority of patients with acute coronary syndromes could result from the fact that intracoronary thrombosis is an intermittent process and that F_{1+2} and fibrinopeptide A have relatively short half-lives. Alternatively, a few patients with unstable angina may exhibit normal plasma concentrations of F_{1+2} and fibrinopeptide A because their symptoms result from poor coronary reserve with otherwise uncomplicated atherosclerotic plaques.

Six months after discharge, patients with acute coronary syndromes who exhibited an uneventful course manifested increased plasma levels of F_{1+2} and greatly reduced or virtually normal plasma levels of fibrinopeptide A. These results are consistent with those of prior studies that showed diminished plasma levels of fibrinopeptide A several days after the onset of acute coronary syndromes.[43,47,48] The normalization of fibrinopeptide A values has been interpreted as demonstrating that coagulation system hyperactivity in these disorders is restricted to the time period during which the coronary thrombosis is generated. However, the data obtained with the F_{1+2} assay, which monitors an earlier step in the coagulation cascade, reveal that abnormalities of the hemostatic mechanism persist long after clinical stabilization in patients with acute coronary syndromes. Indeed, the observation of elevated plasma concentrations of F_{1+2} and normal or slightly elevated plasma levels of fibrinopeptide A signify a hypercoagulable state.

The persistent hypercoagulable state in patients with unstable angina and acute myocardial infarction appears to be independent of the extent of coronary artery disease or drug ingestion. It is suspected that molecular abnormalities of the hemostatic mechanism and blood vessel wall are responsible for the observed hypercoagulable state. The results from trials by Merlini and associates[45] raise the interesting possibility that the increased activity of the hemostatic mechanism may predate the onset of the acute coronary syndrome, and this hypothesis is currently under examination in a large prospective trial (Northwick Park Heart Study II). Finally, the observation that patients with acute coronary syndromes exhibit an increased level of activation of the coagulation system long after clinical stabilization has been achieved has important implications with regard to the pathophysiology and treatment of acute coronary syndromes. It is tempting to speculate that the higher occurrence of cardiac events in patients with unstable angina[49] and myocardial infarction[50] than in those with stable angina may be partially attributable to the persistent hypercoagulable state observed in the first two groups. Indeed, the success of efforts to prevent unstable angina and acute myocardial infarction with warfarin therapy[51,52] may result from the suppression of the persistent activation of the hemostatic mechanism. It is reasonable to propose that detection of the hypercoagulable state with the F_{1+2} assay could identify patients most likely to benefit from prolonged anticoagulant therapy and could provide a means for ascertaining the optimal levels of drug to administer. Prospective trials are needed to test these hypotheses.

The Development of New Anticoagulants as Adjunctive Therapy in Coronary Artery Thrombolysis

The onset of coronary artery thrombosis plays a central role in the development of acute myocardial infarction. The immediate lysis of the arterial thrombus and the subsequent prevention of thrombotic reocclusion are of critical importance in the treatment of this disorder. Indeed, the rapid and sustained reperfusion of the myocardium is a major determinant of overall survival.[53] The ability of thrombolytic agents, such as tissue plasminogen activator (t-PA) and streptokinase, to induce early coronary artery reperfusion is offset by an attendant increase in procoagulant action, as evidenced by increased plasma levels of F_{1+2} and fibrinopeptide A.[54] The addition of heparin and aspirin to thrombolytic regimens atten-

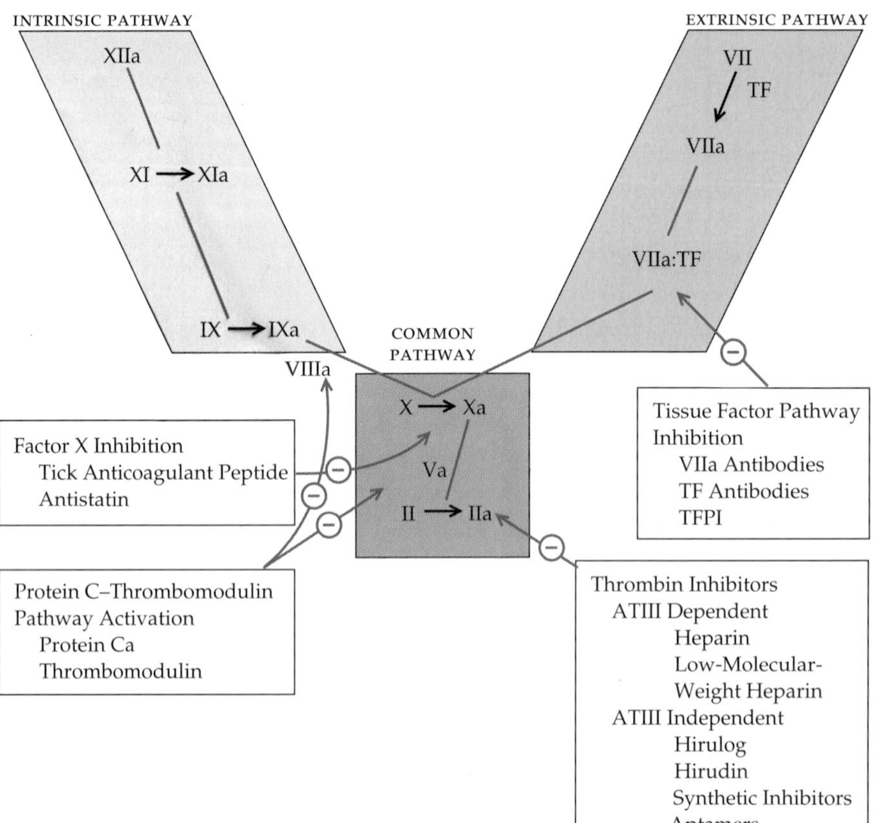

Figure 4 *New anticoagulants and their sites of action. VIIa:TF, factor VIIa–tissue factor complex; ATIII, antithrombin III; TFPI, tissue factor pathway inhibitor.*

uates the increased activity of the coagulation mechanism and improves overall patency rates.[55] However, the most effective regimens achieve adequate reperfusion in only about 55 percent of patients at 90 minutes, and acute arterial thrombotic reocclusion subsequently develops in six percent of patients.[53] The failure of the standard anticoagulant regimen to afford full protection from thrombotic phenomena is largely a result of heparin's inability to inhibit thrombin that is bound to the fibrin clot and factor Xa that is complexed to activated platelets.[56,57] This resistance to therapy is most probably a result of the electrostatic exclusion of the heparin-antithrombin complex from the thrombus or from the neutralization of heparin by local release of inhibitory components from platelets.[58] Heparin-insensitive pools of procoagulants are also exposed during thrombolysis, and they may mediate further deposition of thrombus. These limitations of conventional therapy have prompted the search for new classes of antithrombotic drugs that more completely inhibit the hemostatic mechanism and thereby improve coronary artery patency in patients treated with thrombolytic agents [*see Figure 4*].

Blood-sucking parasites, such as leeches and ticks, have served as important sources for novel anticoagulants. The prototype anticoagulant component is hirudin, a 65-amino-acid protein derived from the leech *Hirudo medicinalis*. Although hirudin was characterized as an antithrombin over 30 years ago, large-scale production of this product for clinical trials has only recently been achieved as a result of the advent of recombinant technology and the design of synthetic analogue peptides. Native and recombinant hirudin (r-hirudin, or CGP 39393) bind tightly and irreversibly to thrombin, forming a one-to-one stoichiometric complex.[59,60] This highly specific interaction blocks all the proteolytic functions of thrombin and leads to inhibition of fibrin and factors Va, VIIIa, and XIIIa generation and to abrogation of thrombin-induced platelet aggregation.[61,62] Detailed structure-function studies of the interaction between hirudin and thrombin have demonstrated that the C-terminal end of hirudin binds to the substrate-recognition site of thrombin, whereas the N-terminal end of hirudin binds to the catalytic center of the enzyme. This information has led to the design of a new class of bivalent thrombin inhibitors known as hirulogs. These synthetic analogues incorporate the aforementioned two binding domains, which are separated by a short linker that is sized to mimic the interatomic distance between the enzyme's substrate recognition site and catalytic center. Hirulog-1 is a 20-amino-acid bivalent peptide that binds reversibly and specifically to thrombin.[63] Hirudin and hirulog directly inhibit thrombin that is bound to fibrin and are not affected by circulating inhibitors, such as platelet factor–4.[57]

In several animal models of arterial thrombosis, hirudin and hirulog have been shown to lead to a greater reduction in fibrin and platelet deposition than has heparin.[64-67] These effects are dose dependent and are not associated with major bleeding complications. In a rat model of t-PA–induced thrombolysis, hirudin and hirulog were superior to heparin in reducing the reocclusion rate.[68] In a dog model of coronary artery thrombotic occlusion, r-hirudin and streptokinase produced a shorter time of reperfusion and a higher patency rate than did heparin and streptokinase.[69] The preliminary clinical evaluation of hirudin and hirulog as adjunctive anticoagulants in patients receiving thrombolytic therapy appears quite promising. In a randomized, open-label trial comparing the effects of hirudin and heparin administration in 246 patients receiving t-PA and aspirin for acute myocardial infarction, hirudin resulted in greater infarction-related artery patency at 18 to 36 hours, decreased rates of reocclusion, fewer in-hospital deaths or reinfarction, and a comparable risk of spontaneous bleeding.[70] Interestingly, plasma levels of fibrinopeptide A in this trial correlated with increased mortality, and plasma concentrations of this marker were significantly reduced in patients treated with hirudin.[71] In a randomized, double-blind study comparing the effects of hirulog and heparin administration in patients receiving streptokinase and aspirin, the patency rate at 90 and 120 minutes was significantly higher in the group receiving hirulog.[72] However, no difference was observed between the two groups with regard to bleeding. In a randomized study comparing the effects of these two agents in 193 patients receiving streptokinase and aspirin for acute myocardial infarction, the administration of higher doses of hirudin resulted in a trend toward decreased mortality and a decrease in serious cardiac events, with no difference in bleeding.[73] The encouraging results of these early studies have provided the impetus for proceeding to large, multicenter phase III trials to definitively compare the relative roles of direct thrombin and heparin administration after thrombolytic therapy (GUSTO-II, OASIS, TIMI-9, and HIT-II). Interestingly, in GUSTO-II and TIMI-9, an early excess of hemorrhagic strokes in patients receiving hirudin in conjunction with thrombolytic therapy prompted a significant dose reduction of this agent. The eventual clinical impact of these thrombin inhibitors will become apparent only when these and other large-scale trials are completed.

Thrombin cleaves fibrinogen in part by recognizing a highly conserved sequence of amino acids centered around an arginine residue on the A-α chain of the substrate. Knowledge about the molecular basis of this interaction has led to the design of a new class of substrate-derived competitive inhibitors of thrombin, in which arginine or a chemical group mimicking this residue is incorporated into a peptide or nonpeptide backbone.[74] Studies using x-ray crystallography to examine thrombin bound to hirudin or its derivatives and to examine earlier synthetic inhibitors of the enzyme have served as starting points for the development of new anticoagulants.[75] Like hirudin, these low-molecular-weight peptide and nonpeptide agents specifically inhibit free as well as thrombus-bound thrombin and are resistant to inactivation by endogenous inhibitors, such as platelet factor 4. From a clinical standpoint, synthetic thrombin inhibitors are particularly attractive because of their rapid onset of action and their potential for oral administration. Although several synthetic inhibitors have been tested in animal models of venous and arterial thrombosis, few data exist concerning their role as adjunctive anticoagulants in the setting of thrombolytic therapy. D-Phe-Pro-Arg-chloromethyl ketone (PPACK) is a peptidyl chloromethyl ketone that irreversibly inactivates thrombin by linking to it covalently and alkylating its active-center histidine.[76] In animal studies, PPACK has been shown to be more effective than heparin in preventing reocclusion in the context of t-PA–induced thrombolysis.[68] Argatroban, an arginine derivative that blocks thrombin's active catalytic site, prevents reocclusion in animal models of thrombolysis.[77] In a phase 1 study of patients with unstable angina, intravenous argatroban resulted in a dose-related increase in activated partial thromboplastin time (aPTT) but had no effect on bleeding time and caused no episodes of spontaneous bleeding.[78] It is noteworthy that cessation of therapy was associated with rebound angina, an effect that has been attributed to uninhibited thrombin activity caused by withdrawal of the drug. The efficacy and safety of argatroban and other synthetic thrombin inhibitors in humans await further clinical study.

Because platelet-bound factor Xa generates thrombin and resists inhibition by the heparin-antithrombin complex, it serves as a logical target for the development of new antithrombotic agents. Two specific factor Xa inhibitors have been described. The tick anticoagulant peptide has been isolated and cloned from the soft tick *Ornithodoros moubata*,[79] and antistatin, a 119-amino-acid polypeptide, has been isolated and cloned from the salivary glands of the Mexican leech *Haementeria officinalis*.[80] The tick and leech proteins are highly selective reversible inhibitors of factor Xa and have dissociation constants in the nanomolar range. The proteins reversibly neutralize free factor Xa and factor Xa that is bound to platelets. In animal models, recombinant tick anticoagulant peptide is superior to heparin in preventing thrombus formation in a prosthetic graft model.[81] In a t-PA–induced animal thrombolysis model, recombinant tick anticoagulant peptide and antistatin were superior to heparin in accelerating thrombolysis and reducing the incidence of thrombotic reocclusion.[82,83] However, the relative efficacy and safety of a thrombin inhibitor (hirudin or hirulog) as compared with a factor Xa inhibitor (recombinant tick anticoagulant peptide or antistatin) in humans who have undergone thrombolysis remain to be established.

A novel class of antithrombins has been discovered by selection for specific thrombin-binding properties of single-stranded DNA. Amplification of these target-bound DNA molecules by polymerase chain reaction has allowed for the identification of a 15-nucleotide consensus sequence, designated an aptamer, which binds to and inhibits the substrate recognition site of thrombin.[84-86] In vitro, these DNA molecules inhibit the generation of fibrinopeptide A and the aggregation of platelets by thrombus-bound thrombin.[87] In a primate model, intravenous infusion of thrombin aptamer was well tolerated and resulted in a dose-dependent prolongation of prothrombin time.[88] It had a short half-life, approximately 100 seconds, which suggests a potential advantage of this agent in clinical situations requiring rapid reversal of anticoagulation. Further studies are needed to determine the antithrombotic potential of these new agents in vivo.

The various thrombin and Xa inhibitors block the action of critical enzymes in the coagulation pathway. Another strategy for suppressing the function of the hemostatic system is to decrease the effective concentrations of specific cofactors, such as factor Va, factor VIIIa, and tissue factor, which regulate the generation of coagulation enzymes.

Infusion of activated protein C selectively proteolyzes cofactors Va and VIIIa and thereby decreases production of factor Xa and thrombin.[23] This natural anticoagulant protein has been isolated from human plasma and has been generated by recombinant techniques. At supraphysiologic levels, both plasma-derived and recombinant activated protein C are effective and safe antithrombotic agents in nonhuman models of arterial thrombosis.[89,90] Purified activated protein C has been infused in normal human subjects without adverse effects.[91] Extensive studies of activated protein C in animal models of coronary artery thrombolysis are currently under way to determine the therapeutic potential of this anticoagulant protein, and human trials are planned for the near future.

The infusion of thrombomodulin would also be expected to generate activated protein C, destroy cofactors Va and VIIIa, and hence suppress in vivo generation of factor Xa and thrombin. Unlike infusion of activated protein C, however, infusion of thrombomodulin has the potential to provide "anticoagulation on demand." Because the mechanism of thrombomodulin's action is wholly dependent on the generation of thrombin in vivo, its therapeutic effect would disappear when thrombin levels fell into the normal range. Therefore, the action of thrombomodulin would be limited to periods of intensive activation of the coagulation mechanism. Hence, one might expect to achieve significant anticoagulation with minimal bleeding complications. Preliminary investigations of thrombomodulin have been completed in rodent models, in which the agent has shown considerable antithrombotic activity. Studies in other animal models are eagerly awaited.

The blockade of tissue factor on the blood vessel wall or on circulating monocytes should reduce the generation of factor VIIa, which in turn would decrease the production of factor Xa and thrombin. The suppression of this pathway has been achieved by infusion of recombinant tissue factor pathway inhibitor, a multivalent, Kunitz-type proteinase inhibitor that inhibits factor Xa as well as the factor VIIa–tissue factor complex.[17,92,93] Alternatively, inhibition of this pathway has also been attained in animal studies by infusion of monoclonal antibodies directed against tissue factor.[94] Such a therapeutic strategy would have great appeal during coronary artery thrombolysis—it would inhibit production of all coagulation enzymes—but it would have little effect on thrombin that is already bound to thrombi.

The detailed understanding of the structure-function relationships of coagulation proteins has led to an explosion in the isolation and design of new drugs that promise to improve on current strategies for anticoagulant therapy. The relative clinical value of thrombin inhibitors, factor Xa inhibitors, activated cofactor inhibitors, and tissue factor inhibitors will ultimately depend on their risk-benefit profiles (especially bleeding complications), which can be established only by large, randomized clinical trials. It is possible that combinations of several antithrombotic agents, each with differing sites of action, will be used to achieve the optimal therapeutic effect. Furthermore, it appears likely that these anticoagulants will be used in conjunction with inhibitors of platelet glycoprotein IIb-IIIa [*see Chapter 11*] as the preferred treatment in coronary artery thrombosis as well as in other arterial and venous thrombotic disorders.

References

1. Griffin JH, Cochrane CG: Human factor XII (Hageman factor). *Methods Enzymol* 45:56, 1976
2. Di Scipio RG, Kurachi K, Davie EW: Activation of human factor IX (Christmas factor). *J Clin Invest* 61:1528, 1978
3. Vehar G, Keyt B, Eaton D, et al: Structure of human factor VIII. *Nature* 312:337, 1984
4. Toole JJ, Knopf JL, Wozney JM, et al: Molecular cloning of a cDNA encoding human antihemophiliac factor. *Nature* 312:342, 1984
5. Spicer EK, Horton R, Bloem L, et al: Isolation of cDNA clones coding for human tissue factor: primary structure of the protein and cDNA. *Proc Natl Acad Sci USA* 84:5148, 1987
6. Morrissey JH, Fakhrai H, Edgington TS: Molecular cloning of the cDNA for tissue factor, the cellular receptor for the initiation of the coagulation protease cascade. *Cell* 50:129, 1987
7. Scarpati EM, Wen D, Broze GJ Jr, et al: Human tissue factor: cDNA sequence and chromosome localization of the gene. *Biochemistry* 26:5234, 1987
8. Mackman N, Morrissey JH, Fowler B, et al: Complete sequence of the human tissue factor gene, a highly regulated cellular receptor that initiates the coagulation protease cascade. *Biochemistry* 28:1755, 1989
9. Downing MR, Butkowski RJ, Clark MM, et al: Human prothrombin activation. *J Biol Chem* 250:8897, 1975
10. Pei G, Powers DD, Lentz BR: Specific contribution of different phospholipid surfaces to the activation of prothrombin by the fully assembled prothrombinase. *J Biol Chem* 268:3226, 1993
11. Doolittle RF: The structure and evolution of vertebrate fibrinogen. *Ann NY Acad Sci* 408:13,1983
12. Henschen A, Lottspeich F, Kehl M, et al: Covalent structure of fibrinogen. *Ann NY Acad Sci* 408:28, 1983
13. van der Logt CP, Reitsma PH, Bertina RM: Intron-exon organization of the human gene coding for the lipoprotein-associated coagulation inhibitor: the factor Xa dependent inhibitor of the extrinsic pathway of coagulation. *Biochemistry* 30:1571, 1991
14. Girard TJ, Warren LA, Novotny WF, et al: Identification of the 1.4 kb and 4.0 kb messages for the lipoprotein-associated coagulation inhibitor and expression of the encoded protein. *Thromb Res* 55:37, 1989
15. Girard TJ, Eddy R, Wesselschmidt RL, et al: Structure of the human lipoprotein- associated coagulation inhibitor gene: intron/exon gene organization and localization of the gene to chromosome 2. *J Biol Chem* 266:5036, 1991
16. Wun T-C, Kretzmer KK, Girard TJ, et al: Cloning and characterization of a cDNA coding for the lipoprotein-associated coagulation inhibitor shows that it consists of three tandem Kunitz-type inhibitory domains. *J Biol Chem* 263:6001, 1988
17. Broze GJ Jr, Warren LA, Novotny WF, et al: The lipoprotein-associated coagulation inhibitor that inhibits the factor VII-tissue factor complex also inhibits factor Xa: insight into its possible mechanism of action. *Blood* 71:335, 1988
18. Foster D, Davie EW: Characterization of a cDNA coding for human protein C. *Proc Natl Acad Sci USA* 81:4766, 1984
19. Beckmann RJ, Schmidt RJ, Santerre RF, et al: The structure and evolution of a 461 amino acid human protein C precursor and its messenger RNA, based upon the DNA sequence of cloned human liver cDNAs. *Nucleic Acids Res* 13:5233, 1985
20. Jackman RW, Beeler DL, VanDeWater L, et al: Characterization of a thrombomodulin cDNA reveals structural similarity to the low density lipoprotein receptor. *Proc Natl Acad Sci USA* 83:8834, 1986
21. Jackman RW, Beeler DL, Fritze L, et al: Human thrombomodulin gene is intron depleted: nucleic acid sequences of the cDNA and gene predict protein structure and suggest sites of regulatory control. *Proc Natl Acad Sci USA* 84:6425, 1987
22. Walker F, Sexton P, Esmon C: The inhibition of blood coagulation by activated protein C through the selective inactivation of activated factor C. *Biochim Biophys Acta* 571:333, 1979
23. Marlar RA, Kleiss AJ, Griffin JH: Mechanism of action of human activated protein C, a thrombin-dependent anticoagulant enzyme. *Blood* 59:1067, 1982
24. Dahlback B, Stenflo J: Inhibitory effect of activated protein C on activation of prothrombin by platelet-bound factor Xa. *Eur J Biochem* 107:331, 1980

25. Rosenberg RD, Damus PS: The purification and mechanism of action of human antithrombin-heparin cofactor. *J Biol Chem* 248:6490, 1973
26. Marcum JA, Mckenney JB, Rosenberg RD: Acceleration of thrombin-antithrombin complex formation in rat hindquarters via heparin-like molecules bound to the endothelium. *J Clin Invest* 74:341, 1984
27. Marcum JA, Rosenberg RD: Heparin-like molecules with anticoagulant activity are synthesized by cultured endothelial cells. *Biochem Biophys Res Commun* 126:365, 1985
28. Marcum JA, Atha DH, Fritze LM, et al: Cloned bovine aortic endothelial cells synthesize anticoagulantly active heparin sulfate proteoglycan. *J Biol Chem* 261:7507, 1986
29. Stern D, Nawroth P, Marcum J, et al: Interaction of antithrombin III with bovine aortic segments: role of heparin in binding and enhanced anticoagulant activity. *J Clin Invest* 75:272, 1985
30. Bauer KA, Kass BL, ten Cate H, et al: Factor IX is activated in vivo by the tissue factor mechanism. *Blood* 76:731, 1990
31. Takahashi I, Kato K, Sugiura I, et al: Activated factor IX-antithrombin III complexes in human blood: quantification by an enzyme-linked differential antibody immunoassay and determination of the in vivo half-life. *J Lab Clin Med* 118:317, 1991
32. Bauer KA, Kass BL, ten Cate H, et al: Detection of factor X activation in humans. *Blood* 74:2007, 1989
33. Bauer KA, Mannucci PM, Gringeri A, et al: Factor IXa-factor VIIIa-cell surface complex does not contribute to the basal activation of the coagulation mechanism in vivo. *Blood* 79:2039, 1992
34. ten Cate H, Bauer KA, Levi M, et al: The activation of factor X and prothrombin by recombinant factor VIIa in vivo is mediated by tissue factor. *J Clin Invest* 92:1207, 1993
35. Bauer KA, Rosenberg RD: The pathophysiology of the prethrombotic state in humans: insights gained from studies using markers of hemostatic system activation. *Blood* 70:343, 1987
36. Bauer KA, Weiss LM, Sparrow D, et al: Aging-associated changes in indices of thrombin generation and protein C activation in humans: normative aging study. *J Clin Invest* 80:1527, 1987
37. Bauer KA, Broekmans AW, Bertina RM, et al: Hemostatic enzyme generation in the blood of patients with hereditary protein C deficiency. *Blood* 71:1418, 1988
38. Johnsson H, Orinius E, Paul C: Fibrinopeptide A (FPA) in patients with acute myocardial infarction. *Thromb Res* 16:255, 1979
39. Mombelli G, Im Hof V, Haeberli A, et al: Effect of heparin on plasma fibrinopeptide A in patients with acute myocardial infarction. *Circulation* 69:684, 1984
40. Eisenberg PR, Sherman LA, Schectman K, et al: Fibrinopeptide A: a marker of acute coronary thrombosis. *Circulation* 71:912, 1985
41. Rapold HJ, Grimaudo V, Declerck PJ, et al: Plasma levels of plasminogen activator inhibitor type I, beta-thromboglobulin, and fibrinopeptide A before, during, and after treatment of acute myocardial infarction with alteplase. *Blood* 78:1490, 1991
42. Neri Serneri GG, Gensini GF, Abbate R, et al: Is raised plasma fibrinopeptide A a marker of acute coronary insufficiency (letter)? *Lancet* ii:982, 1980
43. Theroux P, Latour JG, Leger-Gauthier C, et al: Fibrinopeptide A and platelet factor levels in unstable angina pectoris. *Circulation* 75:156, 1987
44. Kruskal JB, Commerford PJ, Franks JJ, et al: Fibrin and fibrinogen-related antigens in patients with stable and unstable coronary artery disease. *N Engl J Med* 317:1361, 1987
45. Merlini PA, Bauer KA, Oltrona L, et al: Persistent activation of coagulation mechanism in unstable angina and myocardial infarction. *Circulation* 90:61, 1994
46. Bauer KA: Laboratory markers of coagulation activation. *Arch Pathol Lab Med* 117:71, 1993
47. van Hulsteijn H, Kolff J, Briet E, et al: Fibrinopeptide A and beta thromboglobulin in patients with angina pectoris and acute myocardial infarction. *Am Heart J* 107:39, 1984
48. Neri Serneri GG, Gensini GF, Carnovali M, et al: Association between time of increased fibrinopeptide A levels in plasma and episodes of spontaneous angina: a controlled prospective study. *Am Heart J* 113:672, 1987
49. Mulcahy R, Al Awadhi AH, de Buitleor M, et al: Natural history of unstable angina. *Am Heart J* 109:754, 1985
50. The Multicenter Postinfarction Research Group: Risk stratification and survival after myocardial infarction. *N Engl J Med* 309:331, 1983
51. Cohen M, Adams PC, Hawkins L, et al: Usefulness of antithrombotic therapy in resting angina pectoris or non-Q-wave myocardial infarction in preventing death and myocar-

dial infarction (a pilot study from the Antithrombotic Therapy in Acute Coronary Syndromes Study Group). *Am J Cardiol* 66:1287, 1990

52. Smith P, Arnesen H, Holme I: The effect of warfarin on mortality and reinfarction after myocardial infarction. *N Engl J Med* 323:147, 1990
53. The GUSTO Angiographic Investigators: The effects of tissue plasminogen activator, streptokinase, or both on coronary artery patency, ventricular function and survival after acute myocardial infarction. *N Engl J Med* 329:1615, 1993
54. Merlini PA, Cattaneo M, Spinola A, et al: Activation of the hemostatic system during thrombolytic therapy. *Am J Cardiol* 72:59G, 1993
55. Chesebro JH, Badimon JJ, Ortiz AF, et al: Conjunctive antithrombotic therapy for thrombolysis in myocardial infarction. *Am J Cardiol* 72:66G, 1993
56. Bar-Shavit R, Eldor A, Vlodavsky I: Binding of thrombin to subendothelial extracellular matrix: protection and expression of functional properties. *J Clin Invest* 84:1096, 1989
57. Weitz JI, Hudoba M, Massel D, et al: Clot-bound thrombin is protected from inhibition by heparin-antithrombin III but is susceptible to inactivation by antithrombin III-independent inhibitors. *J Clin Invest* 86:385, 1990
58. Beguin S, Lindhout T, Hemker HC: The effect of trace amounts of tissue factor on thrombin generation in platelet rich plasma, its inhibition by heparin. *Thromb Haemost* 61:25, 1989
59. Rydel TJ, Ravichandran KG, Tulinsky A, et al: The structure of a complex of recombinant hirudin and human alpha-thrombin. *Science* 249:277, 1990
60. Stone SR, Hofsteenge J: Kinetics of the inhibition of thrombin by hirudin. *Biochemistry* 25:4622, 1986
61. Lindhout T, Blezer R, Hemker HC: The anticoagulant mechanism of action of recombinant hirudin (CGP 39393) in plasma. *Thromb Haemost* 64:464, 1990
62. Glusa E: Hirudin and platelets. *Semin Thromb Hemost* 17:122, 1991
63. Maraganore JM, Bourdon P, Jablonski J, et al: Design and characterization of hirulogs: a novel class of bivalent peptide inhibitors of thrombin. *Biochemistry* 29:7095, 1990
64. Kelly AB, Marzec UM, Krupski W, et al: Hirudin interruption of heparin-resistant arterial thrombus formation in baboons. *Blood* 77:1006, 1991
65. Sarembock IJ, Gertz SD, Gimple LW, et al: Effectiveness of recombinant desulphatohirudin in reducing restenosis after balloon angioplasty of atherosclerotic femoral arteries in rabbits. *Circulation* 84:232, 1991
66. Heras M, Chesebro JH, Webster MW, et al: Hirudin, heparin, and placebo during deep arterial injury in the pig: the in vivo role of thrombin in platelet-mediated thrombosis. *Circulation* 82:1476, 1990
67. Buchwald AB, Sandrock D, Unterberg C, et al: Platelet and fibrin deposition on coronary stents in minipigs: effect of hirudin vs heparin. *J Am Coll Cardiol* 21:249, 1993
68. Klement P, Borm A, Hirsh J, et al: The effect of thrombin inhibitors on tissue plasminogen activator induced thrombolysis in a rat model. *Thromb Haemost* 68:64, 1992
69. Rigel DF, Olson RW, Lappe RW: Comparison of hirudin and heparin as adjuncts to streptokinase thrombolysis in a canine model of coronary thrombosis. *Circ Res* 72:1091, 1993
70. Cannon CP, McCabe CH, Henry TD, et al: A pilot trial of recombinant desulfatohirudin compared with heparin in conjunction with tissue-type plasminogen activator and aspirin for acute myocardial infarction: results of the Thrombolysis in Myocardial Infarction (TIMI) 5 trial. *J Am Coll Cardiol* 23:993, 1994
71. Scharfstein JS, George D, Burchenal JEB, et al: for the TIMI 5 Investigators: Hemostatic markers predict clinical events in patients treated with rt-PA and adjunctive antithrombotic therapy (abstr). *J Am Coll Cardiol* 23:56A, 1994
72. Lidon RM, Theroux P, Bonan R, et al: Hirulog as adjunctive therapy to streptokinase in acute myocardial infarction (abstr). *J Am Coll Cardiol* 21:419, 1993
73. Lee VL, McCabe CH, Antman EM, et al: for the TIMI 6 Investigators: Initial experience with hirudin and streptokinase in acute myocardial infarction: results of the TMI 6 trial (abstr). *J Am Coll Cardiol* 23:344A, 1994
74. Hauptmann J, Markwardt F: Pharmacologic aspects of the development of selective synthetic thrombotic inhibitors as anticoagulants. *Semin Thromb Hemost* 18:200, 1992
75. Brandstetter H, Turk D, Hoeffken HW, et al: Refined 2.3 Å x-ray crystal structure of bovine thrombin inhibitors formed with the benzamidine and arginine-based thrombin inhibitors NAPAP, 4-TAPAP and MQPA: a starting point for improving antithrombotics. *J Mol Biol* 226:1085, 1992
76. Kettner C, Shaw E: D-Phe-Pro-ArgCH_2Cl. A selective affinity label for thrombin. *Thromb Res* 14:969, 1979

77. Schneider J: Heparin and the thrombin inhibitor argatroban enhance fibrinolysis by infused or bolus-injected saruplase (r-scu-PA) in rabbit femoral artery thrombosis. *Thromb Res* 64:677, 1991

78. Gold HK, Torres FW, Garabedian HD, et al: Evidence for a rebound coagulation phenomenon after cessation of a 4 hour infusion of a specific thrombin inhibitor in patients with unstable angina pectoris. *J Am Coll Cardiol* 21:1039, 1993

79. Waxman L, Smith DE, Arcuri KE, et al: Tick anticoagulant peptide (TAP) is a novel inhibitor of blood coagulation factor Xa. *Science* 248:593, 1990

80. Tuszynski GP, Gasic TB, Gasic GJ: Isolation and characterization of antistatin: an inhibitor of metastasis and coagulation. *J Biol Chem* 262:9718,1987

81. Schaffer LW, Davidson JT, Vlasuk GP, et al: Antithrombotic efficacy of recombinant tick anticoagulant peptide: a potent inhibitor of coagulation factor Xa in a primate model of arterial thrombosis. *Circulation* 84:1741, 1991

82. Mellott MJ, Holahan MA, Lynch JJ, et al: Acceleration of recombinant tissue-type plasminogen activator-induced reperfusion and prevention of reocclusion by recombinant antistatin, a selective factor Xa inhibitor, in a canine model of femoral arterial thrombosis. *Circ Res* 70:1152, 1992

83. Sitko GR, Ramjit DR, Stabilito II, et al: Conjunctive enhancement of enzymatic thrombolysis and prevention of thrombotic reocclusion with the selective factor Xa inhibitor, tick anticoagulant peptide: comparison to hirudin and heparin in a canine model of acute coronary artery thrombosis. *Circulation* 85:805, 1992

84. Bock LC, Griffin LC, Latham JA, et al: Selection of single-stranded DNA molecules that bind and inhibit human thrombin. *Nature* 355:564, 1992

85. Wu Q, Tsiang M, Sadler JE: Localization of the single-stranded DNA binding site in the thrombin anion-binding exosite. *J Biol Chem* 267:24408, 1992

86. Paborsky LR, McCurdy SN, Griffin LC, et al: The single-stranded DNA aptamer-binding site of human thrombin. *J Biol Chem* 268:20808, 1993

87. Li WX, Kaplan AV, Grant GW, et al: A novel nucleotide-based thrombin inhibitor inhibits clot-bound thrombin and reduces arterial platelet thrombus formation. *Blood* 83:677, 1994

88. Griffin LC, Tidmarsh GF, Bock LC, et al: In vivo anticoagulant properties of a novel nucleotide-based thrombin inhibitor and demonstration of regional anticoagulation in extracorporeal circuits. *Blood* 81:3271, 1993

89. Gruber A, Griffin JH, Harker LA, et al: Inhibition of platelet-dependent thrombus formation by human activated protein C in a primate model. *Blood* 73:639, 1989

90. Gruber A, Hanson SR, Kelly AB, et al: Inhibition of thrombus formation by activated recombinant protein C in a primate model of arterial thrombosis. *Circulation* 82:578, 1990

91. Okajima K, Koga S, Kaji M, et al: Effect of protein C and activated protein C on coagulation and fibrinolysis in normal human subjects. *Thromb Haemost* 63:48, 1990

92. Broze GJ Jr, Miletich JP: Isolation of the tissue factor inhibitor produced by HepB2 hepatoma cells. *Proc Natl Acad Sci USA* 84:1886, 1987

93. Haskel EJ, Torr SR, Day KC, et al: Prevention of arterial reocclusion after thrombolysis with recombinant lipoprotein-associated coagulation inhibitor. *Circulation* 84:821, 1991

94. Levi M, ten Cate H, Bauer KA, et al: Inhibition of endotoxin-induced activation of coagulation and fibrinolysis by pentoxifylline or by a monoclonal anti-tissue actor antibody in chimpanzees. *J Clin Invest* 93:114, 1994

Acknowledgments

Figures 1 through 4 Talar Agasyan.

CHAPTER 9

Thrombolytic Agents

Désiré Collen, M.D., Ph.D., H. Roger Lijnen, Ph.D.

Acute myocardial infarction, stroke, and venous thromboembolism have, as their immediate underlying cause, thrombosis of critically situated blood vessels with loss of blood flow to vital organs. One approach to their treatment consists of the pharmacological dissolution of the blood clot via the intravenous infusion of plasminogen activators, which activate the blood fibrinolytic system. This system contains a proenzyme, plasminogen, that is converted to the active enzyme plasmin by the action of plasminogen activators. Plasmin, in turn, digests fibrin to soluble degradation products.

Inhibition of the fibrinolytic system occurs both at the level of the plasminogen activators, by plasminogen activator inhibitors (PAI-1 and PAI-2), and at the level of plasmin, mainly by α_2-antiplasmin. Currently, five thrombolytic agents are available for clinical use: streptokinase, anisoylated plasminogen–streptokinase activator complex (APSAC), two-chain urokinase-type plasminogen activator (tcu-PA), recombinant single-chain urokinase-type PA (rscu-PA, prourokinase), and recombinant tissue-type plasminogen activator (rt-PA). Streptokinase, APSAC, and two-chain urokinase induce extensive systemic activation of the fibrinolytic system, and α_2-antiplasmin serves to inhibit any circulating plasmin. During plasminogen activator therapy, however, α_2-antiplasmin may become exhausted, and as a result, plasmin that is present in the circulation may degrade several plasma proteins. In contrast, the physiologic plasminogen activators, tissue-type plasminogen activator (t-PA) and single-chain urokinase-type plasminogen activator (scu-PA), activate plasminogen preferentially at the fibrin surface. In therapy with these two agents, plasmin, associated with the fibrin surface, is protected from rapid inhibition by α_2-antiplasmin and thus may ef ficiently degrade the fibrin of a thrombus[1] [*see Figure 1*]. Staphylokinase, a protein obtained from *Staphylococcus aureus*, resembles the physiologic plasminogen activators in that it also induces fibrin-specific clot lysis in human plasma in vitro.[2] The mechanism of the fibrin specificity of these three agents is, however, different.

The recognition that early administration of thrombolytic agents in patients with acute myocardial infarction results in recanalization of occluded coronary arteries has provided the basis for large-scale clinical application of thrombolysis in this disease. In clinical trials, reduction of infarct size, preservation of ventricular function, and reduction in mortality have been demonstrated with streptokinase, rt-PA, and APSAC. rt-PA, in combination with intravenous heparin, was found to produce more rapid and more frequent recanalization than that achieved by streptokinase. The international t-PA/streptokinase mortality trial (GISSI-2) and the ISIS-3 study, which used concomitant subcutaneous heparin administration, however, have challenged the hypothesis that early and sustained coronary artery recanalization is the main determinant of clinical outcome.[1] The GUSTO trial, in contrast, has clearly shown a correlation between early patency (which is obtained earlier with an accelerated rt-PA regimen in combination with intravenous heparin than with streptokinase) and reduced mortality.[3]

Nevertheless, all available thrombolytic agents still suffer significant shortcomings, including large therapeutic doses, short plasma half-lives, limited fibrin specificity, reocclusion, and bleeding complications.[1] In this chapter, we review some recent developments toward improved efficacy and fibrin specificity for the thrombolytic agents.

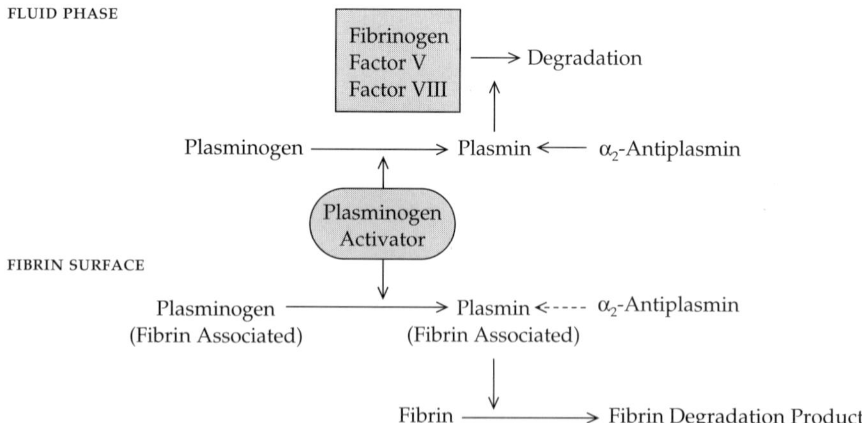

Figure 1 *Schematic representation of the fibrinolytic system. Non–fibrin-specific plasminogen activators (streptokinase, anisoylated plasminogen–streptokinase activator complex, and two-chain urokinase-type plasminogen activator) induce extensive systemic plasminogen activation (fluid phase), and after saturation of α_2-antiplasmin excess plasmin may degrade several plasma proteins including fibrinogen, factor V and factor VIII. Fibrin-specific plasminogen activators (t-PA, scu-PA, staphylokinase) preferentially activate plasminogen at the fibrin surface. Plasmin, associated with the fibrin surface, is protected from rapid inhibition by α_2-antiplasmin and may thus efficiently degrade fibrin.*

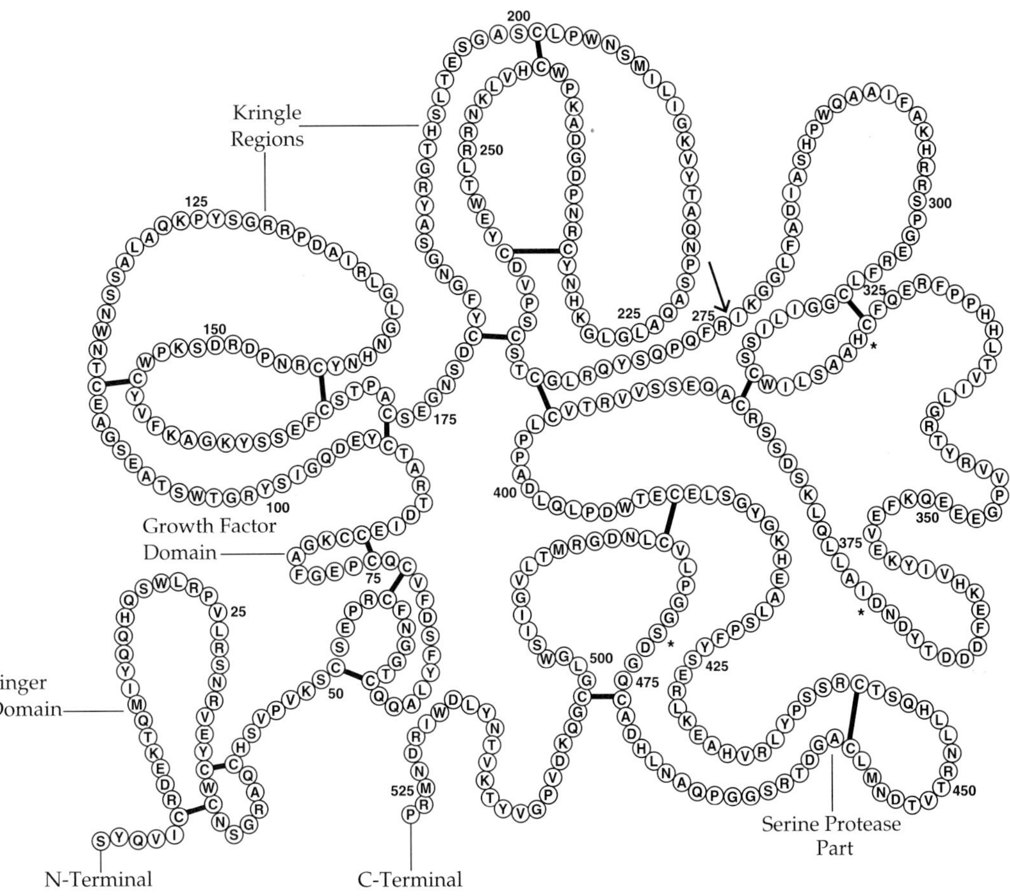

Figure 2 The primary structure of tissue-type plasminogen activator. The amino acids are represented by their single letter symbols and black bars indicate disulfide bonds. The arrow indicates the cleavage site for plasmin. The active site residues are indicated with an asterisk.

Structural-Functional Correlations in the Physiologic Plasminogen Activators t-PA and u-PA

Tissue-type plasminogen activator is a 70-kilodalton serine proteinase, originally isolated as a single polypeptide chain of 527 amino acids [*see Figure 2*].[4] It was subsequently shown that native t-PA contains an N-terminal extension of three amino acids (Gly-Ala-Arg).[5] t-PA is converted by plasmin to a two-chain form by hydrolysis of the Arg^{275}-Ile^{276} peptide bond. The N-terminal region is composed of several domains with homologies to other proteins: a finger domain comprising residues 4–50, a growth factor domain comprising residues 50–87, and two kringles comprising residues 87–176 and 176–262. The region comprising residues 276–527 constitutes the serine proteinase part with the catalytic site, which is composed of His^{322}, Asp^{371}, and Ser^{478}.[4] These distinct domains in t-PA are involved in several functions of the enzyme, including its binding to fibrin, fibrin-specific plasminogen activation, rapid clearance in vivo, and binding to endothelial cell receptors. Binding of t-PA to fibrin is mediated by the finger and second kringle domains. It has been proposed that mainly the second kringle of t-PA is responsible for the stimulatory effect of fibrin on plasminogen activation, although other studies have claimed that both kringles are equivalent in their ability to mediate the stimulation of the catalytic efficiency of t-PA by fibrin.[6]

scu-PA comprises 411 amino acids in a single polypeptide chain and contains the serine proteinase site with the active triad His, Asp, and Ser at positions 204, 255, and 356, respectively[7] [*see Figure 3*]. The molecule contains an N-terminal growth factor domain and a triple-disulfide-bonded kringle structure homologous to the five kringles in plasminogen and the two kringles in t-PA. Conversion of scu-PA to a two-chain form (tcu-PA) occurs after proteolytic cleavage at position Lys^{158}-Ile^{159}. Proteases that cleave the Lys^{158}-Ile^{159} peptide bond in scu-PA include plasmin,[8] kallikrein,[9] trypsin,[9] cathepsin B,[10] human T cell–associated serine proteinase-1,[11] and thermolysin.[12] A fully active tcu-PA derivative is obtained after additional proteolysis by plasmin at position Lys^{135}-Lys^{136}.[13] In addition, a low-molecular-weight form of scu-PA (scu-PA-32k)[14] can be obtained by selective cleavage at position Glu^{143}-Leu^{144}; this cleavage can be obtained with the matrix metalloproteinase Pump-1.[15] In contrast, scu-PA is converted to an inactive two-chain molecule by thrombin[9] after proteolytic cleavage at position Arg^{156}-Phe^{157}. Inactivation of scu-PA by thrombin is strongly enhanced in

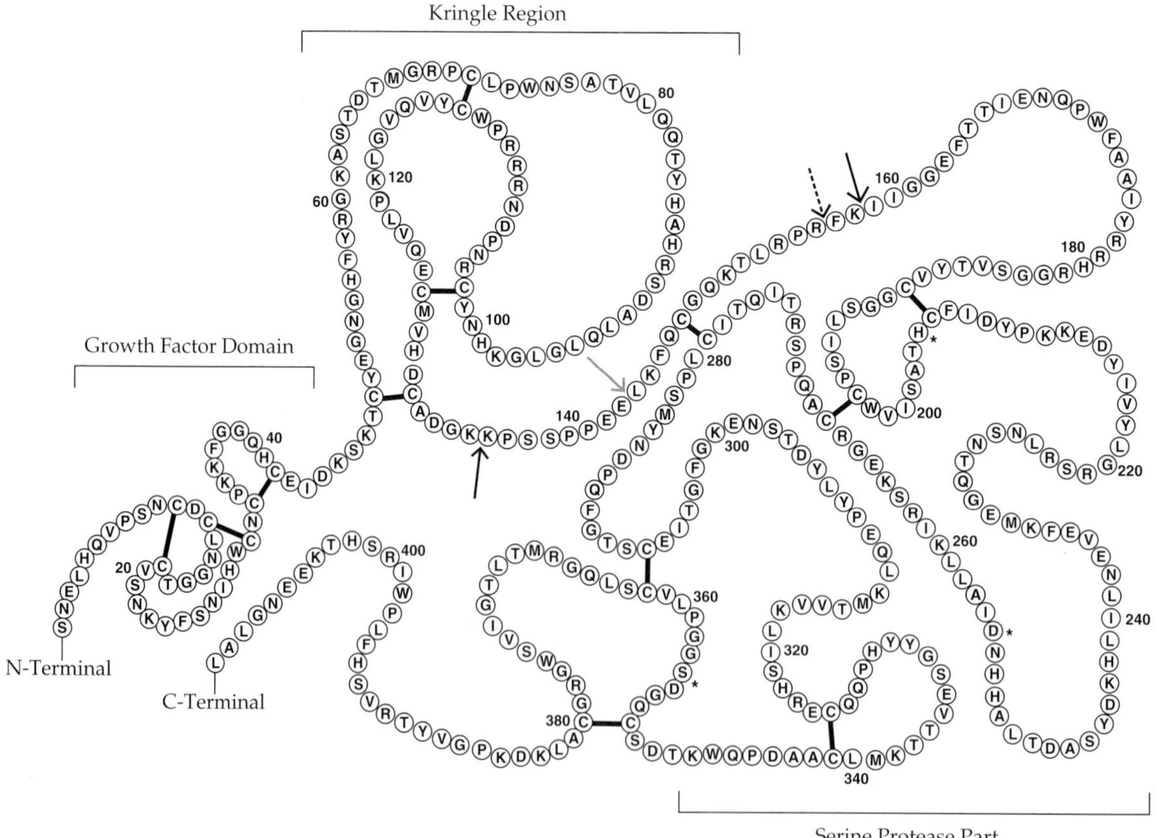

Figure 3 *The primary structure of single-chain urokinase-type plasminogen activator. The amino acids are represented by their single letter symbols, and black bars indicate disulfide bonds. The arrows indicate the cleavage sites for plasmin (solid black), thrombin (dashed black), and Pump-1 (gray). The active site residues are indicated with an asterisk.*

the presence of thrombomodulin,[16] and this effect is dependent on the O-linked glycosaminoglycan of thrombomodulin.[17] This cofactor effect of thrombomodulin on the inactivation of scu-PA by thrombin has been confirmed in a perfused rabbit heart model.[18]

rscu-PA: Mutants and Alternative Administration Schemes

Some approaches to improve the thrombolytic profile of rscu-PA have been attempted. Mutants or variants with improved thrombolytic potency, however, have not yet been reported.

Because clot lysis with scu-PA in plasma is associated with a higher degree of fibrin specificity than clot lysis with tcu-PA, several investigators have constructed mutants of scu-PA in which the plasmin cleavage site was destroyed by site-specific mutagenesis.[6] Such plasmin-resistant mutants of scu-PA (i.e., rscu-PA K158A, rscu-PA K158G), however, have a thrombolytic potency in rabbits with jugular vein thrombosis that is about fivefold lower than that of scu-PA.[19] The thrombolytic potency of such mutants thus appears to be too low to allow their efficient use in humans.

Deletion of the amino acid sequence Arg^{179}–Ser^{184} in u-PA (which is homologous to the PAI-1 binding site of t-PA) has resulted in a urokinase mutant that is resistant to inhibition by PAI-1.[20] No data have been reported on the in vivo fibrinolytic or pharmacokinetic properties of this molecule. In a rabbit model of jugular vein thrombosis, comparable clot lysis was obtained with scu-PA-32k as with tcu-PA (molecular mass, 33 kilodaltons), and was associated with less pronounced systemic breakdown of fibrinogen.[21] scu-PA-32k may thus represent a useful alternative for large-scale production of a single-chain u-PA species by recombinant DNA technology.

Preliminary small clinical trials in patients with acute myocardial infarction have suggested a synergistic interaction between low-dose tcu-PA and scu-PA.[22-24] A multicenter dose-finding trial with scu-PA that was preactivated by administration of urokinase in patients with acute myocardial infarction, however, did not find significant advantages of the combination therapy.[25] Alternatively, some studies have suggested that combination therapy with rscu-PA and rt-PA may allow a substantial reduction in the total dose of thrombolytic agent, while still achieving effective and fibrin-specific coronary artery thrombolysis.[26-28]

Mutants and Variants of t-PA

rt-PA mutants have been constructed with altered pharmacokinetic properties or with altered functional properties, including binding to fibrin and stimulation by fibrin, and resistance to plasma protease inhibitors.[6] rt-PA mutants with deletion of the finger (F), epidermal growth factor (E), and/or kringle 1 (K_1) domains were shown to have a significantly reduced plasma clearance in several animal models. This reduced plasma clearance, however, is frequently associated with a reduced specific thrombolytic activity, resulting in an unchanged or only marginally improved thrombolytic potency.[6]

The pharmacokinetic and thrombolytic properties in animal models of one such mutant, consisting of the kringle 2 (K_2) and protease (P) domains of t-PA (K_2P, BM 06.022, LY 210825), suggested that this molecule, because of its prolonged plasma half-life, may be used for coronary artery thrombolysis by bolus administration.[29-31] In patients with acute myocardial infarction, BM 06.022 was found to be a relatively fibrin-selective compound that did not cause major bleeding complications.[32] Prolonged half-lives have also been obtained by substitution or deletion of one or a few selected amino acids in the finger or growth factor domains.[6] Such mutants may have a specific thrombolytic activity that is better preserved than in domain-deletion mutants. One such t-PA molecule in which Cys^{84} in the growth factor domain is replaced by Ser (half-life in humans of more than 20 minutes, as compared to six minutes for native t-PA) has been used successfully for bolus administration at less than half the dose of native t-PA in a multicenter trial in patients with acute myocardial infarction.[33]

An rt-PA mutant in which Thr^{103} is replaced by Asn and the sequence Lys^{296}-His-Arg-Arg is mutagenized to Ala-Ala-Ala-Ala was found to have both a prolonged half-life and resistance to PAI-1. This mutant was shown to have an increased potency on platelet-rich plasma clots (rich in PAI-1) in animal models.[34] Thus, it appears to be possible to engineer several properties into human t-PA to produce a molecule with an enhanced therapeutic potential.

The t-PA of saliva from the vampire bat *Desmodus rotundus* (bat-PA) was found to constitute a potent and fibrin-specific thrombolytic agent in rabbits and dogs with femoral arterial thrombosis.[35,36] From a family of four *Desmodus* plasminogen activators encoded by four distinct genes, one of the two larger forms (rDSPAα1) was shown to be an efficient and fibrin-specific thrombolytic agent in rats with experimental pulmonary embolism.[37] It remains to be shown in direct comparative studies whether any of these rt-PA mutants or variants offers advantages over wild-type rt-PA for the treatment of thromboembolic disease.

Recombinant Chimeric Plasminogen Activators

Recombinant chimeric plasminogen activators have been constructed primarily with different regions of t-PA and scu-PA, although several alternative combinations have been evaluated.[6] In vivo evaluation in animal models of thrombosis indicated that one of these variants ($K_1K_2P_u$) had a markedly enhanced thrombolytic potency toward venous and arterial thrombi.[38] $K_1K_2P_u$ consists of kringles 1 and 2 of rt-PA (amino acids Ser^1–Gln^3 and Asp^{87}–Phe^{274}) and of the serine proteinase part of rscu-PA (amino acids Ser^{138}–Leu^{411}).[39] The delayed plasma clearance of $K_1K_2P_u$ with relatively preserved specific thrombolytic activity suggested that a significant reduction of the total amount of material required for thrombolytic therapy and its administration by bolus injection may be possible in patients with thromboembolic disease.

A small feasibility study of coronary thrombolysis with $K_1K_2P_u$ has been performed recently in patients with acute myocardial infarction.[40] An intravenous bolus injection of 10 mg was given over five minutes in two patients, and in four patients a second 10-mg bolus was given 15 minutes after the first one. At 30 minutes, all patients were also given 320 mg of aspirin, and a continuous intravenous infusion of heparin (1,000 U/hr) was started. Clot lysis within 30 minutes was not achieved after intravenous injection of a single bolus of 10 mg of $K_1K_2P_u$ in two patients but was obtained in two of the four patients given two 10-mg boluses of $K_1K_2P_u$. Administration of $K_1K_2P_u$ did not induce an overt systemic lytic state in any of the patients, as shown by virtually unchanged levels of fibrinogen and α_2-antiplasmin. In the patients given a single bolus injection, $K_1K_2P_u$-related antigen increased to 2 to 3 μg/ml and disappeared from plasma with an initial half-life of about nine minutes and a terminal half-life of 70 minutes, corresponding to a plasma clearance of approximately 50 ml/min.

Another recombinant plasminogen activator that has recently shown some promise in animal models of thrombosis consists of only the second kringle domain of t-PA linked to the protease domain of scu-PA (K_2tu-PA). In a rabbit model of jugular vein thrombosis, on continuous infusion K_2tu-PA was found to be more potent than both t-PA and scu-PA, without causing more pronounced systemic effects.[41] Upon bolus injection, K_2tu-PA and rt-PA produced comparable degrees of clot lysis, whereas K_2tu-PA was more efficient in inhibiting accretion of new fibrin on the thrombi but did increase the bleeding risk at high doses.[42] Therefore, it remains to be shown whether the prolonged half-life of this molecule, as compared to rt-PA, offers any advantage.

Staphylokinase

Recombinant staphylokinase (STAR), in contrast to streptokinase, induces fibrin-specific clot lysis in human plasma.[2,43] Like streptokinase, STAR forms a stoichiometric complex with plasmin(ogen) that activates other plasminogen molecules.[43,44] Streptokinase and plasminogen produce a complex that exposes the active site in the plasminogen molecule without proteolytic cleavage, whereas generation of plasmin is required for exposure of the active site in the complex with STAR.[45] The fibrin specificity of STAR in human plasma has been explained by rapid inhibition of generated plasmin-STAR complex by α_2-antiplasmin[2,43] and by a greater than 100-fold reduced inhibition rate at the fibrin surface, which may allow preferential plasminogen activation at the fibrin clot.[46] STAR, however, also dissociates in active form from the plasmin-STAR complex following neutralization by α_2-antiplasmin and is recycled.[47] The lack of systemic plasminogen activation by STAR in plasma in the absence of fibrin has been explained by the finding that α_2-antiplasmin prevents generation of active plasmin-STAR complex and thus inhibits plasminogen activation.[48] Fibrin stimulates plasminogen activation by STAR via mechanisms involving the lysine-binding sites of plasminogen, probably by facilitating the generation of plasmin-STAR complex as well as by delaying its inhibition at the clot surface.[48]

STAR has a potency for venous clot lysis in hamsters and rabbits comparable to that of streptokinase.[49] Additional studies in hamsters and dogs have suggested that STAR may be relatively more potent than streptokinase toward platelet-rich clots and potentially less immunogenic.[50] These findings were subsequently confirmed in baboons, in which STAR was shown to have a thrombolytic potency toward jugular vein blood clots comparable to that of streptokinase but to be less immunogenic and less allergenic.[51] Indeed, repeated administration of STAR, in contrast to streptokinase, did not induce resistance to clot lysis in this model. Furthermore, STAR was significantly more efficient than streptokinase for the dissolution of platelet-rich arterial eversion graft thrombi.[51]

These encouraging results have led to the evaluation, on a pilot scale, of the pharmacokinetic, thrombolytic, and immunogenic properties of STAR in patients with acute myocardial infarction.[52] In four of five patients with acute myocardial infarction, 10 mg of STAR given intravenously over 30 minutes was found to induce angiographically documented coronary artery recanalization within 40 minutes. Plasma fibrinogen and α_2-antiplasmin levels were unaffected, and allergic reactions were not observed. However, in these patients, neutralizing antibodies were consistently demonstrable in plasma at 14 to 35 days.[52] Thus, with respect to immunogenicity, the initial observations in humans are not as encouraging as the experience in baboons.

Conclusions

Despite their widespread use in patients with acute myocardial infarction, all currently available thrombolytic agents have a number of significant limitations on their use, including resistance to reperfusion, the occurrence of acute coronary reocclusion, and bleeding complications. Therefore, the quest for thrombolytic agents with a higher thrombolytic potency, specific thrombolytic activity, and/or better fibrin selectivity continues. Several lines of research toward improvement of thrombolytic agents are being explored, including the construction of mutants and variants of plasminogen activators, chimeric plasminogen activators, and plasminogen activators of animal or bacterial origin. Some of these new thrombolytic agents have been evaluated recently in animal models of venous or arterial thrombosis. Pilot studies in patients with acute myocardial infarction have been performed with a few selected agents. Assessment of their relative therapeutic benefit, or lack thereof, will require more detailed dose-finding studies, followed by randomized clinical trials against currently available thrombolytic agents.

References

1. Collen D, Lijnen HR: Basic and clinical aspects of fibrinolysis and thrombolysis. *Blood* 78:3114, 1991
2. Matsuo O, Okada K, Fukao H, et al: Thrombolytic properties of staphylokinase. *Blood* 76:925, 1990
3. The GUSTO Investigators: An international randomized trial comparing four thrombolytic strategies for acute myocardial infarction. *N Engl J Med* 329:673, 1993
4. Pennica D, Holmes WE, Kohr WJ, et al: Cloning and expression of human tissue-type plasminogen activator cDNA in *E. coli*. *Nature* 301:214, 1983
5. Jörnvall H, Pohl G, Bergsdorf N, et al: Differential proteolysis and evidence for a residue exchange in tissue plasminogen activator suggest possible association between two types of protein microheterogeneity. *FEBS Lett* 156:47, 1983
6. Lijnen HR, Collen D: Strategies for the improvement of thrombolytic agents. *Thromb Haemost* 66:88, 1991

7. Holmes WE, Pennica D, Blaber M, et al: Cloning and expression of the gene for pro-urokinase in *Escherichia coli. Biotechnology* 3:923, 1985

8. Günzler WA, Steffens GJ, Ötting F, et al: The primary structure of high molecular mass urokinase from human urine: the complete amino acid sequence of the A chain. *Hoppe Seylers Z Physiol Chem* 363:1155, 1982

9. Ichinose A, Fujikawa K, Suyama T: The activation of pro-urokinase by plasma kallikrein and its inactivation by thrombin. *J Biol Chem* 261:3486, 1986

10. Kobayashi H, Schmitt M, Goretzki L, et al: Cathepsin B efficiently activates the soluble and the tumor cell receptor-bound form of the proenzyme urokinase-type plasminogen activator (Pro-uPA). *J Biol Chem* 266:5147, 1991

11. Brunner G, Vettel U, Jobstmann S, et al: A T-cell-related proteinase expressed by T-lymphoma cells activates their endogenous pro-urokinase. *Blood* 79:2099, 1992

12. Marcotte PA, Henkin J: Characterization of the activation of pro-urokinase by thermolysin. *Biochim Biophys Acta* 1160:105, 1993

13. Günzler WA, Steffens GJ, Ötting F, et al: Structural relationship between human high and low molecular mass urokinase. *Hoppe Seylers Z Physiol Chem* 363:133, 1982

14. Stump DC, Lijnen HR, Collen D: Purification and characterization of a novel low molecular weight form of single-chain urokinase-type plasminogen activator. *J Biol Chem* 261:17120, 1986

15. Marcotte PA, Kozan IM, Dorwin SA, et al: The matrix metalloproteinase Pump-1 catalyzes formation of low molecular weight (pro)urokinase in cultures of normal human kidney cells. *J Biol Chem* 267:13803, 1992

16. de Munk GA, Groeneveld E, Rijken DC: Acceleration of the thrombin inactivation of single chain urokinase-type plasminogen activator (pro-urokinase) by thrombomodulin. *J Clin Invest* 88:1680, 1991

17. de Munk GA, Parkinson JF, Groeneveld E, et al: Role of the glycosaminoglycan component of thrombomodulin in its acceleration of the inactivation of single-chain urokinase-type plasminogen activator by thrombin. *Biochem J* 290:655, 1993

18. Molinari A, Giorgetti C, Lansen J: Thrombomodulin is a cofactor for thrombin degradation of recombinant single-chain urokinase plasminogen activator "in vitro" and in a perfused rabbit heart model. *Thromb Haemost* 67:226, 1992

19. Collen D, Mao J, Stassen JM, et al: Thrombolytic properties of Lys-158 mutants of recombinant single chain urokinase-type plasminogen activator (scu-PA) in rabbits with jugular vein thrombosis. *J Vasc Med Biol* 1:46, 1989

20. Adams DS, Griffin LA, Nachajko WR, et al: A synthetic DNA encoding a modified human urokinase resistant to inhibition by serum plasminogen activator inhibitor. *J Biol Chem* 266:8476, 1991

21. Lijnen HR, Nelles L, Holmes WE, et al: Biochemical and thrombolytic properties of a low molecular weight form (comprising Leu^{144} through Leu^{411}) of recombinant single-chain urokinase-type plasminogen activator. *J Biol Chem* 263:5594, 1988

22. Gulba DCL, Fischer K, Barthels M, et al: Low dose urokinase preactivated natural prourokinase for thrombolysis in acute myocardial infarction. *Am J Cardiol* 63: 1025, 1989

23. Bode C, Schoenermark S, Schuler G, et al: Efficacy of intravenous prourokinase and a combination of prourokinase and urokinase in acute myocardial infarction. *Am J Cardiol* 61:971, 1988

24. Kasper W, Hohnloser SH, Engler H, et al: Coronary reperfusion studies with pro-urokinase in acute myocardial infarction: evidence for synergism of low dose urokinase. *J Am Coll Cardiol* 16:733, 1990.

25. Gulba DC, Bode C, Sen S, et al: Multicenter dose-finding trial for thrombolysis with urokinase preactivated pro-urokinase (TCL 598) in acute myocardial infarction. *Cathet Cardiovasc Diagn* 26:177, 1992

26. Collen D, Van de Werf F: Coronary arterial thrombolysis with low-dose synergistic combinations of recombinant tissue-type plasminogen activator (rt-PA) and recombinant single-chain urokinase-type plasminogen activator (scu-PA) for acute myocardial infarction. *Am J Cardiol* 60:431, 1987

27. Bode C, Schuler G, Nordt T, et al: Intravenous thrombolytic therapy with a combination of single-chain urokinase-type plasminogen activator and recombinant tissue-type plasminogen activator in acute myocardial infarction. *Circulation* 81:907, 1990

28. Kirshenbaum JM, Bahr RD, Flaherty JT, et al: Clot-selective coronary thrombolysis with low-dose synergistic combinations of single-chain urokinase-type plasminogen activator and recombinant tissue-type plasminogen activator. *Am J Cardiol* 68:1564, 1991

29. Jackson CV, Frank JD, Craft TJ, et al: Comparison of the thrombolytic activity of the novel plasminogen activator, LY210825, to anisoylated plasminogen-streptokinase acti-

vator complex in a canine model of coronary artery thrombolysis. *J Pharmacol Exp Ther* 260:64, 1992

30. Martin U, Köhler J, Sponer G, et al: Pharmacokinetics of the novel recombinant plasminogen activator BM 06.022 in rats, dogs, and non-human primates. *Fibrinolysis* 6:39, 1992
31. Nicolini FA, Nichols WW, Mehta JL, et al: Sustained reflow in dogs with coronary thrombosis with K2P, a novel mutant of tissue-plasminogen activator. *J Am Coll Cardiol* 20:228, 1992
32. Müller W, Haerer D, Ellbrück U, et al: Pharmacokinetics and effects on the hemostatic system of bolus application of a novel recombinant plasminogen activator in AMI patients (abstract 63). *Fibrinolysis* 6(suppl 2):26, 1992
33. Kawai C, Hosoda S, Motomiya T, et al: Multicenter trial of a novel modified t-PA, E6010, by i.v. bolus injection in patients with acute myocardial infarction (AMI) (abstract 1630). *Circulation* 86(suppl):I-409, 1992
34. Refino CJ, Paoni NF, Keyt BA, et al: A variant of t-PA (T103N, KHRR-296-299 AAAA) that, by bolus, has increased potency and decreased systemic activation of plasminogen. *Thromb Haemost* 70:313, 1993
35. Gardell SJ, Ramjit DR, Stabilito II, et al: Effective thrombolysis without marked plasminemia after bolus intravenous administration of vampire bat salivary plasminogen activator in rabbits. *Circulation* 84:244, 1991
36. Mellott MJ, Stabilito II, Holahan MA, et al: Vampire bat salivary plasminogen activator promotes rapid and sustained reperfusion without concomitant systemic plasminogen activation in a canine model of arterial thrombolysis. *Arteriosclerosis Thromb* 12:212, 1992
37. Witt W, Baldus B, Bringmann P, et al: Thrombolytic properties of *Desmodus rotundus* (vampire bat) salivary plasminogen activator in experimental pulmonary embolism in rats. *Blood* 79:1213, 1992
38. Collen D, Lu HR, Lijnen HR, et al: Thrombolytic and pharmacokinetic properties of chimeric tissue-type and urokinase-type plasminogen activators. *Circulation* 84:1216, 1991
39. Nelles L, Lijnen HR, Van Nuffelen A, et al: Characterization of domain deletion and/or duplication mutants of a recombinant chimera of tissue-type plasminogen activator and urokinase-type plasminogen activator (t-PA/u-PA). *Thromb Haemost* 64:53, 1990
40. Van de Werf F, Lijnen HR, Collen D: Coronary thrombolysis with $K_1K_2P_u$, a chimeric tissue-type and urokinase-type plasminogen activator: a feasibility study in six patients with acute myocardial infarction. *Coronary Artery Dis* 4:929, 1993
41. Agnelli G, Pascucci C, Colucci M, et al: Thrombolytic activity of two chimeric recombinant plasminogen activators (FK2tu-PA and K2tu-PA) in rabbits. *Thromb Haemost* 68:331, 1992
42. Agnelli G, Pascucci C, Nenci GG, et al: Thrombolytic and haemorrhagic effects of bolus doses of tissue-type plasminogen activator and a hybrid plasminogen activator with prolonged half-life (K2tuPA: CGP 42935). *Thromb Haemost* 70:294, 1993
43. Lijnen HR, Van Hoef B, De Cock F, et al: On the mechanism of fibrin-specific plasminogen activation by staphylokinase. *J Biol Chem* 266:11826, 1991
44. Kowalska-Loth B, Zakrzewski K: The activation by staphylokinase of human plasminogen. *Acta Biochim Pol* 22:327, 1975
45. Collen D, Schlott B, Engelborghs Y, et al: On the mechanism of the activation of human plasminogen by recombinant staphylokinase. *J Biol Chem* 268:8284, 1993
46. Lijnen HR, Van Hoef B, Matsuo O, et al: On the molecular interactions between plasminogen-staphylokinase, α_2-antiplasmin and fibrin. *Biochim Biophys Acta* 1118:144, 1992
47. Silence K, Collen D, Lijnen HR: Interaction between staphylokinase, plasmin(ogen) and α_2-antiplasmin: recycling of staphylokinase after neutralization of the plasmin-staphylokinase complex by α_2-antiplasmin. *J Biol Chem* 268:9811, 1993
48. Silence K, Collen D, Lijnen HR: Regulation by α_2-antiplasmin and fibrin of the activation of plasminogen with recombinant staphylokinase in plasma. *Blood* 82:1175, 1993
49. Lijnen HR, Stassen JM, Vanlinthout I, et al: Comparative fibrinolytic properties of staphylokinase and streptokinase in animal models of venous thrombosis. *Thromb Haemost* 66:468, 1991
50. Collen D, De Cock F, Vanlinthout I, et al: Comparative thrombolytic and immunogenic properties of staphylokinase and streptokinase. *Fibrinolysis* 6:232, 1992
51. Collen D, De Cock F, Stassen JM: Comparative immunogenicity and thrombolytic properties toward arterial and venous thrombi of streptokinase and recombinant staphylokinase in baboons. *Circulation* 87:996, 1993
52. Collen D, Van de Werf F: Coronary thrombolysis with recombinant staphylokinase in patients with evolving myocardial infarction. *Circulation* 87:1850, 1993

Acknowledgments

Figure 1 Talar Agasyan.

Figure 2 Laura Brown. Adapted from "Cloning and Expression of Tissue-Type Plasminogen Activator DNA in *E. coli*," by D. Pennica, W.E. Holmes, W.J. Kohr, et al, in *Nature* 301:214, 1983.

Figure 3 Laura Brown. Adapted from "Cloning and Expression of the Gene for Pro-urokinase in *Escherichia coli*," by W.E. Holmes, D. Pennica, M. Blaber, et al, in *Biotechnology* 3:923, 1985

CHAPTER 10

Antibody Targeting: A Strategy for Improving Thrombolytic Therapy

Edgar Haber, M.D.

In most patients with myocardial infarction, coronary artery occlusion is caused by a thrombus forming on a fissured atherosclerotic plaque. Early reperfusion induced with thrombolytic agents can limit infarct size and reduce left ventricular dysfunction and congestive heart failure, thereby diminishing early and late mortality [*see Chapter 9*]. The most significant limitations of thrombolytic therapy at present include the failure of plasminogen activators to lyse all thrombi (15 to 40 percent of patients do not experience early reperfusion), the delay in restoration of blood flow by more than 45 minutes from the start of thrombolytic therapy, and high rates (five to 25 percent) of early reocclusion after thrombolysis.[1] In addition, intracerebral hemorrhage occurs in 0.3 to 0.7 percent of patients treated. If these limitations can be overcome, thrombolytic therapy certainly will have a more potent effect on reducing the morbidity and mortality from myocardial infarction and, possibly, limiting rates of cerebral infarction and pulmonary embolism.

In the planning of studies aimed at the discovery and development of new thrombolytic agents, properties to be sought in these agents include increased potency and speed of thrombolysis combined with the ability to prevent rethrombosis but not increase rates of hemorrhagic complications. Research in this field has been very active. So far, none of these efforts have produced an agent generally accepted to be superior to those already approved for clinical use. In this chapter, I describe novel approaches for developing agents that dissolve clots or prevent clot formation that are based on the use of antibodies to target the agents to specific components of the thrombus.

Antibody targeting for the treatment or prevention of thrombi entails the engineering of a bifunctional molecule that contains both a highly specific antigen-binding site, which concentrates the molecule at the desired target (the thrombus), and an effector site, which either initiates thrombolysis or prevents additional thrombus formation. The repertoire of potential antibody specificities is extremely large and allows for the selection of monoclonal antibodies that can differentiate among very similar antigens. Thus, it is possible to bind fibrin but not fibrinogen or to recognize the activated form of the platelet receptor glycoprotein IIb-IIIa but not its inactive isomer. This selectivity of antibodies allows the investigator to specify which feature of a thrombus should be targeted. If arterial thrombi that are rich in platelets are to be lysed, antibodies specific for a platelet antigen can be used to concentrate the effector molecule at the thrombus. If new thrombi are to be preferentially lysed, thrombin, which is present in higher concentrations in recently formed thrombi, can be used as a target.

The most practical approach to antibody targeting is to use recombinant DNA methods to create a single molecule containing both an effector molecule and the part of the antibody molecule that contains the antigen-binding site. Not only does this approach avoid the difficulties of chemical cross-linking, but it also may one day enable production of the fusion protein in quantity by fermentation methods.

Antifibrin Antibody–Plasminogen Activator Fusion Proteins

A fusion protein can be created by combining fragments of genomic DNA or messenger RNA coding for segments of the proteins to be joined [*see Figure 1*]. This hybrid gene is then incorporated into a plasmid that has been engineered to effect protein expression in a bacterium, insect cell, or mammalian cell.

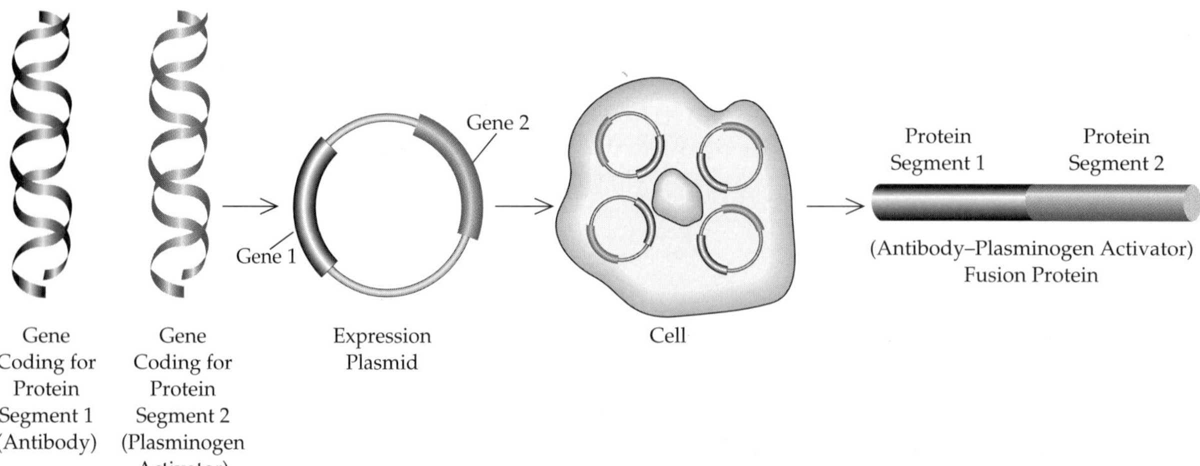

Figure 1 *Fragments of genomic DNA or messenger RNA coding for segments of the proteins to be joined are combined. The hybrid gene is incorporated into a plasmid that effects protein expression in a cell, and the cell generates a fusion protein.*

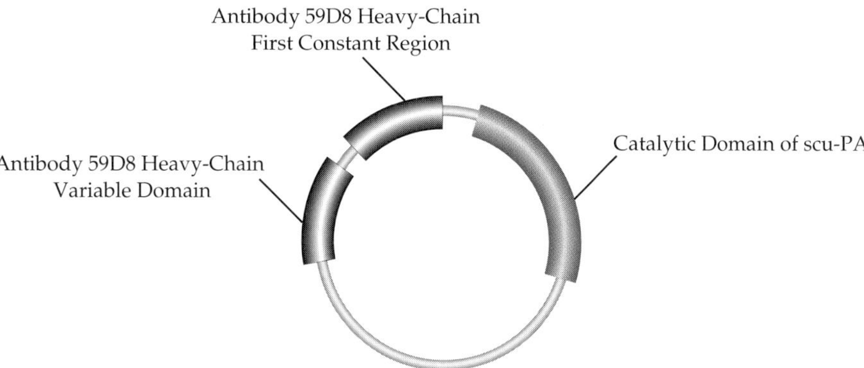

***Figure 2** Expression plasmid for r59D8–scu-PA(32) (32-kilodalton single-chain urokinase-type plasminogen activator). Complementary DNAs coding for the variable region of the heavy chain (V_H) of fibrin-specific antibody 59D8 and the first constant region of the heavy chain, (C_H1), including the hinge, are assembled in a plasmid 5′ of the cDNA coding for the catalytic domain of scu-PA. Because the combined cDNA of this plasmid only codes for a heavy-chain fusion protein, the immunoglobulin light chain must be provided for by transfecting the plasmid into a plasma cell line that produces the 59D8 light chain but no heavy chain. The light chain then assembles with this fusion protein to create the desired Fab–plasminogen activator protein.*

Building on the pioneering work of Neuberger and colleagues[2,3] and on our experience with cross-linked antibody–enzyme model proteins, my research group has used this recombinant technology to create a fusion protein with the activities of antifibrin antibody 59D8 and tissue-type plasminogen activator (t-PA).[4] Methods for generating the 59D8–t-PA protein have been detailed previously.[5,6] t-PA, however, was found not to be an ideal partner in an antibody-targeted fusion protein because the activity of t-PA depends on fibrin binding and is impaired by the presence of an antibody at the N-terminal. We then experimented with single-chain urokinase-type plasminogen activator (scu-PA). DNA coding for the catalytic segment of scu-PA and the fibrin-binding segment of antibody 59D8 was assembled in an expression plasmid that was transfected into a plasma cell already secreting the 59D8 light chain [*see Figure 2*]. The light chain assembled with the chimeric heavy chain (immunoglobulin and plasminogen activator) within the plasma cell, and a molecule was secreted that contained both an antigen-binding site specific for fibrin (from antibody 59D8) and a catalytic site capable of cleaving fibrin (from scu-PA).

The catalytic site of urokinase-type plasminogen activator (u-PA) was selected because u-PA does not require fibrin binding for activation. Because we anticipated that fibrin binding would occur through the fibrin-specific antibody (59D8) portion of the fusion protein, we wanted a plasminogen activator that functioned independently of fibrin binding. The single-chain form, scu-PA, was used because it has the additional advantage of being resistant to inactivation by plasminogen activator inhibitor–1 and α_2-antiplasmin. As it traveled through plasma, a fusion protein containing scu-PA would resist circulating inhibitors and remain incapable of activating circulating plasminogen until it reached the plasmin-rich environment of the thrombus, where it would then become active through cleavage of the plasmin-susceptible Lys^{158}–Ile^{159} peptide bond.[7]

For the recombinant (r) antifibrin–scu-PA protein, we included only the Fab part of the antibody molecule so as to limit the mass of the chimera to its essential components. In a similar vein, the u-PA kringle and growth factor regions were omitted, and only the sequence corresponding to low-molecular-weight (32-kilodalton [kd]) scu-PA was used.[8] (This fragment is reported to be as active in fibrinolysis as the intact molecule.) Initially, the C_H2 domain of the antibody heavy chain and part of the C_H3 domain had been included as a spacer between the antibody and plasminogen activator, but later experience proved that this space was unnecessary (Shaw S-Y. Unpublished data). The r59D8–scu-PA(32) protein contained heavy chain from residues 1 to 351 of antibody 59D8 and, in contiguous peptide sequence, residues 144 to 411 of low-molecular-weight scu-PA.[9]

To evaluate the functional properties of r59D8–scu-PA(32), we compared the specific amidolytic activity and kinetic parameters for activation of plasminogen by plasmin-cleaved r59D8–scu-PA(32) with those of low-molecular-weight two-chain urokinase plasminogen activator (tcu-PA). The specific amidolytic activity of tissue culture–derived scu-PA was 85,000 U/mg. This material was more than 95 percent uncleaved (i.e., single chain) when latent activity was compared with activity after cleavage to high-molecular-weight tcu-PA [scu-PA and r59D8–scu-PA(32) were converted to the two-chain form with plasmin-Sepharose[10,11]]. Given the contribution, on a molar basis, of the 32-kd scu-PA portion of the 103-kd r59D8–scu-PA(32) molecule, the activity of the scu-PA portion was 83,900 U/mg of scu-PA. This is not significantly different from the activity of native scu-PA. In addition, the K_m for activation of plasminogen by the plasmin-cleaved (two-chain) form of r59D8–scu-PA(32) (16.6 μM) did not differ significantly from that of low-molecular-weight tcu-PA (9.1 μM). We also compared the fibrin-binding activity of r59D8–scu-PA(32) (native 32-kd scu-PA does not bind fibrin directly) with that of native 59D8 by measuring the binding of serial dilutions of 59D8 and r59D8–scu-PA(32) to fibrin monomer–coated, 96-well plates. r59D8–scu-PA(32) bound to fibrin in a manner similar to that of native 59D8.

In a human plasma clot lysis assay, r59D8–scu-PA(32) was six times more potent than scu-PA. Furthermore, at equivalent thrombolytic doses, r59D8–scu-PA(32) was more fibrin specific—that is, there was less consumption of fibrinogen and α_2-antiplasmin than with scu-PA. The results were even more striking in vivo when the antibody-targeted plasminogen activator was tested in the rabbit jugular vein model (the in situ formation of a human thrombus in the vein of a rabbit). Compared with scu-PA, r59D8–scu-PA(32) displayed a remarkable 20-fold increase in thrombolytic potency in vivo over the entire dose-response range.[9] r59D8–scu-PA(32) did not cause a decrease in fibrinogen concentration until 83 percent lysis was reached, at which point the fibrinogen concentration was 79±4 percent that of the control.

Runge and colleagues have since studied the in vivo activities of r59D8–scu-PA(32), scu-PA, and t-PA in a baboon model that allows critical comparisons of thrombolytic potency and inhibition of thrombus deposition in relation to both the dose and plasma concentration of each plasminogen activator (Runge MS, et al. Submitted manuscript). In the lysis of thrombi, r59D8–scu-PA(32) was eightfold to 10-fold more potent than rt-PA and 15- to 20-fold more potent than rscu-PA by dose administered, and it was 2.8-fold more potent than rt-PA and 5.6-fold more potent than rscu-PA by plasma concentration. This difference in potency, as calculated by the dose administered in comparison with plasma concentration, is explained by the observation that in the baboon the plasma half-life was 12 times longer for r59D8–scu-PA(32) than for rscu-PA. In an experiment in which pharmacokinetics did not play a role, r59D8–scu-PA(32) was 11 times more potent than scu-PA in the inhibition of thrombin deposition.

Of equally great interest was the observation in the baboon that at equipotent thrombolytic doses, template bleeding times for r59D8–scu-PA(32) were unchanged, whereas those for t-PA and scu-PA were significantly prolonged. Because prolongation of bleeding time apparently reflects the risk of clinical hemorrhage,[12] it will be interesting to determine whether r59D8–scu-PA(32), in addition to being more potent, might also be safer.

D. Collen and coworkers have pursued similar studies with a different fibrin-specific antibody and reached similar conclusions.[13-18] This group engineered an antigen-binding site even smaller than the Fab site used in our r59D8–scu-PA(32) protein, which allowed them to create a single-chain molecule that contained only the light- and heavy-chain variable region (the Fv) of their antibody linked in contiguous peptide sequence to the catalytic site of scu-PA.

Targeting Young Thrombi Using Thrombin-Activated u-PA

Yang and associates have described a fusion protein that contains a fibrin-specific antigen-binding site and a modified scu-PA catalytic domain.[19] The design of this molecule was predicated on the observation that a high concentration of thrombin exists in the vicinity of recently formed intravascular thrombi. Although thrombin is capable of cleaving and inactivating native scu-PA, the u-PA–derived catalytic segment contained in this group's fusion protein (r59D8–scu-PA-T) was modified by site-directed mutagenesis so that the peptide bond normally cleaved by plasmin (to activate urokinase) would now be cleaved by thrombin [*see Chapter 9, Figure 3*]. Thus, a selective thrombin cleavage site in a molecule targeted to fibrin would initiate clot lysis after thrombin activation.

The specific change effected in the u-PA domain was the deletion of Phe[157] and Lys[158] [*see Figure 3*]. According to its design, then, r59D8–scu-PA-T was activated by thrombin but not by plasmin, whereas the fusion protein discussed earlier, r59D8–scu-PA(32), was activated by plasmin but not by thrombin. When activated by thrombin, r59D8–scu-PA-T converted plasminogen to plasmin. In vitro plasma clot lysis assays showed that r59D8–scu-PA-T lysed clots that resulted from the action of thrombin and that heparin and hirudin prevented clot lysis. When incorporated as part of a thrombin-induced clot, only r59D8–scu-PA-T was able to lyse the clot, whereas r59D8–scu-PA(32) and high-molecular-weight scu-PA were ineffective.

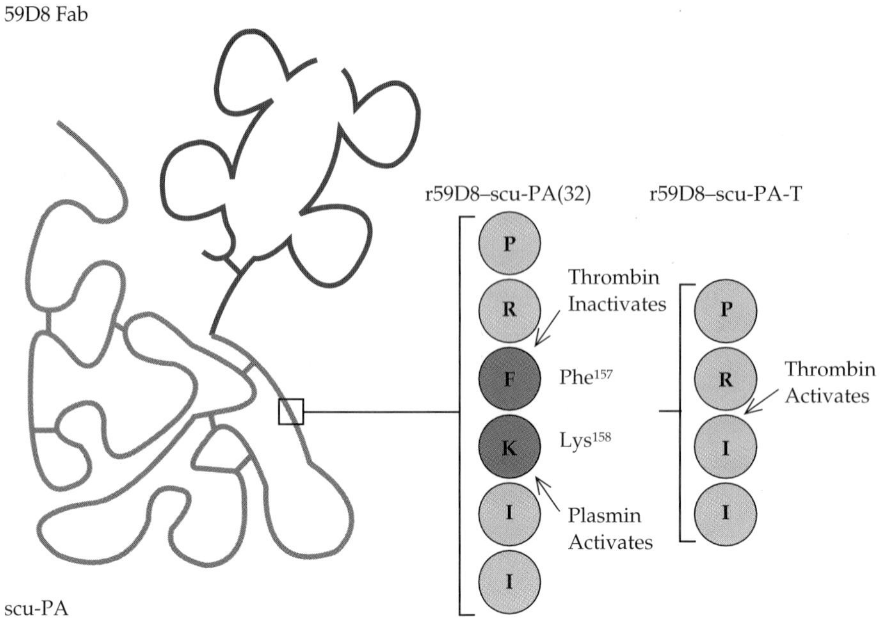

Figure 3 *Activation of r59D8–scu-PA(32) (32-kilodalton single-chain urokinase-type plasminogen activator) and r59D8–scu-PA-T (single-chain urokinase-type plasminogen activator, thrombin cleavable) by plasmin and thrombin.*

These observations suggest that the thrombin-activatable form of 59D8–scu-PA has the potential to selectively lyse fresh clots, which are thrombin rich, more effectively than older clots, which generally do not contain as much thrombin. A clinical event requiring thrombolysis, such as occlusion of a coronary or cerebral artery, usually presents acutely and is the consequence of a very recent thrombus. The therapeutic aim in this situation would be to dissolve the new thrombus but not disturb older thrombi, which might be preventing undesirable hemorrhage, such as at the site of a peptic ulcer. Targetability engendered in fresh thrombi by a high local concentration of thrombin may well be the key to increased plasminogen activator selectivity.

Targeting the Thrombin Inhibitor Hirudin to Fibrin

Bode and associates synthesized a bifunctional molecule that incorporates antifibrin antibody 59D8 and the thrombin inhibitor hirudin.[20] The intent of this design was to inhibit further fibrin deposition at sites of thrombosis while avoiding systemic anticoagulation. An in vitro assay was devised to measure the deposition of fibrin on a preformed clot suspended in plasma. In this model, hirudin is an effective anticoagulant in that it prevents further deposition of fibrin onto the surface of the clot. The 59D8–hirudin conjugate was 10 times as potent as hirudin alone in inhibiting clot deposition, presumably because the fibrin-binding site of the conjugate concentrated hirudin at the surface of the clot. When the 59D8–hirudin conjugate was tested in the baboon thrombosis model discussed in the previous section, the activity of 59D8–hirudin was six times higher than that of unconjugated hirudin (Runge MS. Unpublished data).

A recombinant version of the 59D8–hirudin conjugate also has been produced by methods analogous to those used to produce r59D8–scu-PA(32).[21]

However, a problem specific to hirudin had to be overcome in producing the 59D8–hirudin fusion protein. Because any substitution at the N-terminal of hirudin destroys its activity, a 59D8–hirudin fusion protein would be inactive. Bode and colleagues solved the problem by inserting a peptide sequence that was susceptible to cleavage by factor Xa (a constituent of thrombi) between the antibody segment and the hirudin segment of the fusion protein. In the presence of factor Xa, hirudin could be released from the fusion protein on its arrival at the thrombus and hence become activated.

Targeting a Platelet Receptor

Arterial thrombi contain a high concentration of activated platelets, and platelet-rich thrombi appear to be particularly resistant to thrombolysis. Also, highly platelet-rich thrombi might be a major reason for the failure to obtain reperfusion after thrombolytic therapy, and the accumulation of platelets at thrombi can lead to reocclusion. Platelet aggregation is mediated by fibrinogen binding to the membrane-bound glycoprotein IIb-IIIa receptor[22] [*see Chapter 11*]. An antibody specific for this receptor, 7E3, has been shown to enhance the speed of reperfusion and reduce the rate of reocclusion in animal models of arterial thrombosis.[23,24]

My research group became interested in determining whether the targeting of a plasminogen activator to the glycoprotein IIb-IIIa receptor through 7E3 would enhance the antibody's ability to accelerate clot lysis. We reasoned that a conjugate of 7E3 and u-PA, in addition to blocking access of the glycoprotein IIb-IIIa receptor to fibrinogen by virtue of 7E3's binding to glycoprotein IIb-IIIa, would produce a high local concentration of plasmin that could lyse the bound fibrin molecules responsible for aggregating the platelets.

We conjugated high-molecular-weight tcu-PA to the 7E3 Fab′ by chemical cross-linking.[25] The tcu-PA–7E3 Fab′ conjugate bound purified glycoprotein IIb-IIIa and intact platelets and exhibited plasminogen activator activity. At the concentrations tested, tcu-PA showed very little activity against the clots, whereas the conjugate was 970-fold more active. An equimolar mixture of tcu-PA and 7E3 was no more effective than u-PA alone. The rate of lysis related to the concentration of platelets in the clot, and no enhancement in lysis by the conjugate over u-PA was apparent in clots containing few platelets. Thus, u-PA targeted to glycoprotein IIb-IIIa by conjugation to antibody 7E3 accounted for an improvement in fibrinolytic potency that was substantially greater than that achieved by u-PA and the antibody alone.

Dewerchin and colleagues[26] have also studied several other antibodies to the ligand-induced binding sites on glycoprotein IIb-IIIa in conjugates with recombinant scu-PA. They extended our observations by showing that the conjugates were more effective than scu-PA in the lysis of platelet-rich thrombi in vivo in a hamster model of pulmonary embolism. There is little doubt that the next refinement to platelet targeting will require the construction of a recombinant molecule that contains both a binding site specific for activated platelets and a plasminogen activator catalytic site.

The disadvantage of using 7E3 as a targeting antibody is that it interacts with glycoprotein IIb-IIIa on both activated and resting platelets and thus does not target the thrombus specifically.[22] Some of the antibodies described by Dewerchin and colleagues may be more selective for activated platelets.[26]

Targeting with Bifunctional Antibodies

An alternative to a fusion protein that contains segments of two proteins of different function is a bifunctional antibody that is able to bind both fibrin and a plasminogen activator (without diminishing its enzymatic activity). Such a bifunctional antibody would serve to bring the plasminogen activator into proximity with fibrin, without the need to manipulate the enzyme chemically. We first tested the feasibility of this approach with antibodies to t-PA or u-PA chemically cross-linked to fibrin-specific antibody 59D8.[27,28] A significant enhancement in fibrinolytic activity was demonstrated both in vitro and in vivo with a 59D8–anti-t-PA conjugate[27] and in vitro with a 59D8–anti-u-PA conjugate.[28] A conjugate of the anti-t-PA Fab′ and the Fab′ of 59D8 was also as effective as the intact-antibody conjugate.[29] Sakharov and coworkers have demonstrated a 10-fold enhancement in plasma clot lysis in vitro with cross-linked antibodies specific for fibrin and u-PA.[30]

A better method for producing bispecific antibodies, which avoids the disadvantages of chemical cross-linking, is to use somatic cell fusion to produce bivalent antibodies that possess two different antigen-combining sites. This method was first elaborated in 1983 by Milstein and Cuello[31] and has been applied by my research group in the design of bifunctional antibodies that bind both t-PA and fibrin.[32]

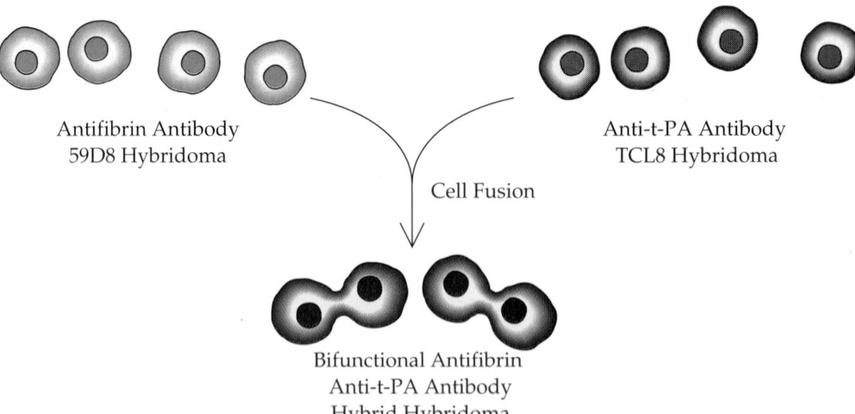

Figure 4 *Hybrid-hybridoma method for generating a bispecific antibody. Two antibody-producing hybridoma lines, one secreting an antibody specific for fibrin and the other secreting an antibody specific for tissue-type plasminogen activator (t-PA), are subjected to somatic cell fusion to produce a hybrid hybridoma. In the fused cells, the light and heavy chains of both antibody types are assorted randomly to form immunoglobulin molecules containing mixtures of chains from both sources. In some molecules, a light and heavy chain from the antifibrin antibody will be paired with a light and heavy chain from the anti-t-PA antibody, producing a bispecific antibody capable of binding both fibrin and t-PA.*

Immunoglobulin G is a symmetrical molecule possessing two antigen-combining sites of the same specificity. Because the component chains of the molecule are assembled after their individual biosyntheses, it is possible to obtain molecules of mixed specificity from cells that are synthesizing two different antibodies.[33] By somatic cell fusion (between a hybridoma line secreting antifibrin antibody 59D8 and another hybridoma line secreting anti-t-PA antibody TCL8), we produced a cell line that secreted a mixture of antibodies. In addition to the antibodies characteristic of the parental lines and inactive immunoglobulins, the hybrid-hybridoma line secreted an antibody that could bind both fibrin and t-PA [*see Figure 4*].

It was anticipated that an antibody specific for both fibrin and t-PA would bind to the fibrin matrix of a thrombus but would also bind to t-PA in plasma, thereby increasing the concentration of t-PA at the surface of the thrombus. This expectation was confirmed by in vitro clot lysis experiments showing that the bispecific antibody enhanced the potency of t-PA 14-fold. When the bispecific antibody was tested in vivo in the rabbit jugular vein model, however, only a 1.6-fold enhancement in fibrinolytic activity was observed.[32] Kurokawa and colleagues have extended this work and by cell fusion produced bispecific antibodies that bind u-PA and fibrin as well as t-PA and fibrin.[34] An immunoconjugate that combined rscu-PA with a bifunctional antibody specific for both scu-PA and fibrin was tested in a baboon venous thrombosis model and showed a fivefold higher thrombolytic potency than unconjugated rscu-PA, a result of both slower clearance from the plasma and fibrin targeting.[35]

The production of bifunctional antibodies by somatic cell fusion is severely limited by product yield. Because the method depends on a random assortment of immunoglobulin chains within the fused cell, none of the products are secreted in large amounts. Recombinant DNA methods have now been developed that efficiently produce molecules that contain two antibody Fv sites of different specificities.[36]

Conclusion

In the decade since the first description of a fibrin-targeted plasminogen activator, there has been considerable progress in antibody targeting.[37] Simple chemical conjugates have evolved into elegant chimeric proteins, the smallest of which comprises only the minimal antigen-binding site, the Fv, and the catalytic site of u-PA.[13] These agents have been more effective than their parent plasminogen activators in a variety of animal models, including one in the baboon that resembles arterial thrombosis in humans. Early studies suggest that safety, as exemplified by diminished effects on hemostasis, may also be enhanced. An antibody specific for a platelet receptor has been used to target a plasminogen activator. In vitro studies suggest that this approach may help dissolve platelet-rich thrombi, which are generally resistant to the available plasminogen activators. The thrombin inhibitor hirudin has been targeted to fibrin, indicating that local, rather than systemic, anticoagulation may be possible. Finally, an alternative to a fusion protein is a bifunctional antibody that can bridge an antigen on a clot and an antigen on a plasminogen activator or an anticoagulant. Bifunctional antibodies as thrombolytic agents are still in an early stage of development. General confirmation of the utility of antibody targeting now awaits clinical studies.

References

1. Collen D: Towards improved thrombolytic therapy. *Lancet* 342:34, 1993
2. Neuberger MS, Williams GT, Fox RO: Recombinant antibodies possessing novel effector functions. *Nature* 312:604, 1984
3. Williams GT, Neuberger MS: Production of antibody-tagged enzymes by myeloma cells: application to DNA polymerase I Klenow fragment. *Gene* 43:319, 1986
4. Schnee JM, Runge MS, Matsueda GR, et al: Construction and expression of a recombinant antibody-targeted plasminogen activator. *Proc Natl Acad Sci USA* 84:6904, 1987
5. Love TW, Runge MS, Haber E, et al: Recombinant antibodies possessing novel effector functions. *Methods Enzymol* 178:515, 1989
6. Love TW, Quertermous T, Zavodny PJ, et al: High-level expression of antibody-plasminogen activator fusion proteins in hybridoma cells. *Thromb Res* 69:221, 1993
7. Declerck PJ, Lijnen HR, Verstreken M, et al: A monoclonal antibody specific for two-chain urokinase-type plasminogen activator: application to the study of the mechanism of clot lysis with single-chain urokinase-type plasminogen activator in plasma. *Blood* 75:1794, 1990
8. Stump DC, Lijnen HR, Collen D: Purification and characterization of a novel low molecular weight form of single-chain urokinase-type plasminogen activator. *J Biol Chem* 261:17120, 1986
9. Runge MS, Quertermous T, Zavodny PJ, et al: A recombinant chimeric plasminogen activator with high affinity for fibrin has increased thrombolytic potency in vitro and in vivo. *Proc Natl Acad Sci USA* 88:10337, 1991
10. Runge MS, Bode C, Matsueda GR, et al: Antibody-enhanced thrombolysis: targeting of tissue plasminogen activator in vivo. *Proc Natl Acad Sci USA* 84:7659, 1987
11. Dewerchin M, Lijnen HR, Van Hoef B, et al: Biochemical properties of conjugates of urokinase-type plasminogen activator with a monoclonal antibody specific for cross-linked fibrin. *Eur J Biochem* 185:141, 1989
12. Gimple LW, Gold HK, Leinbach RC, et al: Correlation between template bleeding times and spontaneous bleeding during treatment of acute myocardial infarction with recombinant tissue-type plasminogen activator. *Circulation* 80:581, 1989
13. Holvoet P, Laroche Y, Lijnen HR, et al: Characterization of a chimeric plasminogen activator consisting of a single-chain Fv fragment derived from a fibrin fragment D-dimer-specific antibody and a truncated single-chain urokinase. *J Biol Chem* 266:19717, 1991
14. Dewerchin M, Vandamme AM, Holvoet P, et al: Thrombolytic and pharmacokinetic properties of a recombinant chimeric plasminogen activator consisting of a fibrin fragment D-dimer specific humanized monoclonal antibody and a truncated single-chain urokinase. *Thromb Haemost* 68:170, 1992
15. Vandamme AM, Dewerchin M, Lijnen HR, et al: Characterization of a recombinant chimeric plasminogen activator composed of a fibrin fragment-D-dimer-specific humanized monoclonal antibody and a truncated single-chain urokinase. *Eur J Biochem* 205:139, 1992
16. Holvoet P, Laroche Y, Lijnen HR, et al: Biochemical characterization of single-chain chimeric plasminogen activators consisting of a single-chain Fv fragment of a fibrin-specific antibody and single-chain urokinase. *Eur J Biochem* 210:945, 1992
17. Holvoet P, Laroche Y, Stassen JM, et al: Pharmacokinetic and thrombolytic properties of chimeric plasminogen activators consisting of a single-chain Fv fragment of a fibrin-specific antibody fused to single-chain urokinase. *Blood* 81:696, 1993
18. Holvoet P, Dewerchin M, Stassen JM, et al: Thrombolytic profiles of clot-targeted plasminogen activators: parameters determining potency and initial and maximal rates. *Circulation* 87:1007, 1993
19. Yang WP, Goldstein J, Procyk R, et al: Design and evaluation of a thrombin-activable plasminogen activator. *Biochemistry* 33:606, 1994
20. Bode C, Hudelmayer M, Mehwald P, et al: Fibrin-targeted recombinant hirudin inhibits fibrin deposition on experimental clots more efficiently than recombinant hirudin. *Circulation* 90:1956, 1994

21. Peter K, Gupta A, Ruef J, et al: A recombinant molecule with high affinity for fibrin exhibits antithrombin activity after cleavage by factor Xa [abstract]. *Circulation* 90:I-348, 1994
22. Coller BS: Platelets and thrombolytic therapy. *N Engl J Med* 322:33, 1990
23. Yasuda T, Gold HK, Fallon JT, et al: Monoclonal antibody against the platelet glycoprotein (GP) IIb/IIIa receptor prevents coronary artery reocclusion after reperfusion with recombinant tissue-type plasminogen activator in dogs. *J Clin Invest* 81:1284, 1988
24. Gold HK, Coller BS, Yasuda T, et al: Rapid and sustained coronary artery recanalization with combined bolus injection of recombinant tissue-type plasminogen activator and monoclonal antiplatelet GPIIb/IIIa antibody in a canine preparation. *Circulation* 77:670, 1988
25. Bode C, Meinhardt G, Runge MS, et al: Platelet-targeted fibrinolysis enhances clot lysis and inhibits platelet aggregation. *Circulation* 84:805, 1991
26. Dewerchin M, Lijnen HR, Stassen JM, et al: Effect of chemical conjugation of recombinant single-chain urokinase-type plasminogen activator with monoclonal antiplatelet antibodies on platelet aggregation and on plasma clot lysis in vitro and in vivo. *Blood* 78:1005, 1991
27. Bode C, Runge MS, Branscomb EE, et al: Antibody-directed fibrinolysis: an antibody specific for both fibrin and tissue plasminogen activator. *J Biol Chem* 264:944, 1989
28. Charpie JR, Runge MS, Matsueda GR, et al: A bispecific antibody enhances the fibrinolytic potency of single-chain urokinase. *Biochemistry* 29:6374, 1990
29. Runge MS, Bode C, Savard CE, et al: Antibody-directed fibrinolysis: a bispecific $(Fab')_2$ that binds to fibrin and tissue plasminogen activator. *Bioconjugate Chemistry* 1:274, 1990
30. Sakharov DV, Sinitsyn VV, Kratasjuk GA, et al: Two-step targeting of urokinase to plasma clot provides efficient fibrinolysis. *Thromb Res* 49:481, 1988
31. Milstein C, Cuello AC: Hybrid hybridomas and their use in immunohistochemistry. *Nature* 305:537, 1983
32. Branscomb EE, Runge MS, Savard CE, et al: Bispecific monoclonal antibodies produced by somatic cell fusion increase the potency of tissue plasminogen activator. *Thromb Haemost* 64:260, 1990
33. Suresh MR, Cuello AC, Milstein C: Bispecific monoclonal antibodies from hybrid hybridomas. *Methods Enzymol* 121:210, 1986
34. Kurokawa T, Iwasa S, Kakinuma A: Enhancement of fibrinolysis by bispecific monoclonal antibodies reactive to fibrin and plasminogen activators. *Thromb Res Suppl* 10:83, 1990
35. Imura Y, Stassen JM, Kurokawa T, et al: Thrombolytic and pharmacokinetic properties of an immunoconjugate of single-chain urokinase-type plasminogen activator (u-PA) and a bispecific monoclonal antibody against fibrin and against u-PA in baboons. *Blood* 79:2322, 1992
36. Huston JS, Keck P, Tai M-S, et al: Single-chain immunotechnology of Fv analogues and fusion proteins. *Immunotechnology*. Gosling JP, Reen D, Eds. Portland Press, London, 1993, p 47
37. Bode C, Matsueda GR, Hui KY, et al: Antibody-directed urokinase: a specific fibrinolytic agent. *Science* 229:765, 1985

Acknowledgments

Figures 1, 2 Talar Agasyan.

Figure 3 Talar Agasyan. Adapted from "Design and Evaluation of a Thrombin-Activable Plasminogen Activator," by W. P. Yang, J. Goldstein, R. Procyk, et al, in *Biochemistry* 33:606, 1994. Used by permission.

Figure 4 Talar Agasyan. Adapted from "Bispecific Monoclonal Antibodies Produced by Somatic Cell Fusion Increase the Potency of Tissue Plasminogen Activator," by E. E. Branscomb, M. S. Runge, C. E. Savard, et al, in *Thrombosis and Haemostasis* 64:260, 1990. Used by permission.

CHAPTER 11

Platelets in Thrombosis and Rethrombosis

Jacek Hawiger, M.D., Ph.D.

Blood platelets are the tiniest corpuscles—14 times smaller than erythrocytes—and they make 14,000 passages through the vascular system during their 10-day life span. They are endowed with an uncanny ability to survey the inner lining of blood vessels for sites of injury. Platelets instantly recognize any discontinuity in the vascular endothelium resulting from a cut (accidental or surgical hemorrhage) or from rupture of an atherosclerotic plaque. Upon encountering the zone of vascular injury, they engage in a series of finely orchestrated steps to seal off the ruptured area through formation of thrombi. This physiologically essential function of platelets in hemostasis can be pathologically subverted when they encounter breaks in cholesterol-rich, atherosclerotic plaques. Then the vigilant and robust response of platelets results in formation of platelet thrombi piling up on the fractured surface of the plaque and leading to a vascular occlusion.

Formation of Platelet-Fibrin Thrombi

Adherence of blood platelets to an atherosclerotic plaque, most likely upon its rupture,[1] is the most frequent underlying cause of thrombotic occlusion in coronary and cerebral arteries, which contributed to over 478,000 and 144,000 deaths, respectively, in the United States in 1991.[2] The exact mechanism of interaction of platelets with an atherosclerotic plaque is poorly understood. Plaque fissuring is an important factor in coronary thrombosis, as illustrated by its occurrence in the majority of patients with sudden cardiac ischemic death.[3] Likewise, the exact mechanisms involved in the reemergence of platelet-fibrin thrombi (rethrombosis) after recanalization of occluded vessels by thrombolytic agents or angioplasty remains unclear. The substantial rate (12 to 43 percent) of reocclusion of coronary arteries following thrombolytic therapy and transluminal coronary angioplasty[4] indicates that formation of platelet and fibrin thrombi takes place even in those pa-

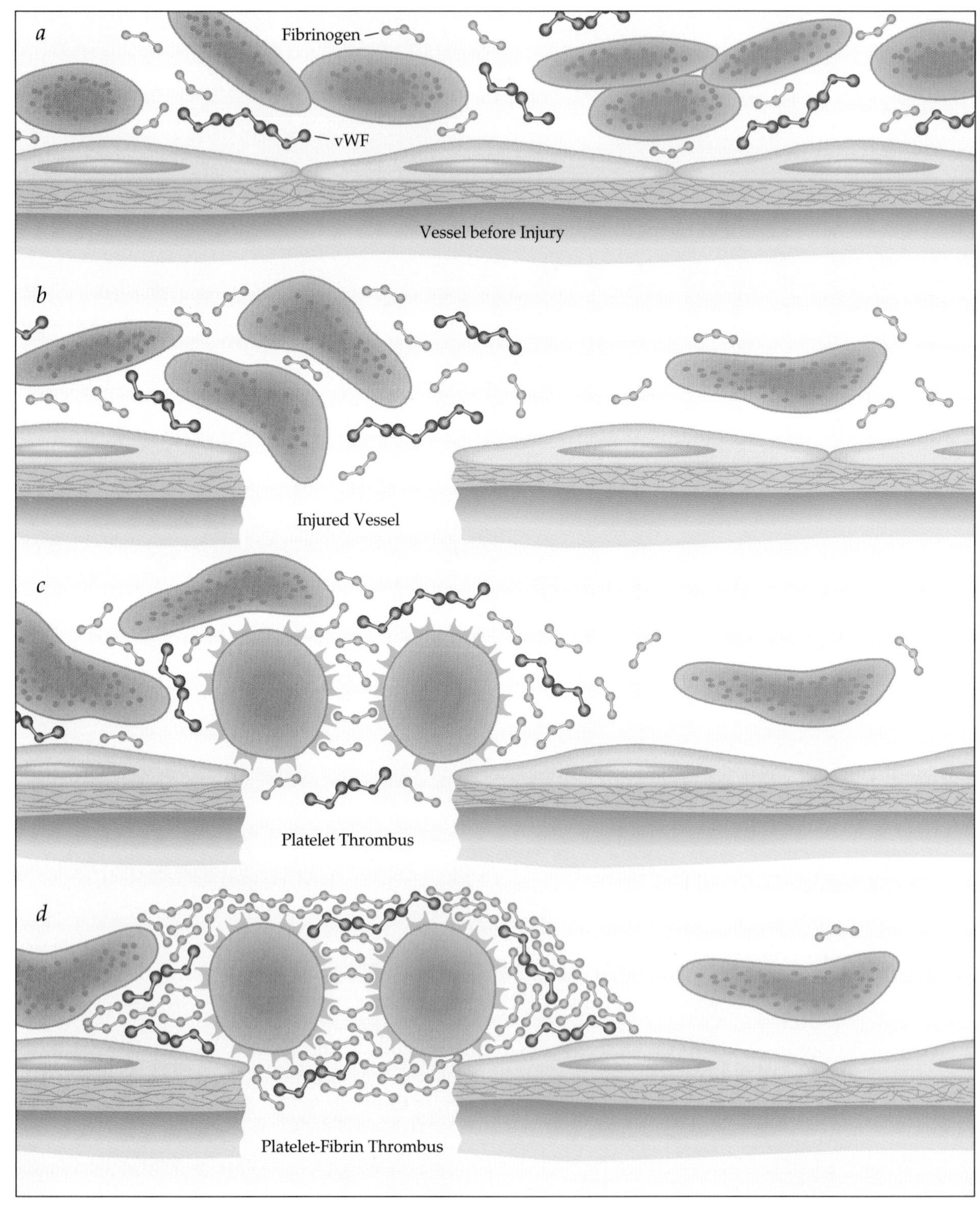

tients who continue to receive heparin and/or platelet inhibitors such as aspirin. The inner aspect of recanalized vessels must provide signals to platelets for rethrombosis. Therefore, measures to inhibit platelet stimulatory pathways that are not affected by aspirin require careful consideration. Fortunately, significant advances have been made in our knowledge of platelet receptors and signal-transducing pathways that give us a better understanding of the molecular mechanisms involved in the formation of platelet thrombi.

Platelet and fibrin thrombi are formed sequentially [*see Figure 1*]. First, platelets interact with adhesive proteins deposited in the subendothelial extracellular matrix exposed in the zone of vascular injury. These adhesive proteins include von Willebrand factor (vWF), collagens, fibronectin, vitronectin, thrombospondin, and laminin. Platelets adhere, change shape from smooth disks to spiny spheres, and spread, forming multiple contact sites with the subendothelial extracellular matrix. Second, more platelets are recruited to the area. Their adherence to each other (aggregation) is mediated by fibrinogen and results in the formation of a platelet thrombus (or a primary hemostatic plug when a vessel wall is cut). Third, while platelets are being activated, thrombin is generated. It can be detected within 45 seconds in a vascular wound caused by venipuncture. Thrombin activates platelets and transforms fibrinogen into a fibrin polymer, forming a network around the platelets and resulting in a platelet-fibrin thrombus, or a secondary hemostatic plug, that is more resistant to the shear stress of the blood flow. A platelet-fibrin thrombus is further consolidated by cross-linking of adjoining fibrin strands by factor XIII (transglutaminase) activated by thrombin. These events take place during the arrest of bleeding (physiologic hemostasis) and when vaso-occlusive thrombi are formed (pathological thrombosis). In both situations, platelets adhere and aggregate in response to vascular injury to form a thrombus.[5]

Whereas the nature of vascular lesions differs (vessel cut as opposed to rupture of atherosclerotic plaque), the common feature of the mechanism of formation of a hemostatic plug and pathological thrombi is the presence of the same type of scaffold supporting the mass of platelets. This scaffold, made of fibrinogen, fibrin, or both, is susceptible to the protein-cutting enzyme plasmin, which is generated in response to the influx of endogenous plasminogen activators (such as tissue-type plasminogen activator and urokinase-type plasminogen activator) or the infusion of exogenous thrombolytic agents [*see Chapter 9*]. Although these activators in supraphysiologic concentrations initiate a process resulting in lysis of pathological thrombi (thrombolysis), the plasminogen activator can also initiate disintegration of

Figure 1 *Formation of platelet-fibrin thrombi. (a) Platelets circulating in a milieu of plasma proteins do not interact with an uninjured vessel wall lined with intact endothelium. Two plasma adhesive proteins, fibrinogen and von Willebrand factor (vWF), remain unbound to platelets. (b) A break in the continuity of the endothelium in an injured vessel triggers signals that attract platelets to the site of injury and induce their anchoring, which is mediated by vWF and its receptors on the activated platelets. (c) Fibrinogen links platelets together to form a thrombus. (d) Thrombin generated at the site of vascular injury transforms fribrinogen into fibrin, which enmeshes the platelet thrombus like a cocoon. The platelet-fibrin thrombus seals off the break in the injured vessel and is more resistant to the hydrodynamic forces of flowing blood.*

a hemostatic plug, which will result in hemorrhage if such a plug seals off breaks in the vascular wall that result from venipuncture or age-related wear of the vascular tree in the brain and elsewhere.

Intravascular and Vascular Signals for Platelets

The signals received by circulating platelets that activate them come from blood and blood vessels. These activating signals are agonists recognized by platelet receptors. The number of agonists that can activate platelets through action on corresponding receptors is astounding considering the tiny dimensions of platelets. Agonists potentially generated at the site of vascular injury and able to activate platelets include adenosine diphosphate (ADP), thrombin, thromboxane A_2, platelet-activating factor (PAF), and epinephrine. With the exception of thrombin, these agonists are small molecules, easily diffusible in the fluid phase of blood and rapidly degraded to less active or inactive molecules. Nevertheless, the agonists generated in blood are potent platelet activators that evoke a rise in intraplatelet calcium concentrations, contraction of the cytoskeleton, and change in platelet shape from a smooth disk to a spiny sphere. Blood signals change inactive receptors capable of recognizing fibrinogen and other adhesive proteins to the active mode, and they induce the platelet storage granules to secrete their constituents, ADP, serotonin, adhesive proteins, and clotting factors, which amplify these intravascular signals. Secreted adhesive proteins include fibrinogen, vWF, and thrombospondin.

The vascular signals (defined as those generated by the vessel wall) that can activate platelets can be derived from an injured endothelium, the subendothelial extracellular matrix, and adventitial structures [*see Chapter 4*]. Normally, the integrity of the endothelium prevents platelets from receiving vascular signals and from displaying adhesive promiscuity toward the subendothelial extracellular matrix. On detachment of or injury to endothelial cells, vWF, collagens, and possibly other matrix components are recognized by platelets, and this recognition is followed by platelet activation. At least two components of the extracellular matrix, vWF and collagen, can measurably activate platelets in vitro.[6,7] The adventitia bears potent platelet-stimulating factors, as shown by experimental insertion of everted blood vessels into the circulation, which leads to a robust formation of vaso-occlusive thrombi strikingly resistant to thrombolytic agents.[8]

Receptors That Sense Signals, Anchor, and Link Platelets

Transmembrane Receptors

As a cellular element, the platelet is endowed with a membrane that bears the highest density of receptors per surface area among the known blood cells. These receptors recognize signals generated in blood and the vascular wall and transmit them to intraplatelet signal transducers. Thrombin and thromboxane A_2 generated at the site of vascular injury are the most potent agonists acting on their respective platelet receptors.[9] Receptors for thrombin and thromboxane A_2 have been cloned and sequenced, and their structures resemble those of the serpentine receptors that span the cell membrane seven times and are coupled to the signal transducers G-protein and phospholipase C. Thrombin not only binds to its seven-transmembrane-segment receptor but also cleaves its extracellular tip. A newly formed N-terminal end folds into the trunk of the thrombin receptor, thereby inducing a steric alteration needed for signaling. Thromboxane A_2, the product of an arachidonic acid cascade that can be blocked by aspirin, is not only a very potent platelet activator but also a vasoconstrictor. It is a short-lived (30 seconds) agonist that acts on a receptor in platelets and vascular smooth muscle.

Epinephrine activates platelets through the alpha$_2$-adrenergic receptor, which also spans the cell membrane seven times and is connected to G-proteins. There is a functional link between alpha$_2$-adrenergic receptors and the fibrinogen receptor integrin $\alpha_{IIb}\beta_3$ (glycoprotein IIb-IIIa complex). The fibrinogen receptor cooperates with alpha$_2$-adrenergic receptors in causing an increase in the intraplatelet level of calcium and alkalinization of the cytoplasm through activation of the Na^+/H^+ antiporter.[10]

Platelet-activating factor is a unique phospholipid-like agonist generated by leukocytes and endothelial cells. It is a potent platelet activator and a vasoconstrictor. Like the receptors for thrombin, thromboxane A_2, and epinephrine, the PAF receptor has seven transmembrane segments characteristic of G-protein and phospholipase-C–coupled receptors.[9]

Adenosine diphosphate, usually derived from the hydrolysis of adenosine triphosphate (ATP) that is abundant in erythrocytes and other cells, is an unusual agonist whose action is directed toward platelets. ADP evokes the rapid change in the shape of platelets from smooth disks to spiny spheres, a change related to the activation of myosin light-chain kinase by a calcium-calmodulin complex. In addition, binding of ADP to its receptor induces a shift in the platelet receptors for fibrinogen and other adhesive proteins from the nonbinding to the binding mode. Functionally, the ADP receptor is assigned to the P_{2t} class of purinergic receptors because of its unique preference for ADP as an agonist, whereas ATP acts as a competitive antagonist.[11] ADP secreted from platelet storage granules, called dense granules, is known to mediate some of the effects of other agonists on platelets, for example, thrombin and collagen.

Adhesive Molecules

Platelets programmed to recognize and seal any breaks in the continuity of the vascular endothelium use sensors that recognize molecular signals in the subendothelial extracellular matrix that have become exposed as a result of endothelial injury or detachment. This set of molecular sensors employed by platelets is made of cell adhesion molecules (CAMs). A number of structurally related CAMs constitute the superfamily of membrane proteins called integrins that mediate the attachment and anchoring of endothelial cells to the vessel wall and the interaction of platelets with the exposed subendothelial extracellular matrix [*see Figure 2 and Figure 3*]. Integrins are calcium-dependent heterodimers composed of two subunits, α and β.[12] Although the members of a distinct group (family) have a common β subunit

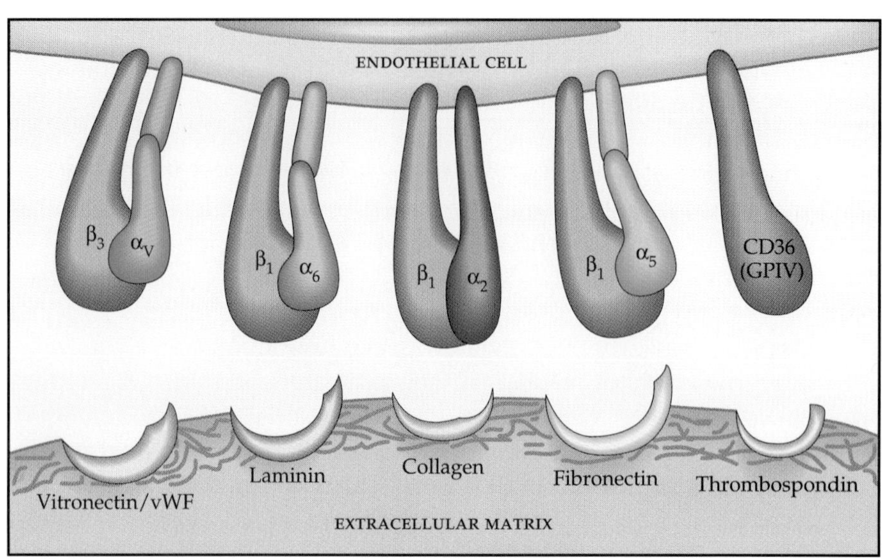

Figure 2 *An endothelial cell is anchored to the vessel wall through multiple receptors interacting with the components of the extracellular matrix. The integrin receptors $\alpha_2\beta_1$, $\alpha_5\beta_1$, $\alpha_6\beta_1$, and $\alpha_v\beta_3$ bind to collagen, fibronectin, laminin, and vitronectin/von Willebrand factor (vWF), respectively. The nonintegrin receptor CD36 (glycoprotein IV [GPIV]) binds to thrombospondin.*

(e.g., β_3 family), the α subunit differs significantly among the members of the same family, thereby contributing to selective interaction with a ligand in the extracellular matrix and in plasma. For example, fibrinogen is recognized by the platelet glycoprotein IIb-IIIa complex, an $\alpha_{IIb}\beta_3$ integrin belonging to the β_3 family [*see Figure 3*]. However, fibrinogen is not recognized by the endothelial vitronectin receptor $\alpha_v\beta_3$ [*see Figure 2*], which bears the same β_3 subunit as the platelet fibrinogen receptor.[13]

In studies discerning the three stages in the interaction of platelets with an injured vessel wall (i.e., adhesion, aggregation, and consolidation of a platelet thrombus), it was established that the initial contact of a platelet with an injured vascular wall is mediated by the interaction of the nonintegrin receptor, glycoprotein Ib, with vWF, an adhesive molecule in the subendothelial extracellular matrix, under high-flow, high-shear conditions [*see Figure 3*]. Under low-flow, low-shear conditions, the initial interaction of platelets with the zone of endothelial injury does not seem to depend on vWF-mediated adhesion.[14] Glycoprotein Ib belongs to a group of leucine-rich proteins encompassing the α_2-glycoprotein.[5,15] Glycoprotein Ib forms a stoichiometric complex with membrane glycoprotein IX. vWF (subunit 240 kd), whose gene has been cloned and sequenced, is a multimeric glycoprotein synthesized in endothelial cells and megakaryocytes.[16] It is stored in the Weibel-Palade bodies, characteristic organelles of endothelial cells, or in platelet α granules. vWF synthesized in endothelial cells is deposited in the subendothelial extracellular matrix and is secreted to plasma. It is not known why vWF multimers in plasma do not react with circulating platelets, whereas those in the subendothelial extracellular matrix engage in adhesive interactions with platelets when exposed to flowing blood. Fibrin monomers promote the interaction of vWF with human platelet glycoprotein Ib, which may provide a functional link between thrombin-induced clotting of fibrinogen and binding of vWF to glycoprotein Ib.[17] Moreover, hydrodynamically stressed human platelets aggregate through the interaction with vWF multimers present in plasma.[18]

vWF can bind to platelets through two distinct mechanisms: the classic pathway involving a nonintegrin receptor, the glycoprotein Ib complex mediating the initial adhesion of platelets to the zone of vascular injury, and the alternative pathway, involving an integrin receptor (β_3 family), the glycoprotein IIb-IIIa complex involved in platelet-thrombus formation (aggregation).[5] A deficiency of the platelet membrane glycoprotein Ib complex in giant platelet syndrome (Bernard-Soulier syndrome) leads to an inability of platelets to properly contact the zone of vascular injury. Thrombin or ADP initiates the alternative receptor pathway for vWF binding to human platelets.[19,20] Platelets from patients with Glanzmann's thrombasthenia, who have a deficiency of glycoproteins IIb and IIIa, do not bind vWF after stimulation with thrombin.[21] Monoclonal antibodies against the glycoprotein IIb-IIIa epitope block binding of vWF, thus affirming the role of glycoprotein IIb-IIIa in the receptor function of platelets.[5]

Other adhesive proteins in the subendothelial (extracellular) matrix are collagens, fibronectin, vitronectin, thrombospondin, and laminin. Together with vWF, they play an important role in maintaining the integrity of endothelial cells by providing anchorage points for endothelial receptors.[5] Once the endothelium is injured and stripped off, these adhesive proteins become attractive sites for platelet receptors [*see Figure 2 and Figure 3*]. Vascular collagens are involved in adhesion of platelets to the subendothelium under the condition of low shear when the presence of vWF is not essential. The platelet integrin $\alpha_2\beta_1$ (glycoprotein Ia-IIa complex, very late antigen–2 [VLA-2]) was shown to be involved in the interaction of platelets with type 1 collagen.[22,23] Fibronectins constitute prototype adhesive molecules in the extracellular matrix and in plasma.[24] They contain a cell adhesion site made of a three-amino-acid motif—arginine (R), glycine (G), and aspartic acid (D). Synthetic peptides containing an RGD motif compete with fibronectins for their receptor, thereby inhibiting adhesion of cells to fibronectin-containing matrix.[25] The fibronectin receptor integrin $\alpha_5\beta_1$, initially identified as VLA-5, is associated with platelet membrane glycoproteins Ic and IIa. This

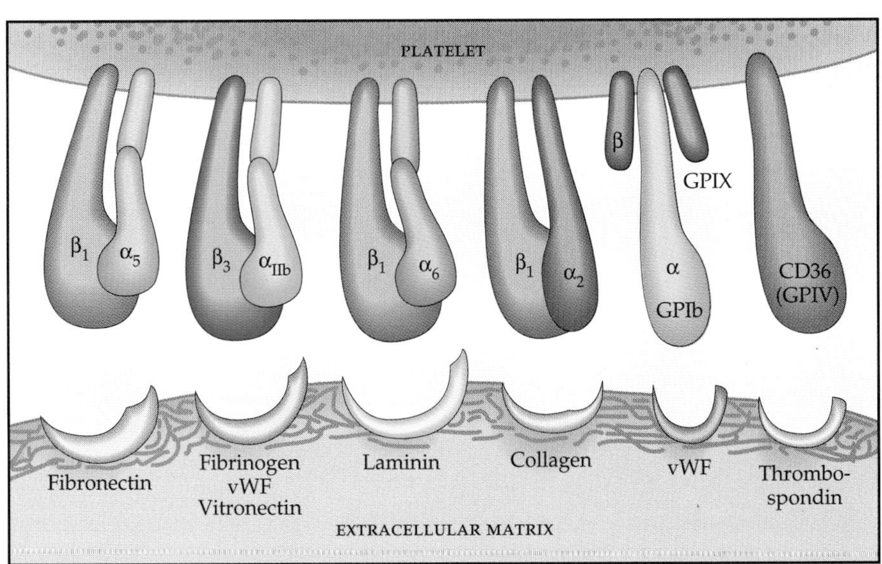

Figure 3 *A platelet binds to extracellular matrix components exposed after endothelial detachment through integrin and nonintegrin receptors similar to those present on endothelial cells. The integrin receptors $\alpha_2\beta_1$, $\alpha_6\beta_1$, $\alpha_5\beta_1$, and $\alpha_{IIb}\beta_3$ bind to collagen, laminin, fibronectin, and fibrinogen/vWF/vitronectin respectively. In addition, the platelet uses glycoprotein Ib-IX complex (GPIb-GPIX) to interact with vWF. The nonintegrin receptor CD36 binds to thrombospondin.*

receptor can mediate platelet adhesion to fibronectin-coated surfaces without a prior activation signal.[26]

The receptor for vitronectin (integrin $\alpha_v\beta_3$) in endothelial cells takes part in the anchoring to vitronectin and vWF in the extracellular matrix.[27] A similar receptor in platelets is activation dependent.[28] Thrombospondin interacts with two receptors on platelets: a nonintegrin glycoprotein IV (designated CD36) and integrin $\alpha_v\beta_3$. Only binding of thrombospondin to integrin $\alpha_v\beta_3$ was inhibited by the peptide RGDS (arginine–glycine–aspartic acid–serine).[29,30] Laminin attached to plastic surfaces promotes adherence of platelets without their activation[31]; antilaminin antibodies inhibit this adherence. A receptor for laminin in nonactivated platelets is the integrin $\alpha_6\beta_1$, a heterodimer VLA-6 composed of glycoproteins Ic and IIa.[32]

The multitude of adhesive proteins in the subendothelial matrix interacting with their receptors on platelets indicates that redundant binding mechanisms exist to mediate the interaction of platelets with the injured vascular wall. Some interactions involve one receptor recognizing multiple ligands, whereas other receptors bind a single ligand. Therapeutically, these interactions can be interrupted by inhibiting the receptors or by blocking the ligand. The latter strategy was employed in a porcine model of coronary thrombosis attenuated by monoclonal antibodies against vWF.[33]

Signal-Transducing Pathways in Platelets

The agonists present in blood or generated at the site of vascular injury stimulate platelet receptors to generate signals transmitted within platelets via signal-transducing pathways. These pathways culminate in a change of platelets from a resting to a functionally active state. As a result, platelets change shape, adhere, aggregate, and secrete the contents of their storage granules.

Platelets carry a rich assortment of biologically active molecules packed into storage granules. Molecules stored in dense granules include a nonmetabolic pool of adenosine nucleotides (ATP and ADP) and guanosine nucleotides (guanosine triphosphate [GTP] and guanosine diphosphate [GDP]), serotonin, Ca^{2+} and Mg^{2+}, and inorganic phosphate. A wider array of small and large proteins are stored in α granules,[34] including heparin-neutralizing factors, adhesive molecules, coagulation factor V, growth factors such as platelet-derived growth factor and transforming growth factor–β, and protease inhibitors such as plasminogen activator inhibitor–1 and α_2-antiplasmin, which regulate fibrinolysis. Secreted molecules interact with other platelets, with plasma proteins, and with cells and the extracellular matrix components in the vessel wall. The secretory response from platelets constitutes an important effector mechanism for the reinforcement of platelet thrombi, regulation of fibrinolysis, promotion of wound healing, and proliferation of atherosclerotic lesions. Genetic deficiencies of platelet storage granules (dense bodies or α granules) are manifested by a bleeding tendency.[35] An acquired defect in the secretion of stored factors can be induced by drugs such as aspirin.

When agonists known to stimulate platelets (ADP, epinephrine, thrombin, and PAF) bind to their respective receptors, they evoke signals transduced by regulatory molecules, such as GTP-binding proteins (G-proteins), and messenger molecules, such as diacylglycerol [*see Figure 4*]. These messenger molecules are generated in platelets because of the activation of a series of enzymes. These enzymes as well as regulatory molecules are cumulatively known as signal transducers. Phospholipase C interacts with seven-transmembrane-segment receptors (e.g., receptors for thrombin and PAF) to generate diacylglycerol and inositol-1,4,5-trisphosphate. Diacylglycerol activates an important signal transducer, protein kinase C, whereas inositol-1,4,5-trisphosphate releases calcium from intraplatelet stores. A rise in calcium triggers a number of signal transducers. Among them, Ca^{2+}-binding protein, calmodulin, activates myosin light-chain kinase involved in cytoskeletal regulation, bringing about the shape change of activated platelets to spiny spheres. The pathway mediated by protein kinase C is important because a number of platelet proteins are phosphorylated (e.g., plekstrin), and functional responses ensue, such as a shift of platelet integrin $\alpha_{IIb}\beta_3$ (glycoprotein IIb-IIIa) into an activated state. This pathway is not blocked by aspirin. Aspirin, however, blocks a pathway mediated by cyclooxygenase, the enzyme that converts arachidonic acid into prostaglandins G_2 and H_2 and then to thromboxane A_2. Arachidonic acid is chiefly generated by phospholipase A_2, an enzyme that splits membrane phospholipids and is regulated by mitogen-activated protein (MAP) kinase.[36] The product of this pathway, thromboxane A_2, is a very potent inducer of platelet secretion and shifts platelet integrins $\alpha_{IIb}\beta_3$ into binding fibrinogen, which mediates aggregation. Although this pathway in platelets is irreversibly blocked by aspirin, other pathways, such as that mediated by protein kinase C, can lead to the same functional responses of platelets manifested by binding of fibrinogen and aggregation despite the presence of aspirin.

Fortunately, these responses of platelets can be attenuated by inhibitory pathways that are triggered by small compounds generated by the vascular endothelium: nitric oxide and prostacyclin (prostaglandin I_2). Inhibitory pathways exercise the negative control imposed by the cyclic nucleotides cyclic adenosine monophosphate (cAMP) and cyclic guanosine monophosphate (cGMP) [*see Figure 4*]. Cyclic AMP is elevated when inhibitors such as prostacyclin and adenosine interact with their receptors. Cyclic GMP is generated when nitric oxide, known as endothelium-derived relaxing factor, interacts with platelets.[34] An additional control mechanism is provided by phosphatases, which are able to dephosphorylate signal transducers.

The multiple signal-transducing pathways provide redundancy and diversity in the ways platelets respond to stimuli. Multiple pathways pose a challenge for effective inhibition of platelet activation because pharmacological blockade of one signal-transducing pathway may not be sufficient for a complete inhibition of platelet function, as observed with aspirin.

Role of Fibrinogen in Formation and Organization of Platelet Thrombi

Platelet thrombus formation depends on the bridging of platelets by fibrinogen, the most abundant intercellular adhesion molecule in plasma. Studies of afibrinogenemia, a disorder characterized by prolonged bleeding

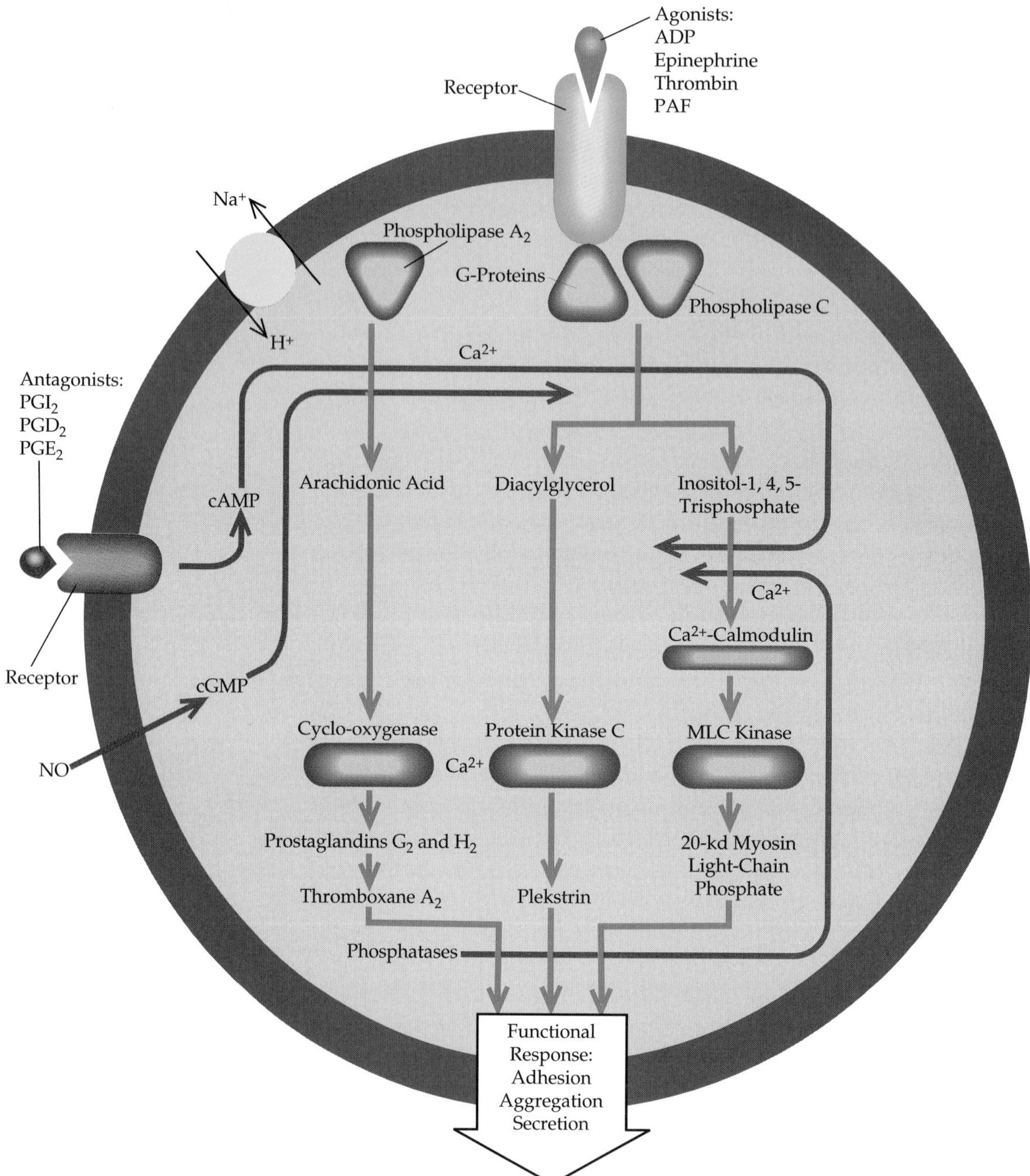

Figure 4 *Signal transducing pathways in platelets. Several signal transducers relay signals generated by binding of agonists adenosine diphosphate (ADP), epinephrine, thrombin, and platelet activating factor (PAF) to their receptors. The signal transducers (shown in blue) include G-proteins, phospholipases A_2 and C, cyclo-oxygenase, protein kinase C, and myosin light-chain (MLC) kinase, among others. The messenger molecules calcium, diacylglycerol, and inositol-1,4,5-trisphosphate mediate signaling events, culminating in the functional response manifested in adhesion, aggregation, and secretion. Platelet antagonists represented by prostacyclin (PGI_2), prostaglandin D_2 (PGD_2), prostaglandin E_2 (PGE_2), and nitric oxide (NO) induce inhibitory pathways mediated by cAMP and cGMP, respectively. Together with platelet phosphatases, the platelet antagonists negatively regulate platelet activation. The green arrows indicate stimulation. The red arrows indicate inhibition.*

time and abnormal aggregation of platelets,[37] provided key evidence for the role of fibrinogen in platelet function in vivo and in vitro. In fact, not only the fibrinogen present in plasma but also that stored in platelet α granules is essential for aggregation of platelets.[38] In ligand-binding experiments, approximately 40,000 to 50,000 molecules of ^{125}I-labeled fibrinogen bound to each thrombin- or ADP-stimulated platelet.

The main role of platelet agonists such as ADP, thrombin, and epinephrine is to activate receptors for fibrinogen on the platelet membrane,[5] converting them from the nonbinding to binding mode and enabling platelet aggregation to begin. As a result, dimeric fibrinogen molecules bind to activated receptors and link together two platelets, which are then joined by more platelets through a snowball effect to produce an aggregate composed of 10 or more platelets. The platelet receptor for fibrinogen is made up of a complex of two membrane glycoproteins, denoted glycoprotein IIb-IIIa, which belong to the integrin β_3 family; the complex is coded $\alpha_{IIb}\beta_3$. The genes for glycoprotein IIb-IIIa have been cloned, and the amino acid sequences of both glycoproteins have been deduced.[39] The $\alpha_{IIb}\beta_3$ complex is defective in patients with Glanzmann's thrombasthenia, a genetically determined bleeding disorder in which platelets do not bind fibrinogen and do not aggregate.[39] Monoclonal antibodies against the glycoprotein IIb-IIIa complex can induce a thrombasthenic-like state by blocking the binding of fibrinogen to human platelets.[40]

Structure-Function of Fibrinogen

Until the early 1980s, the location of the region on the fibrinogen molecule responsible for interaction with the exposed platelet receptor was unknown. Human fibrinogen is composed of three pairs of nonidentical chains (α, β, and γ) that are linked by a series of disulfide bonds and arranged in three main structural domains, one central E and two distal D; this complex structure posed a significant challenge to unraveling the structure-function relationship of fibrinogen.[41] The essential role of the γ chain in the interaction of human fibrinogen with activated platelet receptors has been established, and the C-terminal sequence of the γ chain, HHLGGAKQAGDV, encompassing residues 400 to 411, was pinpointed by my research group as the platelet receptor recognition site.[42,43] This site, so far not identified on other adhesive proteins, confers ligand specificity on human fibrinogen. Findings from our studies on truncated fibrinogen peptides were corroborated by studies with a series of analogues containing replacements for residues deleted in previous experiments.[44]

Further support for the essential role of the C-terminal segment of the fibrinogen γ chain in interactions with platelets came from studies of two natural fibrinogen variants with distinctive γ-chain ends resulting from alternative splicing.[41] The platelet receptor recognition site occurs in the predominant variant of the fibrinogen γ chain. A minor γ-chain species, the variant γ', has an elongated and highly charged sequence, and its ability to interact with platelets is diminished.[45] This variant does not occur in the platelet pool of fibrinogen.

The powerful application of molecular biology in the elegant series of experiments conducted by Earl Davie's group on the γ chain of recombinant human fibrinogen reaffirmed the essential role of the C-terminal end of the

γ chain of human fibrinogen in interactions with receptors on ADP-stimulated platelets.[46] Moreover, mutagenesis experiments incisively disproved the functional significance of the two RGD sequence motifs on the α chain of human fibrinogen in mediating platelet aggregation. What really matters in the fibrinogen-platelet interaction is the presence of two sticky ends made of the C-terminal segments of the two γ chains [*see Figure 5*]. The geometric arrangement of these tight linkages apparently involves a parallel, rather than perpendicular, orientation to the plane of the platelet membrane. Because the gaps between platelets in the closely packed aggregate in vivo are 100 to 300 Å wide,[47] a parallel orientation seems more consistent with the dimensions of fibrinogen.[48] Either way, parallel or perpendicular, each half of the fibrinogen molecule is endowed with one domain able to interact with platelet receptors, thus fulfilling the bivalency requirement for linking two platelets together, which is necessary for formation of platelet aggregates. Electron microscopic analysis of the topology of fibrinogen domains interacting with isolated glycoprotein IIb-IIIa complex indicates that one fibrinogen molecule can interact with two glycoprotein IIb-IIIa complexes.[49] With two contact points provided by one fibrinogen molecule, receptors on platelets can be ligated by fibrinogen in both *trans* (fibrinogen molecule bridging two platelets) and *cis* (fibrinogen bound to receptors on the same platelet) interactions [*see Figure 5*].

Finally, fibrinogen bound to platelet receptors can be the target for three enzymes that modify its properties: thrombin, factor XIIIa, and plasmin. Thrombin transforms fibrinogen into fibrin, and factor XIIIa, activated by thrombin, cross-links fibrin at its adhesive ends on the γ chain or through other sites on the α chain.[50] The molecular bridges made by fibrinogen's linking platelets together are thus transformed into tightly cross-linked fibrin scaffolding less prone to disruption by plasmin generated in response to endogenous plasminogen activators or infusion of exogenous thrombolytic agents (i.e., streptokinase or tissue-type plasminogen activator).

Interaction of Fibrinogen with Platelet Receptors

The search for complementary binding sites on the platelet $\alpha_{IIb}\beta_3$ that interact with the γ chain of human fibrinogen took a cross-linking approach with radiolabeled synthetic peptides. As a result, a binding site was localized between residues 294 and 314 of glycoprotein IIb (α_{IIb} integrin). A synthetic peptide analogue of this site corresponding to residues 296 to 306 was inhibitory when tested in ^{125}I-fibrinogen binding and platelet aggregation assays.[51]

Although the RGD-containing sequences on the α chain of human fibrinogen are not required for its interaction with platelet receptors,[46] the site in β_3 integrin between residues 109 and 171 does interact with RGD peptides.[52] A point mutation within this site (Asp^{119}→Tyr) results in a loss of binding of fibrinogen in the Cam variant of Glanzmann's thrombasthenia.[53] Apparently, this site influences the binding function of the glycoprotein IIb site that interacts with γ chain peptides.

The central mechanism controlling the binding of fibrinogen to its platelet receptor is the platelet's shift from the nonbinding to the binding mode. Fibrinogen is abundantly available in plasma at all times but cannot reach platelet receptors without a signal generated by vascular injury. It appears that activation of platelets with ADP and thrombin opens the gate composed of the regulatory sites on glycoprotein IIIa that in resting platelets prevent access of bulky fibrinogen to its binding site(s) on glycoprotein IIb (α_{IIb}).[5] Experimentally, it was possible to cleave portions of glycoprotein IIIa, and possibly glycoprotein IIb, with proteolytic enzymes and thereby allow fibrinogen to bind to its platelet receptor without a need for ADP-mediated activation.[54]

The negative regulation of the fibrinogen receptor involves cAMP- or cGMP-mediated reactions. An increase in levels of cAMP induced by prostacyclin or of the nonprostanoid forskolin correlates with inhibition of binding of fibrinogen and vWF to activated platelets, which is paralleled by inhibition of platelet aggregation.[5,19] Infusion of prostacyclin in humans slows the formation of a hemostatic plug, as measured by bleeding time.[55] Prostacyclin also reduces the adhesive interaction of platelets with artificial surfaces. The rise of cGMP levels induced by nitric oxide–generating compounds also exerts negative regulation on the fibrinogen receptor.[56]

In some patients with afibrinogenemia, the formation of platelet thrombi appears to be normal, suggesting that other proteins substitute for the missing fibrinogen in achieving platelet aggregation. Our studies indicated that vWF binds to ADP-treated normal platelets and mediates their aggregation.[57] In vitro aggregation of platelet-rich plasma from afibrinogenemic patients has been reported to depend on binding of vWF to platelet membrane glycoproteins IIb and IIIa.[58] Thus, platelet aggregates (thrombi) can

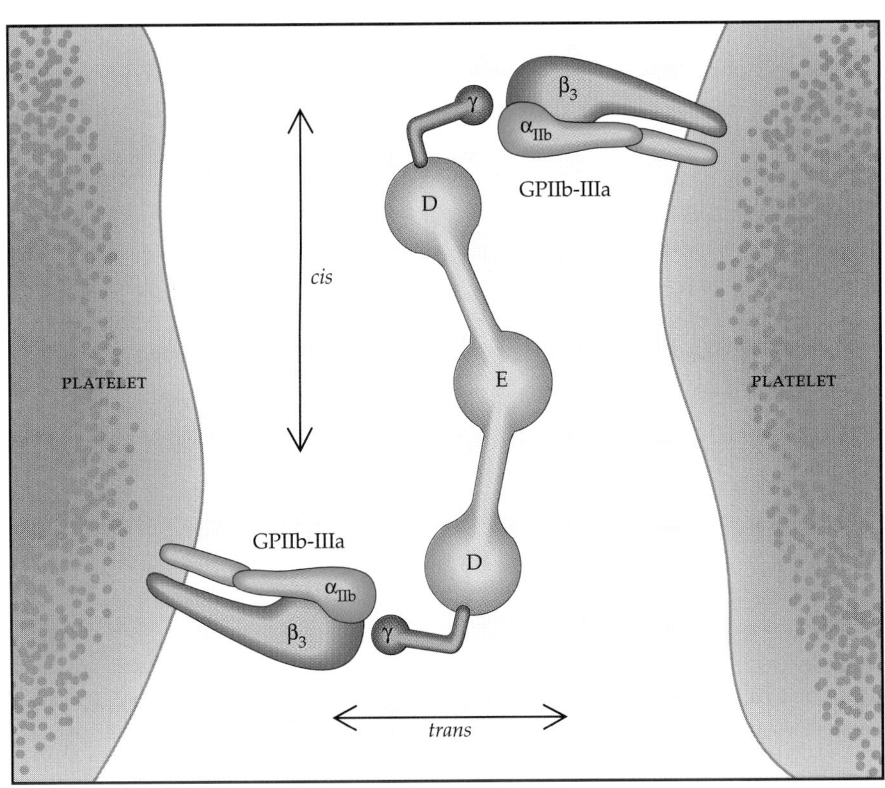

Figure 5 *The molecular bridging of receptors on two platelets by fibrinogen. Sticky ends of fibrinogen located in the C-terminal domain of the γ chain interact with the α_{IIb} subunit of glycoprotein IIb-IIIa (GPIIb-IIIa) on two adjoining platelets, engaging fibrinogen in* trans *interaction. Alternatively, fibrinogen may bind to two neighboring receptors on the same platelet, engaging them in* cis *interaction. Fibrinogen is depicted as a trinodular structure observed in electron microscopy as having two globular D domains and one central E domain. The γ chain segment recognizing the platelet receptor has the sequence His-His-Leu-Gly-Gly-Ala-Lys-Gln-Ala-Gly-Asp-Val.*

be formed in vitro in a fibrinogenemic plasma or in vivo in patients with congenital afibrinogenemia and acquired hypofibrinogenemia. This finding means that during thrombolytic therapy, when fibrinogen levels are low, the alternative mechanism of platelet aggregation mediated by vWF can be operational and may contribute to early rethrombosis.

Pathological platelet thrombi can form in response to shear stress in small arteries and arterioles that are narrowed by atherosclerosis or vascular spasm. Unusually large vWF multimers derived from stressed endothelial cells are exceptionally effective in mediating shear-induced platelet aggregation.[18] Aspirin does not inhibit shear-induced platelet aggregation, indicating that aspirin-insensitive pathways of platelet stimulation are operational in binding large vWF forms to platelets stressed by shear forces.[59]

Aspirin Inhibition of Signal-Transducing Pathways

Soon after the development of the in vitro platelet aggregation method to study platelet function, three groups of investigators independently reported that aspirin inhibits aggregation.[60-62] Subsequently, Vane[63] and Smith and Willis[64] demonstrated that aspirin blocks platelet synthesis of prostaglandin. Cyclo-oxygenase, the key signal transducer in the arachidonic acid pathway of platelet stimulation, is the target for irreversible inhibition by aspirin [*see Figure 4*].[65]

In the Veterans Administration Cooperative Study, aspirin treatment reduced the rates of acute myocardial infarction and death in men with unstable angina.[66] The United States Physicians' Health Study thrust aspirin into the mainstream of preventive antithrombotic therapy by demonstrating that it is effective in the primary prevention of heart attacks in men.[67] In the Second International Study of Infarct Survival (ISIS-2) trial, aspirin was shown to reduce mortality and reinfarction rates in patients with acute myocardial infarction treated with the thrombolytic agent streptokinase.[68] However, the observation that aspirin is only 48 to 50 percent effective in preventing strokes and heart attacks can be attributed to the fact that aspirin-induced blockade of cyclo-oxygenase is not sufficient for ablation of thrombus (aggregate) formation when the potency of the agonist (e.g., thrombin or collagen) is high. Highly potent agonists can induce other pathways of platelet activation.

Platelet Receptor Blockade and the New Generation of Antiplatelet Drugs

Elucidation of the molecular mechanism by which fibrinogen recognizes platelet receptors led to a new approach to prevent platelet thrombi. This approach gained in significance because it is based on inhibition of the final step in a sequence of events leading to the binding of fibrinogen to platelet integrin receptors. Irrespective of the agonists stimulating signal-transducing pathways in platelets, the induction of fibrinogen binding to platelet receptors constitutes the common step. The blockade of fibrinogen receptors is therefore the logical way to prevent platelet thrombi from forming.

Synthetic peptide analogues of platelet receptor recognition domains on human fibrinogen and antibodies against the fibrinogen receptor inhibit platelet-adhesive receptors no matter which agonists are involved with platelet activation pathways.[20,40] Synthetic peptides simply occupy the exposed binding sites on the platelet glycoprotein IIb-IIIa complex for fibrinogen, vWF, and other adhesive proteins. Thus, identification of the C-terminal segment of the γ chain of human fibrinogen as a domain responsible for its interaction with receptors on activated platelets resulted in the development of analogues of the native sequence encompassing residues γ 400 to 411 and in the application of an antipeptide antibody against γ 385–411.[43] Alternatively, RGD peptides representing a sequence of the cell adhesion site of fibronectin can also inhibit binding of fibrinogen to platelet integrin $\alpha_{IIb}\beta_3$.[25]

Current evidence indicates that the peptide γ 400–411 can reversibly inhibit the formation of a hemostatic plug in rabbit mesenteric artery.[44] In ex vivo experiments using whole human blood pumped through a Baumgartner chamber at controlled flow conditions, the synthetic peptide γ 400–411 and peptide RGDS completely inhibited platelet thrombus formation.[69] The antibody against the C-terminal domain of the γ chain of human fibrinogen is also effective in blocking the interaction of human platelets with fibrinogen absorbed to a synthetic polymer surface, whereas several monoclonal antibodies directed toward other epitopes of human fibrinogen were less inhibitory or without effect.[70]

The γ-chain sequence used for the design of a new class of platelet-adhesive receptor blockers is selective for the integrin $\alpha_{IIb}\beta_3$ on activated platelets.[5] The dodecapeptide γ 400–411, which has a sequence unique for fibrinogen, did not cause any measurable effect on the integrity of human endothelial cell monolayers (detachment or attachment) in vitro.[71] In contrast, peptides containing the RGDS sequence caused detachment of human endothelial cells from the extracellular matrix.[27,71] The inhibitory effect of tetrapeptide RGDS on the adhesive receptors in endothelial cells may have detrimental consequences on the integrity of the vascular endothelium in vivo, and thus, endothelial healing in the zone of vascular injury following thrombolysis or angioplasty may be interrupted. Recently, natural peptides containing the RGD sequence were identified in several snake venoms, such as those of the green tree viper (trigramin) and the viper *Echis carinatus* (echistatin). These naturally occurring proteins, denoted disintegrins, blocked platelet integrin $\alpha_{IIb}\beta_3$ in vitro and the formation of platelet thrombi in rat mesenteric artery.[72] Their effect on endothelial cells is unclear.

A series of monoclonal antibodies against the glycoprotein IIb-IIIa complex of platelet membrane (e.g., 7E3) has been developed.[40] These antibodies interfere with platelet spreading and thrombus formation ex vivo and with platelet-mediated occlusion of coronary arteries in dogs and Dacron vascular grafts in baboons.[73,74] They have been tested in human phase III clinical trials for the prevention of thrombosis after angioplasty.[75] The limit on repeated use of these antibodies and their observed in vitro effect on the detachment of endothelial cells indicate the need for developing synthetic integrin blockers that are more platelet selective.

Such peptides and nonpeptide mimetics will constitute a new generation of antithrombotic agents.

Synthetic peptides and monoclonal antibodies that block platelet integrin receptors irrespective of the agonist-induced pathways of platelet activation offer a new approach to antithrombotic therapy. Nevertheless, antithrombotic therapy can influence the physiologically important hemostatic mechanisms that seal off the breaks in the vasculature. Thus, the targeting of new therapeutic agents to thrombi associated with atherosclerotic plaques in occluded arteries will ultimately lead to effective methods for the treatment and prevention of thrombosis and rethrombosis.

References

1. Fuster V, Stein B, Ambrose JA, et al: Atherosclerotic plaque rupture and thrombosis: evolving concepts. *Circulation* 82(suppl II):II-47, 1990
2. American Heart Association: *Health and Stroke Facts: 1994 Statistical Supplement*. American Heart Association, Dallas, 1993
3. Davies MJ, Thomas A: Thrombosis and acute coronary-artery lesions in sudden cardiac ischemic death. *N Engl J Med* 310:1137, 1984
4. Lange RA, Willard JE, Hillis LD: Southwestern Internal Medicine Conference: restenosis: the Achilles heel of coronary angioplasty. *Am J Med Sci* 306:265, 1993
5. Hawiger J: Adhesive interactions of blood cells and the vascular wall. *Hemostasis and Thrombosis: Basic Principles and Clinical Practice*, 3rd ed. Colman RW, Hirsh J, Marder VJ, et al, Eds. J.B. Lippincott Co., Philadelphia, 1994, p 762
6. Sakariassen KS, Muggli R, Baumgartner HR: Measurement of platelet interaction with components of the vessel wall in flowing blood. *Methods Enzymol* 169:37, 1989
7. Kroll MH, Harris TS, Moake JL, et al: Von Willebrand factor binding to platelet GPIb initiates signals for platelet activation. *J Clin Invest* 88:1568, 1991
8. Jang I-K, Gold HK, Ziskind AA, et al: Differential sensitivity of erythrocyte-rich and platelet-rich arterial thrombi to lysis with recombinant tissue-type plasminogen activator: a possible explanation for resistance to coronary thrombolysis. *Circulation* 79:920, 1989
9. Hawiger J: Repertoire of platelet receptors. *Methods Enzymol* 215:131, 1992
10. Banga HS, Simons ER, Brass LF, et al: Activation of phospholipases A and C in human platelets exposed to epinephrine: role of glycoproteins IIb/IIIa and dual role of epinephrine. *Proc Natl Acad Sci USA* 83:9197, 1986
11. Cusack NJ, Hourani SM: Subtypes of P_2 purinoceptors: studies using analogues of ATP. *Ann NY Acad Sci* 603:172, 1990
12. Hynes RO: Integrins: versatility, modulation and signaling in cell adhesion. *Cell* 68:11, 1992
13. Cheresh DA, Berliner SA, Vincente V, et al: Recognition of distinct adhesive sites on fibrinogen by related integrins on platelets and endothelial cells. *Cell* 58:945, 1989
14. Weiss HJ, Turitto VT, Baumgartner HR: Effect of shear rate on platelet interaction with subendothelium in citrated and native blood: I. Shear-dependent decrease of adhesion in von Willebrand's disease and the Bernard-Soulier syndrome. *J Lab Clin Med* 92:750, 1978
15. Lopez JA, Chung DW, Fujikawa K, et al: Cloning of the α chain of human platelet glycoprotein Ib: a transmembrane protein with homology to leucine-rich α 2-glycoprotein. *Proc Natl Acad Sci USA* 84:5615, 1987
16. Sadler JE, Shelton-Inloes BB, Sorace JM, et al: Cloning and characterization of two cDNAs coding for human von Willebrand factor. *Proc Natl Acad Sci USA* 82:6394, 1985
17. Loscalzo J, Inbal A, Handin RI: Von Willebrand protein facilitates platelet incorporation in polymerizing fibrin. *J Clin Invest* 78:1112, 1986
18. Moake JL, Turner NA, Stathopoulos NA, et al: Involvement of large plasma von Willebrand factor (vWF) multimers and unusually large vWF forms derived from endothelial cells in shear stress-induced platelet aggregation. *J Clin Invest* 78:1456, 1986
19. Fujimoto T, Ohara S, Hawiger J: Thrombin-induced exposure and prostacyclin inhibition of the receptor for factor VIII/von Willebrand factor on human platelets. *J Clin Invest* 69:1212, 1982

20. Timmons S, Kloczewiak M, Hawiger J: ADP-dependent common receptor mechanism for binding of von Willebrand factor and fibrinogen to human platelets. *Proc Natl Acad Sci USA* 81:4935, 1984
21. Ruggeri ZM, Bader R, de Marco L: Glanzmann thrombasthenia: deficient binding of von Willebrand factor to thrombin-stimulated platelets. *Proc Natl Acad Sci USA* 79:6038, 1982
22. Hemler ME, Crouse C, Takada Y, et al: Multiple very late antigen (VLA) heterodimers on platelets: evidence for distinct VLA-2, VLA-5 (fibronectin receptor) and VLA-6 structures. *J Biol Chem* 263:7660, 1988
23. Santoro SA: Identification of a 160,000 dalton platelet membrane protein that mediates the initial divalent cation-dependent adhesion of platelets to collagen. *Cell* 46:913, 1986
24. Hynes RO, Yamada KM: Fibronectins: multifunctional modular glycoproteins. *J Cell Biol* 95:369, 1982
25. Ruoslahti E, Pierschbacher MD: New perspectives in cell adhesion: RGD and integrins. *Science* 238:491, 1987
26. Piotrowicz RS, Orchekowski RP, Nugent DJ, et al: Glycoprotein Ic-IIa functions as an activation-independent fibronectin receptor on human platelets. *J Cell Biol* 106:1359, 1988
27. Chen CS, Thiagarajan P, Schwartz SM, et al: The platelet glycoprotein IIb/IIIa-like protein in human endothelial cells promotes adhesion but not initial attachment to extracellular matrix. *J Cell Biol* 105:1885, 1987
28. Thiagarajan P, Kelly KL: Exposure of binding sites for vitronectin on platelets following stimulation. *J Biol Chem* 263:3035, 1988
29. Asch AS, Barnwell J, Silverstein RL, et al: Isolation of the thrombospondin membrane receptor. *J Clin Invest* 79:1054, 1987
30. Lawler J, Hynes RO: An integrin receptor on normal and thrombasthenic platelets that binds thrombospondin. *Blood* 74:2022, 1989
31. Ill CR, Engvall E, Ruoslahti E: Adhesion of platelets to laminin in the absence of activation. *J Cell Biol* 99:2140, 1984
32. Sonnenberg A, Modderman PW, Hogervorst F: Laminin receptor on platelets is the integrin VLA-6. *Nature* 336:487, 1988
33. Bellinger DA, Nichols TC, Read MS, et al: Prevention of occlusive coronary artery thrombosis by a murine monoclonal antibody to porcine von Willebrand factor. *Proc Natl Acad Sci USA* 84:8100, 1987
34. Hawiger J: Platelet secretory pathways: an overview. *Methods Enzymol* 169:191, 1989
35. White JG: Inherited abnormalities of the platelet membrane and secretory granules. *Hum Pathol* 18:123, 1987
36. Lin L-L, Wartmann M, Lin AY, et al: $cPLA_2$ is phosphorylated and activated by MAP kinase. *Cell* 72:269, 1993
37. Weiss HJ, Rogers J: Fibrinogen and platelets in the primary arrest of bleeding. *N Engl J Med* 285:369, 1971
38. Tollefsen DM, Majerus PW: Inhibition of human platelet aggregation by monovalent antifibrinogen antibody fragments. *J Clin Invest* 55:1259, 1975
39. Phillips DR, Charo IF, Parise LV, et al: The platelet membrane glycoprotein IIb-IIIa complex. *Blood* 71:831, 1988
40. Coller BS, Peerschke EI, Scudder LE, et al: A murine monoclonal antibody that completely blocks the binding of fibrinogen to platelets produces a thrombasthenic-like state in normal platelets and binds to glycoproteins IIb and/or IIIa. *J Clin Invest* 72:325, 1983
41. Doolittle RF: Fibrinogen and fibrin. *Annu Rev Biochem* 53:195, 1984
42. Hawiger J, Timmons S, Kloczewiak M, et al: Gamma and alpha chains of human fibrinogen possess sites reactive with human platelet receptors. *Proc Natl Acad Sci USA* 79:2068, 1982
43. Kloczewiak M, Timmons S, Lukas TJ, et al: Platelet receptor recognition site on human fibrinogen: synthesis and structure-function relationship of peptides corresponding to the carboxy-terminal segment of the gamma chain. *Biochemistry* 23:1767, 1984
44. Kloczewiak M, Timmons S, Bednarek MA, et al: Platelet receptor recognition domain on the gamma chain of human fibrinogen and its synthetic peptide analogues. *Biochemistry* 28:2915, 1989
45. Peerschke EIB, Francis CW, Marder VJ: Fibrinogen binding to human blood platelets: effect of γ chain carboxyterminal structure and length. *Blood* 67:385, 1986

46. Farrell DH, Thiagarajan P, Chung DW, et al: Role of fibrinogen α chain sites in platelet aggregation. *Proc Natl Acad Sci USA* 89:10729, 1992
47. Shirasawa K, Chandler AB: Fine structure of the bond between platelets in artificial thrombi and in platelet aggregates induced by adenosine diphosphate. *Am J Pathol* 57:127, 1969
48. Moon DG, Shainoff JR, Gonda SR: Electron microscopy of platelet interactions with heme-octapeptide-labeled fibrinogen. *Am J Physiol* 259(pt 4):C611, 1990
49. Weisel JW, Nagaswami C, Vilaire G, et al: Examination of the platelet membrane glycoprotein IIb-IIIa complex and its interaction with fibrinogen and other ligands by electron microscopy. *J Biol Chem* 267:16637, 1992
50. Cottrell BA, Strong DD, Watt KWK, et al: Amino acid sequence studies on the α-chain of human fibrinogen: exact location of cross-linking acceptor sites. *Biochemistry* 18:5405, 1979
51. D'Souza SE, Ginsberg MH, Matsueda GR, et al: A discrete sequence in a platelet integrin is involved in ligand recognition. *Nature* 350:66, 1991
52. D'Souza SE, Ginsberg MH, Burke TA, et al: Localization of an Arg-Gly-Asp recognition site within an integrin adhesion receptor. *Science* 242:91, 1988
53. Loftus JC, O'Toole TE, Plow EF, et al: A β_3 integrin mutation abolishes ligand binding and alters divalent cation-dependent conformation. *Science* 249:915, 1990
54. Niewiarowski S, Budzynski AZ, Morinelli TA, et al: Exposure of fibrinogen receptor on human platelets by proteolytic enzymes. *J Biol Chem* 256:917, 1981
55. FitzGerald GA, Friedman LA, Miyamori I, et al: A double blind placebo controlled crossover study of prostacyclin in man. *Life Sci* 25:665, 1979
56. Mendelsohn ME, O'Neill S, George D, et al: Inhibition of fibrinogen binding to human platelets by S-nitroso-*N*-acetylcysteine. *J Biol Chem* 265:19028, 1990
57. Fujimoto T, Hawiger J: Adenosine diphosphate induces binding of von Willebrand factor to human platelets. *Nature* 297:154, 1982
58. De Marco L, Girolami A, Zimmerman TS, et al: Von Willebrand factor interaction with the glycoprotein IIb/IIIa complex: its role in platelet function as demonstrated in patients with congenital afibrinogenemia. *J Clin Invest* 77:1272, 1986
59. Moake JL, Turner NA, Stathopoulos NA, et al: Shear-induced platelet aggregation can be mediated by vWF released from platelets, as well as by exogenous large or unusually large vWF multimers, requires adenosine diphosphate, and is resistant to aspirin. *Blood* 71:1366, 1988
60. Weiss HJ, Aledort LM: Impaired platelet connective tissue reaction in man after aspirin ingestion. *Lancet* ii:495, 1967
61. Evans G, Packham MA, Nishizawa EE, et al: The effect of acetylsalicylic acid on platelet function. *J Exp Med* 128:877, 1968
62. Zucker MB, Peterson J: Inhibition of adenosine diphosphate-induced secondary aggregation and other platelet functions by acetylsalicylic acid ingestion. *Proc Soc Exp Biol Med* 127:547, 1968
63. Vane JR: Inhibition of prostaglandin synthesis as a mechanism of action for aspirin-like drugs. *Nature* [*New Biol*] 231:232, 1971
64. Smith JB, Willis AL: Aspirin selectively inhibits prostaglandin production in human platelets. *Nature [New Biol]* 231:235, 1971
65. Roth GJ, Majerus PW: The mechanism of the effect of aspirin on human platelets: I. Acetylation of a particular fraction protein. *J Clin Invest* 56:624, 1975
66. Lewis HD Jr, Davis JW, Archibald DG, et al: Protective effects of aspirin against acute myocardial infarction and death in men with unstable angina: results of Veterans Administration cooperative study. *N Engl J Med* 309:396, 1983
67. Steering Committee of the Physicians' Health Study Research Group: Final report on the aspirin component of the ongoing Physicians' Health Study. *N Engl J Med* 321:129, 1989
68. ISIS-2 (Second International Study of Infarct Survival) Collaborative Group: Randomised trial of intravenous streptokinase, oral aspirin, or both, or neither among 17187 cases of suspected myocardial infarction: ISIS-2. *Lancet* ii:349, 1988
69. Weiss HJ, Hawiger J, Ruggeri ZM, et al: Fibrinogen-independent platelet adhesion and thrombus formation on subendothelium mediated by glycoprotein IIb-IIIa complex at high shear rate. *J Clin Invest* 83:288, 1989
70. Shiba E, Lindon JN, Kushner L, et al: Antibody-detectable changes in fibrinogen adsorption affecting platelet activation on polymer surfaces. *Am J Physiol* 260:C965, 1991
71. Chen CS, Hawiger J: Reactivity of synthetic peptide analogs of adhesive proteins in regard to the interaction of human endothelial cells with extracellular matrix. *Blood* 77:2200, 1991

72. Gould RJ, Polokoff MA, Friedman PA, et al: Disintegrins: a family of integrin inhibitory proteins from viper venoms. *Proc Soc Exp Biol Med* 195:168, 1990
73. Yasuda T, Gold HK, Fallon JT, et al: Monoclonal antibody against the platelet glycoprotein (GP) IIb/IIIa receptor prevents coronary artery reocclusion after reperfusion with recombinant tissue-type plasminogen activator in dogs. *J Clin Invest* 81:1284, 1988
74. Hanson SR, Pareti FI, Ruggeri ZM, et al: Effects of monoclonal antibodies against the platelet glycoprotein IIb/IIIa complex on thrombosis and hemostasis in the baboon. *J Clin Invest* 81:149, 1988
75. Kleiman NS, Ohman EM, Califf RM, et al: Profound inhibition of platelet aggregation with monoclonal antibody 7E3 Fab after thrombolytic therapy: results of the Thrombolysis and Angioplasty in Myocardial Infarction (TAMI) 8 pilot study. *J Am Coll Cardiol* 22:381, 1993

Acknowledgments

Studies conducted in our laboratory and described in this chapter were supported by grants HL-30648 and HL-33014 from the National Heart, Lung, and Blood Institute. The assistance of Carol Walter in the preparation of this manuscript and Edna Kunkel in drawing the illustrations are acknowledged. Many laboratories have contributed to the remarkable progress encompassing the field of platelets and the vascular wall. The author regrets that several original references had to be omitted from this text due to constraints of space.

Figures 1, 2, 3, 5 Edna Kunkle. Adapted by Dimitry Schidlovsky.

Figure 4 Edna Kunkle. Adapted by Dana Burns-Pizer.

CHAPTER 12

Molecular Mechanisms of Cardiac Hypertrophy

Radovan Zak, Ph.D.

One characteristic of the growth process that accompanies ontogeny is the precise size relationship between the whole and its parts that results in predictable ratios of organ to body size. The functional load placed on an organ clearly plays an important role in determining its proper size, as has been shown in animal experiments and clinical studies. Thus, sustained use of a muscle that exceeds its normal work load leads to its enlargement, whereas its disuse leads to atrophy. Similarly, the loss of one kidney is functionally compensated by the enlargement of the other one.

The relationship between functional load and organ size can also be noticed during evolution, because the size of the heart depends on the degree of exertion associated with the life-style of an animal. Moreover, domestication resulting in sedentary life or breeding for speed is accompanied by appropriate changes in heart size.[1] However, it should be recognized that during development, the growth of organs is regulated even before their function becomes fully established. The functional demand then must be viewed as modulating this basic growth rate so that the final size of the organ will be above a genetically determined minimum. This chapter describes some of the characteristics of cardiac growth induced by hemodynamic demands and analyzes how these demands are translated into the language of mechanisms that regulate genes.

Relationship Between Heart Growth and Hemodynamic Load

The paramount need for the proper rate of systemic circulation is met by the heart's ability to adapt promptly to acutely as well as chronically altered hemodynamic demands. On a short-term basis, the heart is able to cope with the altered load by its ability to change the perfusion pressure via the Frank-Starling mechanism. When the change in load is repeated or long-lasting, either because of a different pattern of physical activity or because of pathological changes in the cardiovascular system, a second mechanism becomes activated, resulting in altered activities of genes that eventually adjust the heart size to new demands.

Changes in Heart Size Due to Altered Load

Although this chapter focuses on cardiac hypertrophy, it is safe to assume that the reduction of cardiac size seen during decreased hemodynamic load represents similar regulatory phenomena. Many models of cardiac hypertrophy have been developed,[2] each having unique advantages as well as drawbacks that must be carefully examined depending on the nature of the intended study. Of particular concern should be the necrotic changes of the heart that accompany most models of acute cardiac overload. These necrotic changes might lead not only to temporal disorganization of cellular structures but also to proliferation of connective tissue cells with consequent accumulation of collagen. The increase of nonmuscle cells should be considered whenever nuclear activities are to be studied.

The available animal models of cardiac hypertrophy include increased pressure overload, such as aortic or pulmonary artery stenosis, or renal hypertension.[2] Volume overload can be produced by surgical procedures eliciting aortic insufficiency or arteriovenous fistula as well as by nonsurgical techniques such as iron deficiency anemia or pacing bradycardia. Models of multiple causes of overload include hyperthyroidism, carbon monoxide exposure, simulated high altitude, administration of catecholamines, and enforced exercise. Moreover, there are several genetic models of heart overload, including spontaneously hypertensive salt-sensitive rats and cardiomyopathic hamsters. Recently, transgenic models of hypertrophy have been introduced that include lines carrying mouse-protamine-1–simian virus 40 (SV40) T antigen or atrial natriuretic factor–SV40 T antigen constructs that develop SV40-specific rhabdomyosarcoma in the right atrium. In addition, heart enlargement caused by cell hyperplasia was described with c-*myc* as a transgene.[3] Advancement in microsurgery has made it possible to produce stable pressure overload in mice, which offers the possibility to examine the expression of specific transgenes in overloaded hearts.[3] However, one should remember that cardiac dynamics in the mouse heart, with its 600 beats/min, is likely to differ from that in larger species, especially humans, with their much slower heart rates.

As in vitro models of altered cardiac growth, retrograde perfusion of nonworking as well as working isolated hearts has been used. Moreover, hypertrophy of isolated cells in cultures has been studied using cells derived from hearts of neonatal and adult animals. These studies have been especially useful in determining the role of humoral factors and of mechanical loading, whether in the form of passive stretch or actively developed isometric tension.[2]

Cellular Features of Cardiac Growth

Normal myocardial tissue can be viewed as comprising two cell types: cardiomyocytes of the contractile compartment, which form the bulk of tissue protein, and cells of the support compartment, which include smooth muscle cells as well as nonmyocytes such as endothelial cells and fibroblasts (which contribute two thirds of the heart tissue nuclei). In an evaluation of the cellular features of cardiac growth, it must be remembered that the proliferative characteristics of individual cell types differ markedly. Moreover, it appears that cross signaling between cardiomyocytes and nonmuscle cells is likely to play an important role in growth regulation.[4] Studies of isolated, purified cell populations thus must be viewed as providing only a partial insight into the growth process.

The cellular basis of cardiac enlargement involves the hypertrophy of existing cardiomyocytes as well as their proliferation (hyperplasia).[1] The relative contribution of these processes changes with the age of the animal, with cellular hypertrophy taking place mainly in the adult. The trend of decreasing rate in myocyte proliferation is clearly noticeable in the late fetal period, so that at birth only two percent of cells are still dividing in the rat heart and at three postnatal weeks, less than one percent of cells show mitosis. On the other hand, the timing of the loss of proliferative potential differs between species, in humans occurring substantially later than in small laboratory animals.

The mitotic activity of cardiomyocytes is, in general, reflected in the rate of labeled thymidine incorporation into DNA and in the activity of DNA polymerase. However, these measures of DNA synthesis cannot be automatically equaled with hyperplasia, because DNA synthesis could be caused by multinucleation, increased DNA content of nuclei (polyploidy), and DNA repair. Additional markers of cell proliferation are to be used to make the assessment of mitotic activity more accurate. Several such markers have become available and include proliferating cell nuclear antigen (PCNA, cyclin), which is a DNA polymerase-δ auxiliary protein expressed only within the G_1–S phases of the mitotic cycle and is absent in nondividing cells.[5] In the heart, PCNA is detectable only in myocytes of prenatal and early postnatal rats and is absent in the adult heart. Despite the great promise of these new approaches to evaluate a cell's mitotic activity, their rigorous validation in terms of the actual cell number in the heart still has to be done.

Present data indicate that the imposition of work overload on the heart produces cellular responses that depend on the extent of ongoing DNA synthesis.[2] Thus, in neonatal animals in which thymidine labeling is relatively high, cardiac enlargement takes place through cell proliferation as well as hypertrophy of existing myocytes. In contrast, in the adult animal only hypertrophy occurs, and indication of cell division is seen only when the overload is prolonged. The occurrence of cell death and damage, however, complicates interpretation of these experiments. Nevertheless, it is safe to conclude that no sharp or absolute demarcation exists between the stages when cells synthesize DNA and when they do not. Thus, in humans and other large animals, DNA synthesis leading to polyploidy is common even at the age when the hearts are mitotically quiescent. Moreover, growth factors and tumor-promoting agents are able to stimulate DNA synthesis in cultures of nonproliferating myocytes derived from hearts of adult rats.

Hemodynamic Load as a Determinant of Cardiac Phenotype

The changes in hemodynamic load of the heart result not only in the altered overall rate of organ growth but also in phenotypic changes. Thus, the compensatory growth reflects the change in the rate of genes expressed as well as the reprogramming of their repertoire [*see Figure 1*], resulting in an enlarged organ and also altered phenotype and hence changed properties of the heart. The molecular basis for these changes resides in the polymorphism of proteins constituting the cardiac cell. With few exceptions, these proteins exist as a family of closely related proteins called isoforms.[2] Individual members of a given family show slight divergence in amino acid sequence, with resulting difference in properties between isoforms. In the overloaded heart, it is not uncommon to see one isoform replacing the other. Therefore, in an evaluation of the growth process, the expression of individual genes must be evaluated in addition to the sum of all gene products. Besides the switches in isoform expression, the properties of the overloaded heart can also be altered via discoordinated expression of a set of genes encoding individual organelles, such as the changed mitochondrial to myofibrillar ratio, which might have a profound effect on energy supply and demand.

Phenotypic Transitions Due to Altered Load

Almost all proteins constituting myocardial cells that have been investigated in some detail have been found to belong to isoform families ranging in size from two, such as the troponin C family, to at least eight, such as the myosin heavy chains. In some isoform families, this diversity is generated by the expression of different genes, as in the troponin C family and myosin heavy chains. In other instances, this diversity is achieved by alternative splicing of gene transcripts, as seen in

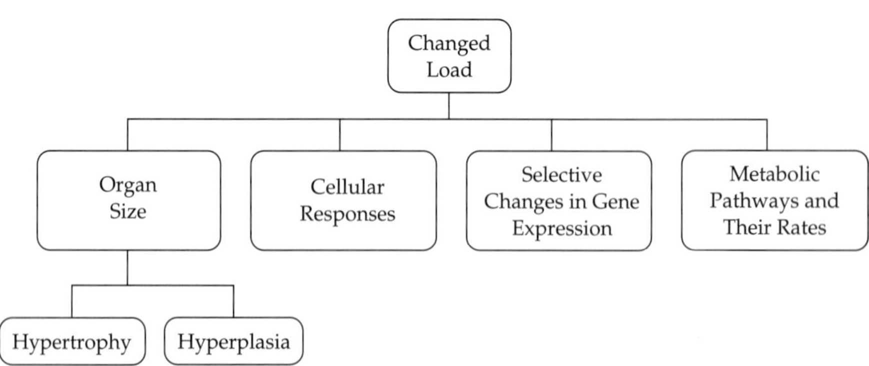

Figure 1 *Adaptive options of the heart during functional overload. The heart might respond to increased work load by increasing its size through enlargement of existing myocytes (hypertrophy) or by increasing their number (hyperplasia). Various subsets of genes might be modulated so that the ratios of cellular constituents might change. In addition, by selective regulation of specific genes, the isoform composition of the heart changes. Consequently, the product of adaptive growth is not only an enlarged heart but also a heart of altered phenotype and, hence, changed properties.*

families of tropomyosin or troponin T. From a pool of all the isoforms, only a subset is expressed at any given time, depending on the developmental, metabolic, and functional state of the heart.

MYOFIBRILLAR PROTEINS

Myosin isoforms (isomyosins) in the heart have been studied extensively.[2] Their multiplicity arises from the association between α and β cardiac myosin heavy chains, products of two separate genes that form two homodimers and one heterodimer. The myosin heavy chains in the atria and ventricles are indistinguishable by amino acid sequence and by complimentary DNA analysis. In contrast, the two classes of light chains, myosin light chain–1 and –2, differ between atria and ventricles. Consequently, there are two subfamilies of cardiac myosins: ventricular and atrial. The ventricular isoforms have been investigated most thoroughly, partly because they are easily distinguishable by electrophoresis in the native state. Various models of cardiac hypertrophy have shown the redistribution of isomyosins in favor of the β homodimer (V3 isomyosin). Enforced exercise of both normal and hypertensive animals resulted in isomyosin shift toward the α homodimer (V1). Changes in human hearts during hemodynamic overload have also been investigated, and the results are, in general, similar to those found in animal studies. The repression of α cardiac myosin heavy chain by increased work load was noticed in patients with stenosis and insufficiency of the mitral valve. However, human hearts, like hearts from any species of large body size, differ from those of small laboratory animals. For example, in rats the α cardiac myosin heavy chain constitutes close to 90 percent of total cardiac myosin heavy chains, whereas in humans it constitutes only 10 percent. This most likely reflects differences in basal metabolic rates and heart rates seen in animals of different body sizes.

In models in which the hemodynamic load is altered by manipulation of the thyroid state, the results differ from those already described. The hyperthyroidism induces the expression of α cardiac myosin heavy chain and reciprocal down-regulation of β cardiac myosin heavy chain, whereas hypothyroidism produces opposite changes. Although the action of thyroid hormone on the heart undoubtedly has a peripheral component caused by the increased oxygen utilization, its effect on the expression of myosin heavy chains can be demonstrated under nonworking conditions. Thus, the reciprocal changes in α cardiac myosin heavy-chain and β cardiac myosin heavy-chain expression were demonstrated in cultured myocytes and in "empty" beating heterotransplanted heart.[6] The action of thyroid hormone on cardiac myosin heavy-chain expression is a direct one because a thyroid-responsive element has been identified in the 5′ region of the α cardiac myosin heavy-chain gene. The effect of thyroid hormone is mediated through binding to a nuclear *trans*-activating factor, identified as thyroid receptor–α_1, that belongs to the steroid hormone and retinoic acid superfamily of DNA-binding proteins.[7]

The changes in myosin light-chain expression in hypertrophied hearts were also investigated, especially in humans.[8] Both atria and ventricles of fetal heart express myosin light chain–1 that is identical to that of skeletal muscles of the fetal stage. Postnatally, the ventricles completely repress this "embryonic/atrial" isoform, whereas the atria retain it during the entire life. In hearts with congenital malformation that result in increased work load, this postnatal repression of the embryonic/atrial myosin light chain–1 is delayed. Similarly, this myosin light chain appears in hearts with acquired valvular disease, and correction of the lesion leads to its repression.

Although myosin expression in the overloaded heart has been studied most extensively, other phenotypic markers also have been investigated [*see Table 1*]. It is evident that phenotypic transitions result in a substantial remodeling of all cellular compartments.[2,9]

Sarcoplasmic Reticulum

Several messenger RNAs (mRNAs) encoding components of sarcoplasmic reticulum, such as Ca^{2+}-adenosine triphosphatase (ATPase), ryanodine receptor, and phospholamban, are decreased in the late stage of hypertrophy and in failing hearts. Opposite changes take place in thyrotoxic hearts, whereas no change in either failing or thyrotoxic hearts was found for calse-

Table 1 Isoform Switches in Compensatory State of Hypertrophy

Constituent	*Change*	*mRNA*	*Protein*
Myofibrils			
α Cardiac myosin heavy chain	↓	+	+
β Cardiac myosin heavy chain	↑	+	+
Myosin light chain–1			
Embryonic/atrial	↑	+	+
Ventricular	↓		
α-Skeletal actin	0→	+	
β-Tropomyosin	0→	+	
Sarcoplasmic reticulum			
Ca^{2+}-ATPase, slow/cardiac (SERCA 2a)	↓	+	+
Ryanodine receptor (RYR 2)	↓	+	+
Phospholamban, slow/cardiac	↓	+	+
Na^+ - Ca^{2+} exchanger	↑	+	+
Extracellular matrix			
Collagen type III	↑	+	+
Plasma membrane			
β_1-Adrenergic receptor	↓		+
Na^+, K^+-ATPase			
Subunit α_2	↓	+	+
Subunit α_3	↑	+	+
Sarcoplasmic enzymes			
Creatine kinase BB	↑		+
Lactic dehydrogenase M	↑		+

↑—increase in isoform after overload. ↓—decrease in isoform after overload. 0→—isoform not present before overload. +—mRNA or protein was analyzed.

questrin mRNA coding for protein involved in calcium storage within terminal cisternae.[10]

Mitochondrial Constituents

A particularly important aspect of the growth process is maintenance of the balance between energy production by mitochondria and its consumption by myofibrils and ionic pumps, as indicated by the proportionate increase in mitochondrial ribosomal RNA and total RNA contributed by cytosolic ribosomes. Consequently, the mitochondrial mass as well as the amount of cytochrome c oxidase accumulates proportionally to other cell organelles, especially during the stage of developing hypertrophy.[11] During the later stages, however, myofibrils accumulate disproportionately faster than mitochondria, which might eventually contribute to energy imbalance. The biosynthesis of mitochondria is a complex process because some of their key constituents, such as cytochrome c oxidase, are multisubunit complexes with some subunits encoded by the nuclear genome and some by the mitochondrial one. In the normal heart, the expression of the two genomes is well coordinated. After overload, however, this coordination is lost; whereas the nuclearly encoded mRNAs follow changes seen in other cytoplasmic RNAs, the mRNAs transcribed from mitochondrial genes transiently lag behind, indicating that different mechanisms are involved in the transcriptional regulation of the two genomes.[11]

Cytoskeletal Changes

Reorganization of cytoskeletal markers in myocytes is another change found in overloaded hearts, where disproportionate regulation of gene activities results in an elevated density of microtubules and the amount of polymerized tubulin.[12]

Extracellular Matrix

Another way by which overload can produce structural changes of the myocardium is by disproportionate responses of muscle and nonmuscle cells. The acute overload of the heart results in increased proliferation of connective tissue cells, with consequent accumulation of total collagen and a change in its constituting types. The mRNA encoding the fibrillar collagen types I and III, which are products of cardiac fibroblasts, shows transient activation, reaching its peak at three days of overload.[13]

Capillary Density

The effects of overload on angiogenesis are of particular interest because of the heart's dependence on oxygen delivery. Like the proliferative response of cardiomyocytes, coronary angiogenesis is age dependent.[14] Capillary growth keeps pace with the increased cardiac mass when the growth stimulus is produced in young subjects, and in hearts of adult animals the response is slower, often resulting in decreased capillary density. Nevertheless, even in adult hearts, the ability for capillary growth and fibroblast proliferation is not lost entirely or irreversibly but can be activated to various degrees depending on the type of hemodynamic overload.

Expression of Hypertrophy-Related Phenotype

The response of myocytes to many forms of intervention is accompanied by expression of some genes that are usually quiescent in the mature heart,[15-17] including the proto-oncogenes c-*fos* and c-*myc* and those expressing α-skeletal actin, β-tropomyosin, and atrial natriuretic factor. Moreover, β cardiac myosin heavy-chain expression is upregulated, and in hearts with congenital valvular disease, the elimination of embryonic/atrial myosin light chain–1 is retarded. Because all the aforementioned genes are also expressed in fetal and neonatal hearts, they are referred to as fetal genes. The significance of this phenotype is not clear. The common feature of fetal and hypertrophic heart is relative low partial pressure of oxygen and the need for efficient assembly of nascent proteins because of rapid growth. It is of interest that hypertrophy caused by exercise or thyrotoxicosis is not accompanied by re-expression of fetal genes. Moreover, some genes, such as the β cardiac myosin heavy-chain gene, are also expressed preferentially in old animals. Whatever the significance of hypertrophy phenotype, it is a convenient marker of heart overload.

Gene Expression During Phenotypic Transitions

The phenotypic changes described in the preceding section were assessed by quantitation of either a given isoform or its mRNA. Such data by themselves, although indicative of adaptive changes of the heart, do not provide information about the steps at which the gene is regulated. The expression of a protein-encoding gene is a highly complex process that involves four broad categories of events:

1. Transcriptional steps that include conformational changes in chromatin structure, followed by steps leading to initiation of transcription.
2. Processing of nascent mRNA and transport of mature mRNA from the nucleus into the cytoplasm, where it undergoes regulated degradation.
3. Translational steps, including the association of cytoplasmic mRNA with ribosomes to form translationally active complexes as well as the processes leading to polypeptide initiation, elongation, and termination.
4. Processing of the final product, a protein, including its degradation.

The level of either a protein or its mRNA at any given moment, referred to as its steady-state level, is thus determined by the balance between its rates of synthesis and degradation. Because determination of these rates is quite laborious, and because no assumption can be made about the principal step of gene regulation, it is advantageous to dissect the overall pathway of gene expression into subsets of possible regulatory events. The most convenient dissection point lies between transcription and translation. By determining whether the observed change in the amount of a protein or its synthetic rate corresponds to a change in the amount of corresponding mRNA, one can tell whether the predominant regulatory steps involve pretranslational events or translational and posttranslational steps. A close agreement between the changes in protein and mRNA amounts indicates that it is the steady-state level of mRNA that is responsible for altered gene expression, not the efficiency of message translation. The correlation between change in mRNA and protein, however, does not tell which of the steps that precedes translation is modulated; it could include initiation of transcription, RNA polymerase II activity, or degradation of cytoplasmic mRNA, as well as nuclear nascent mRNA. All these events could be responsible for determining the level of mRNA.

Several studies geared to elucidating the key regulatory step in gene expression have been attempted using the thyroid hormone[18] and pressure-induced models of hypertrophy.[19] In general, an agreement between measurements of α and β cardiac myosin heavy-chain mass or rate of synthesis and the abundance of their respective mRNAs has been found, indicating pretranslational control as being the main regulatory step. To identify the actual step involved, studies have also measured the in vitro transcription rate. In thyroid[20] and pressure-induced[21] models of hypertrophy, the transcription rate of myosin heavy chains and of sarcomeric actins was found to be primarily responsible for the changes in mRNA levels. Posttranscriptional regulation—namely, selection of a polyadenylation site and alternative splicing resulting in inclusion or excision of a single codon—has also been found to be involved, at least after manipulation of the thyroid state of the animal.[22]

Functional Consequences of Phenotypic Changes

The changes in cardiac phenotype caused by hemodynamic overload before the onset of heart failure have well-defined functional consequences.[9] There are no major abnormalities in the concentration of high-energy compounds, and the maximal rate of myocardial oxygen consumption remains unchanged because the activity of cytochrome c oxidase, a rate-limiting factor for oxidative capacity, increases in proportion to heart size. This increased activity, however, might not be sufficient to satisfy the oxygen demand of the hypertrophied heart during exercise. Moreover, decreased coronary reserve with increased coronary vascular resistance might have compounding detrimental effects.

In the energy-utilizing processes, changes are observed even under resting conditions, as documented by the increased duration of the action potential. There are no changes in the membrane density of the Na^+,K^+-ATPase; however, the isoform shift in the subunit composition of the complex favors the low-affinity α_3 isoform at the expense of α_2, which might lead to increased sodium gradient with resulting elevation in intracellular calcium concentration.[23] In addition, the mechanical overload is associated with increased sodium influx closely matched by enhanced Na^+-Ca^{2+} exchange activity and the amount of mRNA encoding the exchanger.[24] The load-induced increase in sodium influx is thus likely to lead to increased myocardial calcium concentration, which could be reflected in increased contractility.

In the contractile cycle, a decrease in maximum unloading shortening velocity is well documented. In small laboratory animals, this change is explained by a shift toward the β cardiac myosin heavy chain containing V3 isomyosin that has lower ATPase activity than the V1 isoform. The consequence of this change is a decrease in the amount as well as rate of tension-independent heat liberation. This, in turn is associated with a decrease in calcium cycling per beat, caused by a decrease in sarcoplasmic Ca^{2+}-ATPase, ryanodine receptor, and phospholamban. In terms of cardiac function, these changes lead to increased efficiency of cross-bridge cycle (i.e., fewer ATP molecules are hydrolyzed per given tension developed) and in slowing of the relaxation (i.e., decreased rate of calcium removal).[10] The contractile properties of the hypertrophic heart could also be altered because of cytoskeletal remodeling; the increased mass of microtubules, forming dense arrays parallel to myofibrils, is likely to impede sarcomere motion.[12] In addition, the changes in the collagen matrix due to fibrosis and altered collagen type lead to increased stiffness of the heart.

Signals Coupling the Hemodynamic Load to Gene Activity

Many putative signals linking the hemodynamic load to the activity of cardiac genes have been investigated. Most of the mechanistic studies have focused on the transcriptional events, as described in this section. However, the initiation of transcription is only the first step in the complex pathway of gene expression. Certainly, transcription plays an important role in phenotypic transitions, especially when a new gene product is induced—for instance, after myogenic differentiation. However, the situation in most genes expressed in the mature heart is more complex because the respective mRNAs and their translation products are already present and only their levels change because of overload. It is thus likely that in addition to transcriptional initiation, other steps of gene expression are targets of regulatory events, including altered rates of protein degradation.[7]

General Features of Transcriptional Control

The expression of genes transcribed by RNA polymerase II is determined by multiple sequence-specific DNA–protein interactions that occur in the regulatory region of the gene.[7,17] The promoter and enhancer sequences (*cis*-regulatory elements) that mediate basal and/or an inducible transcription may contain overlapping target sites for sequence-specific *trans*-acting factors. Specific DNA-binding protein, alone or in complex with accessory proteins, binds to these nucleotide sequences. Different proteins may share an evolutionary relationship and can bind to a common sequence, such as CCAAT. However, there are factors specific for gene expression of a given cell type and for a response to specific agents such as steroid hormones, growth factors, heat shock, and heavy metals. In addition, it has been shown that a single protein can bind to different DNA sequences, thus suggesting a remarkable flexibility in the DNA–protein interaction. Furthermore, a modification (e.g., phosphorylation) of preexisting factor(s) also could alter either the DNA-binding properties and *trans*-acting capacity or their interaction with other proteins or even with the RNA polymerase II itself.

Several *cis*-regulatory elements and their respective transcription factors that appear to mediate skeletal-muscle-specific gene expression

Table 2 Signaling Mechanisms Postulated to Trigger Cardiac Hypertrophy

Sensors of mechanical work
Perturbations of cell structures
Adrenergic neuroeffectors
Energy utilization and generation
Primary signals generated by sensors
Ionic equilibrium: Na^+ influx = ↑ Ca^{2+} via Na^+ - Ca^{2+} exchanger; Ca^{2+} influx
Humoral factors
Myocytes: angiotensin II; transforming growth factor–β_1
Nonmyocytes: endothelin-1; non–muscle cell conditioned medium
Epinephrine, norepinephrine
NAD/NADH* → ADP-ribosylation
Intracellular signals
Ca^{2+}; inositol triphosphate; 1,2-diacylglycerol; cAMP
Biochemical effectors: protein kinase cascade
Protein kinase A, protein kinase C, calmodulin, mitogen-activated protein kinase, S6 kinase
Biological responses: change in gene activity
Induction of transcription factors
Immediate early genes (c-*fos*, c-*jun*, *erg*1)
Induction of growth factors
Transforming growth factor–β_1
Activation of transcription factors (phosphorylation)
Fos/Jun transcription factor: cAMP–responsive-element-binding protein

*NAD/NADH—ratio of oxidized nicotinamide adenine dinucleotide (NAD) to its reduced form (NADH).

have been identified. These include sequences referred to as E-box or MEF-1 elements, which interact with a class of transcription factors that contain a helix-loop-helix structure. So far, several such myogenic factors have been identified, such as MyoD, myogenin, and myf5. Regulatory mechanisms for the expression of myofibrillar genes in cardiac myocytes are more obscure because the helix-loop-helix factors are absent. Multiple positive and negative *cis*-acting elements and their respective binding factors, however, have been reported in the regulation of α and β cardiac myosin heavy-chain gene expression in skeletal and cardiac muscle backgrounds. Moreover, several *cis* elements that are required for cardiac-specific gene expression have been identified in troponin T and myosin light chain–2 genes.[17]

Search for Signals Regulating Cardiac Compensatory Growth

The fidelity and effectiveness of mechanisms by which the heart and other muscles adjust their size to functional demands have attracted the attention of investigators for many years. The challenge is to identify the load sensor(s) and signal(s) linking the external load, essentially a mechanical phenomenon, with the activity of the genetic apparatus. Whatever these sensors and feedback effectors are, they must be able to regulate the overall gene activity, resulting in more or less proportionate enlargement of the heart. Moreover, at the same time, their action has to be gene specific because individual genes respond to overload with different kinetics, magnitude, and direction of changes.

For the purpose of analysis, one can conceptualize the function-growth relationship as consisting of the following steps: recognition of mechanical work by a sensor that generates a load-dependent signal; transformation of this signal into a cytoplasmic message; transformation of this message to the biochemical effector; and, finally, a biological response (i.e., altered gene expression) [*see Table 2*].

Sensors of Mechanical Work and Their Signals

By dissecting the events of cardiac function, one can envision several steps as possibly sensing the mechanical work load: (1) perturbation of cell structures by mechanical forces associated with systolic wall stress and/or coronary flow, (2) adrenergic neuroeffectors, and (3) rate of ATP utilization and its metabolic correlates. Remarkable progress has been made in the studies of the first two mechanisms. Thus, a number of stretch-activated channels, cation selective as well as nonselective, have been found in diverse cell types.[25] In the heart, the best documented of the stretch-activated channels is the stretch- and ionophore-induced sodium influx into cultured myocytes, which increases protein and RNA radiolabeling. Furthermore, with only a few hours' delay, the Na^+ influx is followed by an increase in mRNA coding for the Na^+-Ca^{2+} exchanger, which is reflected eventually in enhanced exchanger activity in overloaded hearts.[24] The temporarily elevated Na^+ concentration might retard the efflux of Ca^{2+} and thus increase the intracellular concentration of this second messenger. Although the properties of the cardiac sodium stretch-activated channel have not been evaluated directly, it has been shown in *Xenopus* oocytes that in order to respond to membrane perturbation, a stretch-activated channel requires coupling with underlying cytoskeleton.[26]

Another example of a stretch-induced signaling molecule is angiotensin II. It has been known for some time that the renin-angiotensin system is also present in the myocardium,[27] with angiotensin II being localized in membrane-limited vesicles within the cytoplasm of ventricular myocytes.[28] Angiotensin II is released into the growth medium from cultured embryonic myocytes in response to mechanical stretch. Taken together with the general growth-promoting effects of angiotensin II seen in cultured cells, these data indicate the presence of a novel autocrine regulation in the heart. Its physiologic relevance can be shown by treatment of overloaded hearts with angiotensin-converting enzyme inhibitor, which prevents the development of hypertrophy.

It is important to keep in mind that hypertrophy of cardiac myocytes also can be regulated by paracrine mechanisms because nonmuscle cells are abundant in the heart and are likely to experience similar mechanical forces as myocytes. Examples of such mechanisms might include endothelin-1[3] and a factor present in non–muscle cell conditioned medium.[4] The latter factor is present in growth media conditioned by nonmyocytes derived from embryonic heart and might belong to the transforming growth factor–β family of growth factors. Whatever the regulatory mechanism, it is well documented that protein synthesis and growth of both cultured cells and perfused hearts are enhanced when stretch is applied to them.[16]

As for the adrenergic neuroeffectors, the plasma level of catecholamines has been found to be increased after hemodynamic overload; nevertheless, some aspects of their involvement in triggering cardiac hypertrophy are controversial.[29] Thus, infusion of norepinephrine has been shown to induce substantial cardiac enlargement that was diminished either by alpha or beta blockers and abolished by their combination.[30] Moreover, reduction of work load by verapamil did not have any effect on the development of hypertrophy. On the other hand, another study showed that the load-induced hypertrophy appeared to be independent of both alpha- and beta-adrenergic activity.[31] In cultured quiescent embryonic myocytes, alpha but not beta agonists induced protein synthesis, whereas in adult myocytes, both classes of agonists increased protein synthesis in the absence of contractile activity. Nevertheless, the effect was larger when the cells were actively beating, especially in the case of beta agonists, indicating the synergistic effects of loading and catecholamines on protein synthesis.[32] Examples of the putative metabolic sensor are nicotinamide adenine dinucleotide (NAD)/reduced NAD (NADH)-dependent adenosine diphosphate (ADP) ribosylation of nonhistone proteins and moderate hypoxia[33]; the latter was shown to increase protein synthesis in cultured cells.

Cytoplasmic Messenger Systems

Despite the lack of direct evidence for increased cellular concentration of ionized calcium after overload, there are at least four known mechanisms that might lead to such a change. These include the Na^{+}-Ca^{2+} exchanger, stretch-activated calcium channel, beta-adrenergic receptor–mediated influx through L-type channels, and mobilization from sarcoplasmic reticulum via inositol 1,4,5-trisphosphate. There is strong evidence for hypertrophic stimuli to be associated with the hydrolysis of phosphatidylinositol by phospholipase C.[3] This, in turn, leads to generation of inositol 1,4,5-trisphosphate and 1,2-diacylglycerol, the activator of protein kinase C. The level of cyclic adenosine monophosphate (cAMP) has been also shown to increase in a stretch-dependent manner in both beating and arrested myocytes, and its elevated level correlated well with protein synthesis.[34] This change, however, is only transient, because in later stages of hypertrophy, the adenylate cyclase–cAMP system appears to be impaired.[29]

Protein Kinase Cascade

The increase in protein kinase C activity by various interventions known to induce the expression of the "hypertrophy" phenotype, such as alpha-adrenergic agonists, endothelin-1, and stretch, is well documented.[3] The increase in protein kinase C activity caused by stretch seems to be independent of calcium or sodium influx through stretch-activated channels.[16,28] However, the mobilization of intracellular calcium is likely to occur because the level of inositol trisphosphate is rapidly and substantially increased by stretch.[35]

As for the participation of angiotensin II in the cascade of hypertrophy-regulating events, it is known that its effects are mediated by the angiotensin receptor AT_1 with consequent generation of phospholipid-derived second messengers.[36] This leads to an increased intracellular concentration of ionized calcium and an activation of several protein kinases, such as protein kinase C, mitogen-activated protein (MAP) kinase, and tyrosine-specific kinase. The activity of the last enzyme is critically dependent on calcium mobilization.[37] Moreover, stretch-activated MAP kinase is involved in phosphorylation and activation of yet another enzyme of the cascade, the S6 kinase, which, in turn, phosphorylates the S6 protein of ribosomal subunit 40 with consequent increase in the efficiency of protein synthesis.[16] Needless to say, the list of kinases and their targets will be extended in the future.

Response in the Signaling Pathway—Activation of Gene Expression

Whatever the elements of the signaling pathway initiated by sensors of mechanical work might be, the result is an activation of specific cardiac genes and eventual heart enlargement. This effect might be mediated either by induction of transcription factors that are normally absent or present in low amounts or by phosphorylation and activation of existing ones. The first instance includes the induction of immediate early gene expression, c-*fos*, c-*myc*, c-*jun*, and *egr*1, of which the changes in c-*fos* are quantitatively far more pronounced than those in the other ones.[16] The other example of this mechanism is the induction of the gene encoding transforming growth factor–β1 (TGF-β1) as seen in myocytes treated with angiotensin II.[36] There might be synergism between these two responses because a variety of growth factors induce intermediate early gene expression with similar kinetics, as seen after cardiac overload.[3,15,38]

An example of activation of existing factors is the phosphorylation of Jun, the product of the proto-oncogene c-*jun* by the action of MAP kinase.[16] Jun together with Fos forms the heterodimeric transcription factor AP-1. This might be yet another example of synergism in regulatory mechanisms: the growth stimulus might lead to induction of c-*fos* expression as well as to activation of existing Jun. Indeed, the AP-1 binding motif has been identified in the promoter region of some genes induced by the hypertrophic stimulus (e.g., atrial natriuretic factor gene), but not in others (e.g., skeletal α-actin). Because of the great number of genes and the apparent lack of common themes in regulatory sequences between them, it is not surprising that the signal transduction pathway is so complex. The existence of multiple signaling pathways acting synergistically and in combination then could be the basis not only for the gene-specific responses but also for the broad range of phenotypic options specifically induced by a given type of overload.[39] This view is supported by demonstrations that different sets of genes are upregulated in neural cells depending on which pathway of calcium entry was activated. Apparently, a single messenger can produce a distinct pattern of genes expressed depending on the kinetics of its entry and on the threshold concentration it reaches within the cytoplasm.[40] It thus appears unlikely that a single key regulatory signal governs the responses of all genes in all types of overload. The challenge of future investigations will then be to elucidate the cross-talk and point of convergence between individual pathways.

References

1. Zak R: Cell proliferation during cardiac growth. *Am J Cardiol* 31:211, 1973
2. Bugaisky LB, Gupta M, Gupta MP, et al: Cellular and molecular mechanisms of cardiac hypertrophy. *The Heart and Cardiovascular System*, 2nd ed. Fozzard HA, et al, Eds. Raven Press, New York, 1992, p 1621
3. Chien KR, Knowlton KU, Zhu H, et al: Regulation of cardiac gene expression during myocardial growth and hypertrophy: molecular studies of an adaptive physiological response. *FASEB J* 5:3037, 1991
4. Lang CS, Hartogensis WE, Simpson PC: β-Adrenergic stimulation of cardiac non-myocytes augments the growth-promoting activity of non-myocyte conditioned medium. *J Mol Cell Cardiol* 25:915, 1993
5. Baserga R, Rubin R: Cell cycle and growth control. *Crit Rev Eukarocyte Gene Expression* 3:47, 1993
6. Korecky B, Zak R, Schwartz K, et al: Role of thyroid hormone in regulation of isomyosin composition, contractivity, and size of heterotypicaly isotransplanted rat heart. *Circ Res* 60:824, 1987
7. Shimizu N, Camoretti-Mercado B, Jakovcic S, et al: RNA transcription in heart muscle. *The Heart and Cardiovascular System*, 2nd ed. Fozzard HA, et al, Eds. Raven Press, New York, 1992, p 1525
8. Sutsch G, Brunner UT, von Schulthess C, et al: Hemodynamic performance and myosin light chain-1 expression of the hypertrophied left ventricle in aortic valve disease before and after valve replacement. *Circ Res* 70:1035, 1992
9. Swynghedauw B: Remodeling of the heart in chronic pressure overload. *Basic Res Cardiol* 86(suppl1):99, 1991
10. Alpert NR, Periasamy M, Arai M, et al: The regulation of calcium cycling in stressed hearts. *Cardiac Adaptation in Heart Failure*. Holtz J, et al, Eds. Steinkopff Verlag, Darmstadt, 1992
11. Wiesner RJ, Achenbrenner V, Ruegg V, et al: Coordination of nuclear and mitochondrial gene expression during the development of cardiac hypertrophy in rats. *Am J Physiol* 267:C229, 1994
12. Tsutsui H, Ishihara K, Cooper G: Cytoskeletal role in the contractive dysfunction of hypertrophied myocardium. *Science* 260:682, 1993
13. Chapman D, Weber KT, Eghbali M: Regulation of fibrillar collagen types I and III and basement membrane type IV collagen gene expression in pressure overloaded rat myocardium *Circ Res* 67:787, 1990
14. Tomanek RJ: Age as a modulator of coronary capillary angiogenesis. *Circulation* 86:320, 1992
15. Parker TG, Schneider MD: Growth factors, proto-oncogenes, and plasticity of the cardiac phenotype. *Annu Rev Physiol* 53:179, 1991
16. Komuro I, Yazaki Y: Control of cardiac gene expression by mechanical stress. *Annu Rev Physiol* 55:55, 1993
17. Chien KR, Zhu H, Knowlton KV, et al: Transcriptional regulation during cardiac growth and development. *Annu Rev Physiol* 55:77, 1993
18. Everett AW, Sinha AM, Umeda PK, et al: Regulation of myosin synthesis by thyroid hormone: relative change in the alpha- and beta-myosin heavy chain mRNA levels in rabbit heart. *Biochemistry* 23:1596, 1984
19. Izumo S, Lompre AM, Matsuoka R, et al: Myosin heavy chain messenger RNA and protein isoform transitions during cardiac hypertrpohy. *J Clin Invest* 79:970, 1987
20. Umeda PK, Darling DS, Kennedy JM, et al: Control of myosin heavy chain expression in cardiac hypertrophy. *Am J Cardiol* 59:49A, 1987
21. Boheler KR, Chassagne C, Martin X, et al: Cardiac expression of α- and β-myosin heavy chains and sarcomeric α-actins are regulated through transcriptional mechanisms. *J Biol Chem* 267:12979, 1992
22. Sindhwani R, Ismail-Beigi F, Leinwand LA: Post-transcriptional regulation of rat α cardiac myosin heavy chain gene expression. *J Biol Chem* 269:3272, 1994

23. Charlemagne D, Orlowski J, Oliviero P, et al: Alteration of Na-K-ATPase subunit mRNA and protein levels in hypertrophied rat heart. *J Biol Chem* 269:1541, 1994
24. Kent RL, Rozich JD, McCollam PL, et al: Rapid expression of the cardiac Na^+-Ca^{2+} exchanger in response to pressure overload. *Am J Physiol* 265:H1024, 1993
25. Sachs F: Mechanical transduction by membrane ion channels. *Mol Cell Biochem* 104:57, 1991
26. Hamil OP, McBride DV: Rapid adaptation of the mechanosensitive channel in *Xenopus* oocytes. *Proc Natl Acad Sci USA* 89:7462, 1992
27. Baker KM, Booz GW, Dostal DE: Cardiac action of angiotensin II: role of an intracardiac renin-angiotensin system. *Annu Rev Physiol* 54:227, 1992
28. Sadoshima J, Xu Y, Slayter HS, et al: Autocrine release of angiotensin II mediates stretch-induced hypertrophy of cardiac myocytes in vitro. *Cell* 75:977, 1993
29. Gupta MP, Gupta M, Zak R: The dynamic state of cardiac phenotype: modulation by the β-adrenergic system. *The Adapted Heart.* Nagano M, et al, Eds. Raven Press, New York, 1994, p 365
30. Zierhut W, Zimmer HG: Significance of myocardial α- and β-adrenoreceptors in catecholamine-induced cardiac hypertrophy. *Circ Res* 65:1417, 1988
31. Cooper G, Kent RL, Uboh CE, et al: Hemodynamic versus adrenergic control of cat right ventricular hypertrophy. *J Clin Invest* 75:1403, 1985
32. Clark WA, Rudnick SJ, LaPres JJ, et al: Signal mechanisms for hypertrophy and atrophy in cultured adult heart cell. *Circ Res* 73:1163, 1993
33. Zak R: Factors controlling cardiac growth. *Growth of the Heart in Health and Disease.* Zak R, Ed. Raven Press, New York, p 165, 1984
34. Xenophontos XP, Watson PA, Chua BH, et al: Increased cyclic AMP content accelerates protein synthesis in rat heart. *Circ Res* 65:647, 1989
35. Dassouli A, Sulpice J-C, Roux S, et al: Stretch-induced inositol triphosphate and tetrakisphosphate production in rat cardiomyocytes. *J Mol Cell Cardiol* 25:973, 1993
36. Sadoshima J, Izumo S: Molecular characterization of angiotensin II–induced hypertrophy of cardiac myocytes and hyperplasia of cardiac fibroblasts. *Circ Res* 73:413, 1993
37. Huckle WR, Prokp CA, Dy RC, et al: Angiotensin II stimulates protein-tyrosine phosphorylation in a calcium-dependent manner. *Mol Cell Biol* 10:6290, 1990
38. Simpson PC: Proto-oncogenes and cardiac hypertrophy. *Annu Rev Physiol* 51:189, 1988
39. Jacob R: The functional ambivalence of adaptive processesæ considerations based on the example of the hemodynamically overloaded heart. *Basic Res Cardiol* 86(suppl 3):3, 1991
40. Bading H, Ginty, DD, Greenberg ME: Regulation of gene expression in hippocampal neurons by distinct calcium signaling pathways. *Science* 260:181, 1993

Acknowledgment

Figure 1 Talar Agasyan.

CHAPTER 13

Gene Mutations That Cause Familial Hypertrophic Cardiomyopathy

Christine E. Seidman, M.D., Jonathan G. Seidman, Ph.D.

Familial hypertrophic cardiomyopathy (FHC) is an inherited disease of heart muscle that is characterized by unexplained cardiac hypertrophy and myocyte disarray. The first clinical description of the disease appeared in 1869,[1] and over the ensuing 125 years, FHC has been the focus of numerous clinical reports, pathophysiological studies, and most recently, molecular genetic investigations. Various names have been affixed to the condition, including hypertrophic obstructive cardiomyopathy, asymmetric septal hypertrophy, and idiopathic hypertrophic subaortic stenosis. Given the diversity of clinical manifestations of the disease and the spectrum of different gene defects that cause it, the more general descriptor familial hypertrophic cardiomyopathy is most appropriate and is used here.

The considerable efforts by clinicians and researchers to understand FHC have been disproportionate to its estimated prevalence of 19.7 per 100,000 individuals.[2] This attention may be accounted for by the serious sequelae of the condition, particularly the high incidence of sudden death in affected individuals. FHC is the most common cause of death among young athletes who die suddenly.[3] Although athletes are at no greater risk for this condition than are others in the general population sudden death in individuals considered to be among society's most physically fit has prompted substantial media reporting of FHC.[4] The pattern of disease inheritance and the difficulties associated with the accurate diagnosis of this condition, particularly in prepubescent children, have also heightened medical attention to FHC. Further, the recognition that other cardiovascular diseases can produce a hypertrophic phenotype that is similar to that seen in FHC has led to the hope that a more complete understanding of this rare disease may provide important insights into other, more common conditions. Recently, mutations in three genes have been demonstrated to cause FHC. These findings provide the opportunity for improved diagnosis and management and should help elucidate cellular pathways that link a genotype to a pathologic phenotype. Definition of the latter may assist in the development of therapeutics for FHC and for cardiac hypertrophy that occurs secondary to other diseases.

Clinical Features of Familial Hypertrophic Cardiomyopathy

Detailed reviews of the clinical features of FHC are presented in cardiovascular texts[5] and in consensus reports on FHC.[6] This chapter summarizes only those pathophysiological and clinical findings of FHC that specifically relate to recent molecular genetic studies.

Increased cardiac mass accompanied by myocyte disarray defines the pathology of FHC [*see Figures 1a and 1b*]. Left ventricular hypertrophy can be either focal and subtle or widespread and massive. Although it is classically defined as asymmetric, concentric hypertrophy is common in FHC, and the left ventricular free wall is virtually always involved. The histologic manifestations of FHC include increased myocyte size with abnormal intracellular and intercellular architecture [*see Figures 1c and 1d*]. Myocyte disarray is a cardinal feature of this condition, and like the cardiac hypertrophy of FHC, both the extent and location of the disarray vary considerably between patients.

Disease symptoms may be absent or when present can be mild or debilitating, stable or progressive. Dyspnea and angina occur commonly, and palpitations may be transient or protracted, resulting in dizziness and syncope. Sudden death occurs in both clinically symptomatic and asymptomatic patients and may be the presenting sign of the disease. Endocarditis, atrial fibrillation, congestive heart failure, and thromboemboli occur in FHC, further increasing its morbidity and mortality. The annual mortality in affected individuals has been reported to be as high as four percent[7]; however, in many individuals long-term survival is excellent.[8] It has been generally recognized that children with hypertrophic cardiomyopathy are at higher risk for sudden death; however, neither the distribution nor the severity of cardiac hypertrophy appears to predict which adults are at risk for premature death. Identification of the precise gene defect that causes the condition has permitted a new approach to risk stratification.

Hypertrophic cardiomyopathy is typically diagnosed by physical examination, 12-lead electrocardiography, two-dimensional echocardiography, and Doppler ultrasonography.[5] Physical and electrocardiographic findings may suggest the presence of FHC, but the diagnosis requires the demonstration of increased myocardial mass, usually by echocardiography. Previous studies[9,10] have attempted to define the degree of hypertrophy required for diagnosis (often based on the ratio of the interventricular septum and left ventricular free wall); however, in an individual at risk for FHC, the finding of any unexplained hypertrophy should be considered to be indicative of disease. In the absence of confounding conditions, such as systemic hypertension or valvular heart disease, diagnosis of hypertrophic cardiomyopathy in adults that is derived from results of standard noninvasive imaging is generally accurate. However, in prepubescent children, diagnosis can be more difficult because cardiac hypertrophy may not be manifested.[11] The recent application of ultrasonographic tissue characterization (backscatter imaging) to the study of cardiomyopathies[12] may be particularly valuable for diagnosing FHC because such a technique may identify altered cellular architecture (myocyte disarray) that precedes the development of hypertrophy.

Genetic Causes of Familial Hypertrophic Cardiomyopathy

Considerable progress has been made in our understanding of the molecular basis of FHC. Genetic linkage analyses initially demonstrated that the disease is genetically heterogeneous[13]; that is, mutations in different genes can produce the same phenotype. At present, three gene mutations have been identified in individuals with FHC, and evidence exists for at least one more. Mutations in the genes encoding β cardiac myosin, α-tropomyosin,

a

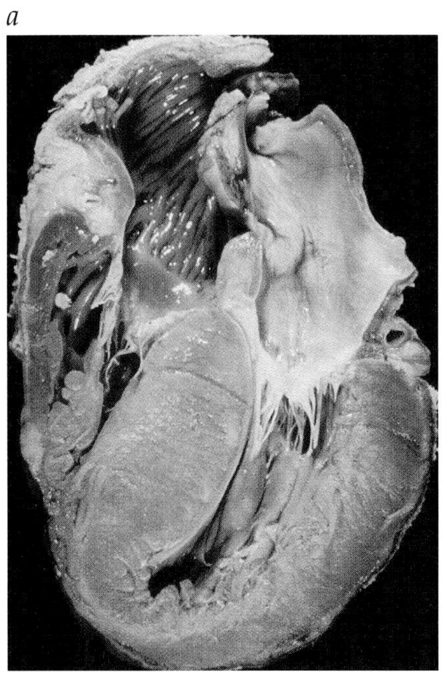

b

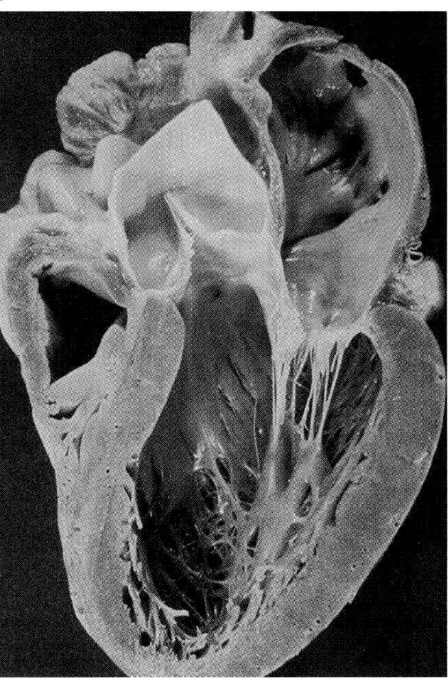

c

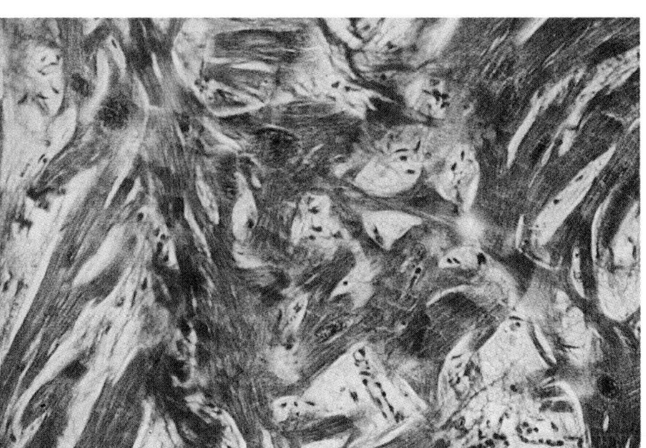

d

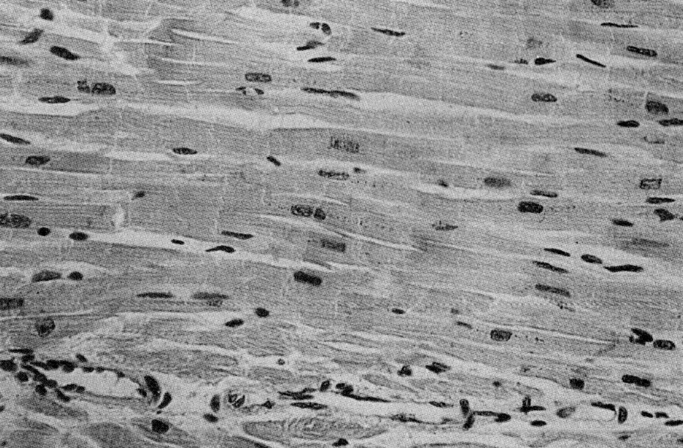

Figure 1 *The gross and cellular pathology of familial hypertrophic cardiomyopathy (FHC). Gross anatomic findings of a heart from an individual with hypertrophic cardiomyopathy (a) compared with findings in a heart from an unaffected person (b) reveal the increased mass of the left ventricle walls and the regions of fibrosis in the affected heart. Tissue section (c) from a patient with a hypertrophic cardiomyopathy (Masson-Wright trichrome stain) demonstrates myocyte and myofibrillar disarray in contrast to the normal myocyte architecture (hematoxylin-eosin stain) present in an unaffected individual (d).*

and cardiac troponin T appear to account for as much as 70 percent of FHC. Because these three FHC genes encode sarcomeric proteins, FHC can be considered a disease of the sarcomere.

Clinical Genetics of Familial Hypertrophic Cardiomyopathy

Hypertrophic cardiomyopathy can be familial and transmitted as an autosomal dominant trait, or it can be sporadic, in which neither of the parents of an affected individual has the disorder. Genetic analyses have demonstrated that de novo mutation of the β cardiac myosin heavy chain gene can cause sporadic hypertrophic cardiomyopathy, which, in one reported case, was transmitted to an offspring.[14] Collectively, these data suggest that sporadic and familial hypertrophic cardiomyopathies are both clinically and genetically related; de novo germ line mutations that cause sporadic disease can be transmitted to successive generations, thereby initiating new familial disease.

Estimates of the percentage of familial versus sporadic disease vary, but at least 50 percent of affected individuals have inherited hypertrophic cardiomyopathy from an affected parent.[15] Clinical evaluations in multiple large pedigrees have demonstrated that FHC is transmitted as an autosomal dominant trait with a high degree of penetrance. That is, approximately half of the first-degree adult relatives of an affected individual also have hypertrophic cardiomyopathy. Three large families in which the disorder has been transmitted in multiple generations are shown in Figure 2. Clinical evaluations (physical examination, 12-lead electrocardiography, and two-dimensional echocardiography) of the 96 adult members of family A revealed hypertrophic cardiomyopathy in 27 individuals.[16] These affected individuals have a 50 percent chance of transmitting FHC to each offspring, regardless of the child's sex. In contrast, the offspring of an unaffected individual are at no risk for developing the disease.

The pattern of inheritance in familial and sporadic hypertrophic cardiomyopathies indicates that all offspring of an affected individual should be clinically evaluated for this disease. Unfortunately, clinical studies are complicated by the age-related penetrance of FHC. That is, an individual who has inherited an FHC mutation may not develop signs or symptoms of disease until after puberty, a fact that necessitates longitudinal evaluations for accurate assessment of disease status.

Genetic Linkage Studies

Recognition of the autosomal dominant mode of transmission of FHC has allowed the definition of the chromosome location of disease genes by cosegregation (or linkage) analysis. This method is particularly useful for the identification of disease-causing genes when the biochemical defect resulting from a gene mutation is unknown. The technique first involves the screening of polymorphisms (variations in DNA sequence) scattered throughout the genome until a polymorphism is identified that is closely linked to the disease in a particular kindred. The genomic location of the linked polymorphism defines the chromosome location of the disease gene. A polymorphism on chromosome 14q1 (q1 denotes a region on the long arm of the chromosome) was coinherited with disease status in all affected family members of family A [*see Figure 2*], indicating the map location of an FHC locus[16]; the map location was designated cardiomyopathy, hypertrophic locus 1 (*CMH1*). Statistical analyses indicated a likelihood of greater that 2,000,000,000:1 (Lod score greater than 9) that an FHC gene was located on chromosome 14.

Definition of the map location of a disease gene permits the evaluation of candidate genes for potential disease-causing mutations. Candidate genes are defined as those that map to the disease locus and are expressed in the tissue that manifests the disease phenotype. Knowledge of the map location of a disease gene is also essential for the positional cloning of novel genes that may be involved in the pathology. By 1989, fewer than 20 genes had been mapped to chromosome 14q1; these included the genes encoding angiogenin, cathepsin G and cathepsin G–like 2, cytotoxic T cell–associated esterase 1, four transfer RNAs, the α and δ chains of the T cell receptor, and the cardiac myosin heavy-chain polypeptides. Because the α and β cardiac myosin heavy-chain genes mapped to chromosome 14q1 and encoded important cardiac sarcomeric proteins, they were considered to be candidates for mutations that might cause FHC. Subsequent analyses demonstrated that missense mutations in the β cardiac myosin heavy-chain gene cause approximately 40 percent of all cases of FHC.

Genetic linkage studies also suggested that not all FHC was caused by β cardiac myosin-heavy chain gene mutations. That is, in some families (e.g., families MI and BA [*see Figure 2*]), polymorphisms on chromosome 14q1 (particularly polymorphisms within the β cardiac myosin heavy-chain gene) were not coinherited with FHC. These findings demonstrated that FHC is genetically heterogeneous.[13] To define the chromosome location of other disease genes, families with FHC that was not linked to *CMH1* were identified, clinically characterized, and genetically studied. The identification of other FHC loci was expedited by improvements in the human genome map. Over the past five years, highly informative polymorphisms have been identified and mapped in the human genome: most of these are dinucleotide, trinucleotide, and tetranucleotide sequences that occur as tandem repeats. The number of repeats at a particular genomic location varies considerably between individuals; therefore, these markers of chromosome location are highly polymorphic. These short, tandem repeat sequences can be readily characterized by polymerase chain reaction amplification; the sequences permit definition of the genomic location of a disease gene within a year of acquisition of DNA samples from family members. Using the hundreds of short, tandem repeat sequences that are scattered throughout the genome, investigators identified the chromosome locations of three other FHC genes on chromosome 1q3 (*CMH2*[17]), chromosome 15q2 (*CMH3*[18]), and chromosome 11 (*CMH4*[19]). Further, because these studies identified families with FHC that do not have mutations at any of these loci, the chromosome location of at least one other FHC gene remains unknown (Seidman CE, Seidman JG, unpublished data). Estimates of the fraction of disease that maps to each FHC loci are imprecise, but preliminary analyses suggest that mutations in each of these genes cause fewer than 20 percent of all cases of FHC.

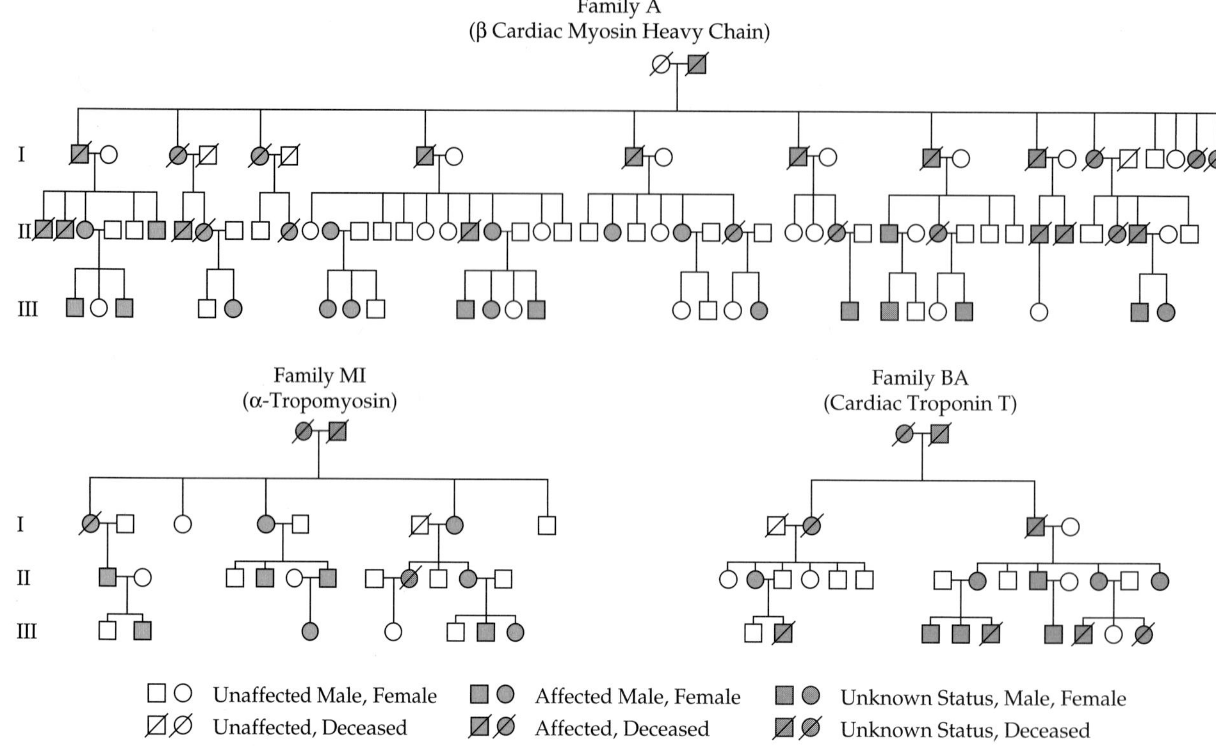

Figure 2 *Pedigrees of three kindreds with hypertrophic cardiomyopathy, which segregates as an autosomal dominant trait. The mutated genes (β cardiac myosin heavy chain [top], α-tropomyosin [bottom left], and cardiac troponin T [bottom right]) that cause FHC in each family are provided in parentheses. Note the presence of affected individuals in every generation and the equal sex distribution among affected individuals.*

Familial Hypertrophic Cardiomyopathy Is a Disease of the Sarcomere

The sarcomere is the major functional and structural unit of contraction in striated muscle and is composed of thick and thin filaments. Of the eight known components of the thick filament, myosin heavy and light chains are most abundant. The thin filament is formed from actin, α-tropomyosin, and troponin molecules I, C, and T. Because mutations within the β cardiac myosin heavy-chain gene that mapped to chromosome 14 were demonstrated to cause FHC, other sarcomeric genes were potential candidate genes for FHC linked to other loci. Analyses of genes that encode cardiac sarcomeric proteins in families with FHC that does not map to the β cardiac myosin heavy-chain gene (i.e., families BA and MI [*see Figure 2*]) have led to the identification of disease-causing mutations in cardiac troponin T (*CMH2*, on chromosome 1) and α-tropomyosin (*CMH3*, on chromosome 15). The mutated gene responsible for FHC linked to chromosome 11 (*CMH4*) is still unknown.

Familial Hypertrophic Cardiomyopathy Is Caused by β Cardiac Myosin Heavy-Chain Gene Mutations

More than 20 myosin heavy-chain genes are in the human genome. However, two genes, designated α and β cardiac myosin heavy-chain genes, encode myosins that are made in large amounts in cardiac tissues. In humans, α cardiac myosin heavy-chain genes are expressed during embryonic development and in the adult atria. In the adult ventricle, myosin heavy-chain polypeptides are derived primarily from the β cardiac myosin heavy-chain gene. Both α and β cardiac myosin heavy-chain genes are organized in a tandem array, separated by fewer than 5,000 base pairs,[20,21] on chromosome 14q1, precisely where the *CMH1* locus was mapped. Because of their pattern of expression and their genetic location, and because mutations in these genes might be expected to cause myocyte and myofibrillar disarray, the cardiac myosin heavy-chain genes were excellent candidates for mutations that could cause FHC at *CMH1*.

Disease-causing mutations can be classified as involving either rearrangement of the disease gene (i.e., insertions, deletions, translocations, or inversions) or point mutations (i.e., single nucleotide changes that alter the encoded amino acid). To date, only two rearrangements of the cardiac myosin heavy-chain genes have been reported, a deletion of the 3′ end of the gene[22] and an α/β hybrid myosin heavy-chain gene.[23] The latter rearrangement probably arose from mispairing and homologous recombination within the α and β cardiac myosin heavy-chain genes but appears not to cause FHC; affected individuals with the hybrid gene also have a missense mutation in the nonrearranged β cardiac myosin heavy-chain gene that alone can cause FHC.[24] Thus, cardiac myosin heavy-chain gene rearrangements do not commonly cause FHC. In contrast, 19 different missense mutations[25,26] that cause FHC have been identified in the β cardiac myosin heavy-chain gene [*see Figure 3*]. These mutations appear to cause approximately 40 percent of cases of FHC.[24]

The nucleotide sequence changes found in β cardiac myosin heavy-chain genes are considered disease-causing mutations for five reasons:

1. Studies of affected and unaffected members of large families demonstrate a strict concordance between disease status and genotype. For example, the FHC mutation in family A [*see Figure 2*], designated Arg403Gln [*see Figure 3*], is present only in affected members[27]; unaffected members are homozygous for the normal arginine residue at 403. The odds of this association's occurring in family A as a result of chance are less than 1:17,000,000.
2. These missense mutations have never been identified in more than 200 unrelated and unaffected individuals, thereby demonstrating that these are not common polymorphisms.
3. These mutations alter the encoded amino acid residue and typically affect regions of the polypeptide that have been conserved throughout vertebrate evolution.
4. Most of these mutations alter the charge of the encoded amino acid. Because individuals with FHC caused by conservative mutations appear to have a better prognosis, nonconservative mutations may perturb myosin function more significantly than those that do not affect charge.
5. β Cardiac myosin heavy-chain gene missense mutations and hypertrophic cardiomyopathy have arisen de novo simultaneously in two families, providing compelling evidence that these mutations cause FHC.

Identification of FHC-causing mutations from many families has demonstrated little evidence of a strong founder effect[28]; that is, a different mutation is found in nearly all families, suggesting that FHC families do not share a distant common ancestor. This finding further implies that strategies to define the genetic defect that causes FHC in a given family must be comprehensive rather than restricted to analyses of previously identified mutations. Ribonuclease A protection assays, single-strand conformation polymorphisms, denaturing gradient gel electrophoresis, and direct DNA sequencing techniques have each been used to identify FHC mutations.

Application of these techniques to analyses of the β cardiac myosin heavy-chain gene has been hampered by the size of the gene (40 exons spanning approximately 30,000 base pairs [*see Figure 3*]), the size of the transcribed message and protein (a 6,000–base pair mRNA and a 2,000-amino-acid polypeptide), and the heterozygous state of all affected individuals. However, because almost all of the mutations identified to date are located in the region of the gene that encodes the head or the head-rod junction of the molecule, restricting mutation screens to the amino terminal half of the gene may be appropriate. Although considerable effort and expense are expended on the identification of the disease-causing mutation responsible

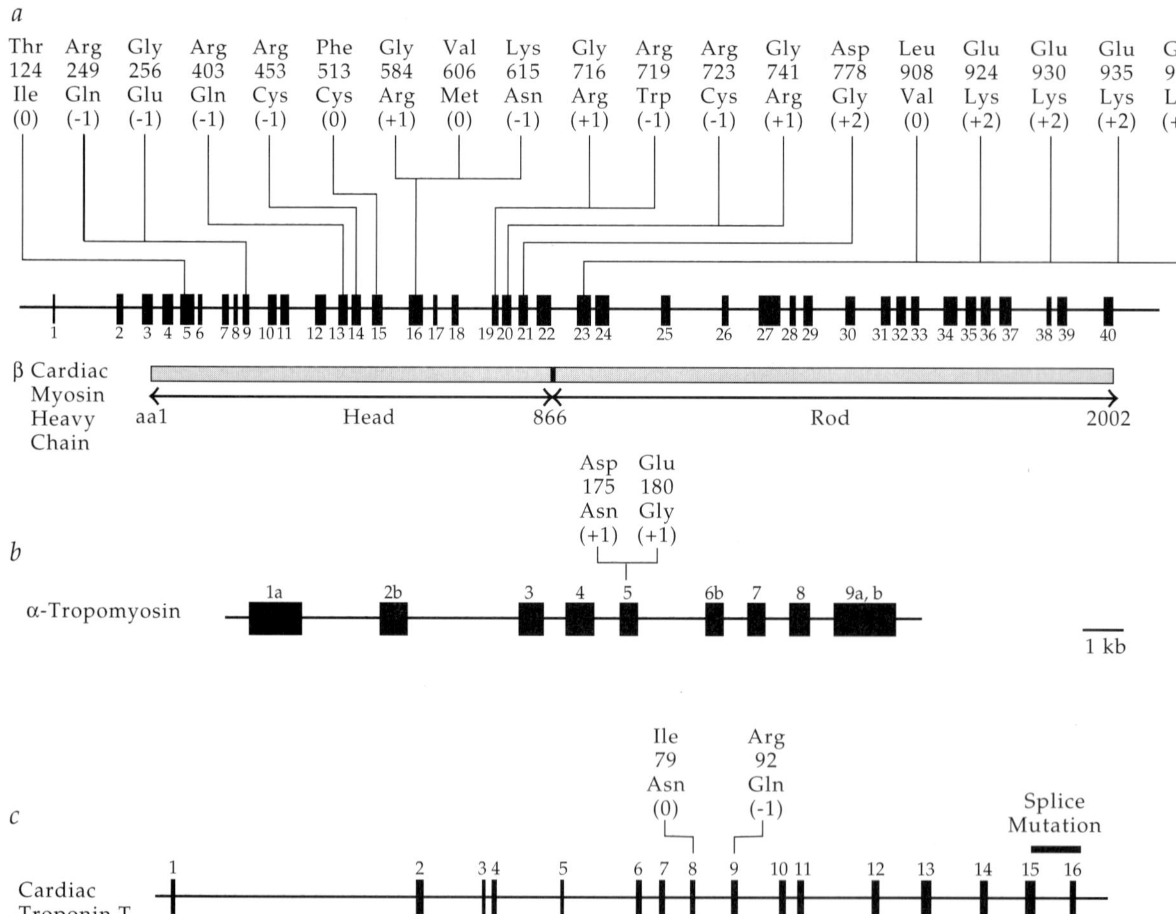

Figure 3 *The spectrum of gene mutations that cause FHC. Missense mutations in the β cardiac myosin heavy chain (a), α-tropomyosin (b), and cardiac troponin T genes (c) are shown along with the resultant change in the amino acid (three-letter code) and charge (in parenthesis). Only those exons that encode striated muscle α-tropomyosin are shown. The genomic structure of the rat cardiac troponin T gene is shown (c), and the human mutations that cause FHC are indicated.*

for FHC in an individual, such data permit gene-based diagnosis in all other family members and provide information that may assist in treatment.

Familial Hypertrophic Cardiomyopathy Is Caused by Mutation in Thin Filament Genes

Until recently, the only known FHC-causing mutations were those identified in the β cardiac myosin heavy-chain gene. However, because genetic linkage studies had demonstrated that FHC is a genetically heterogeneous disorder, mutations in other genes must exist that cause this phenotype. Two models were considered to explain the genetic heterogeneity of FHC. One possibility was that gene defects that disrupted sarcomeric structure and function would cause myocyte disarray and hypertrophy. This model implied that other FHC genes, like the β cardiac myosin heavy-chain gene, would encode sarcomeric proteins. An alternative possibility was that the hypertrophic phenotype was a common pathology that accompanied any perturbation of myocyte function. This model suggested that other FHC genes would encode proteins whose only common feature was their expression in the myocardium.

Linkage between FHC and DNA polymorphisms had identified that *CMH2* is on chromosome 1q3.[17] At least four sarcomeric protein genes are encoded in the vicinity of *CMH2*: skeletal actin, cardiac troponin T, troponin I, and myosin-binding protein H. These genes were each considered candidates for mutations that might cause FHC. However, detailed analyses in affected members of three kindreds with FHC linked to the *CMH2* locus failed to identify mutations in skeletal actin, troponin I, or myosin-binding protein H genes.[29] In contrast, mutation screens[29] of the cardiac troponin T gene of affected individuals from these three families revealed differences between these sequences and those of the troponin T gene derived from unaffected individuals [*see Figure 3*]. Affected members of two families have a missense mutation in exon 8 (Ile79Asn) or exon 9 (Arg92Gln: family BA [*see Figure 2 and Figure 3*]) that alters residues that have been highly conserved during vertebrate evolution. Affected members of a third family have a mutation in the 5′ splice sequence of intron 15, causing a failure in exon splicing in genomic RNA that results in a defective mRNA; this failure is predicted to cause aberrant cardiac troponin T mRNA transcripts. As with the β cardiac myosin heavy-chain missense mutations, mutations in the cardiac troponin T gene are considered to be disease causing based on the concordance between genotype and phenotype in FHC families, the absence of these sequence variations in unaffected individuals, and the predicted effect that each mutation would produce on the structure of the encoded polypeptide. Further, because cardiac troponin T is expressed only in the myocardium, these mutations are predicted to cause a cardiac-specific phenotype.

The FHC gene at the *CMH3* locus on chromosome 15 is α-tropomyosin.[29] Two missense mutations (Asp175Asn and Glu180Gly [*see Figure 3*]) have been identified that segregate with disease status in two different families and are not found in unaffected individuals. Both mutations predict nonconservative amino acid substitutions in residues that have been strictly conserved during vertebrate evolution. Although each mutation occurs in exon 5, the pathophysiology produced by the two mutations appears to be quite different. Affected individuals with the Glu180Gly mutation have considerably less cardiac hypertrophy than do those with the Asp175Asn mutation. The average left ventricular wall thickness in individuals with the Asp175Asn mutation (family MI [*see Figure 2*]) was 19 ± 4.7 mm. In contrast, the average left ventricular wall thickness found in individuals with the Glu180Gly mutation was 10.1 ± 4.2 mm. Although such differences are unlikely to affect survival, these findings suggest that the hypertrophic phenotype may partly reflect genotype.

The FHC-causing mutations in α-tropomyosin and troponin T are expected to alter the structure and function of the thin filament in cardiac muscle [*see Figure 4*]. The two troponin T missense mutations are located in a region that is involved in calcium-insensitive binding to α-tropomyosin,[30] whereas the splice mutation should affect the C-terminal, which binds α-tropomyosin in a calcium-dependent fashion.[31] Both missense mutations in α-tropomyosin occur in the domain involved in calcium-dependent binding to troponin T.[32] Because the α-tropomyosin isoform found in cardiac tissue is abundant in other striated muscle, the cardiac-specific phenotype produced by these mutations may reflect interactions that are specific for cardiac troponin T. Recent studies have identified five additional mutations in the cardiac troponin T gene that cause FHC.[33] Clinical evaluations revealed that the extent of cardiac hypertrophy produced by these different mutations (as assessed by maximum left ventricular wall thickness) is significantly less than that produced by β cardiac myosin heavy-chain mutations.

The recognition that β cardiac myosin heavy-chain, cardiac troponin T, and α-tropomyosin gene mutations can all cause FHC has implications for our understanding of the molecular cause of this condition. These data strongly support the concept that FHC is a disease of the sarcomere [*see Figure 4*]. β Cardiac myosin heavy chain is a major component of the thick filament, and cardiac troponin T and α-tropomyosin are major components of the thin filament. We anticipate that other FHC genes, including at least one encoded on chromosome 11 at *CMH4*, will also encode sarcomeric proteins. Whether defects in any cardiac protein or only in those proteins specific to the sarcomere can cause hypertrophy remains unknown. Mutations in sarcomeric proteins that are expressed in other striated muscles would be recognized as a cause of FHC only if the resulting phenotype was cardiac-specific. In contrast, a sarcomeric gene defect that significantly disrupts skeletal as well as cardiac muscle would be expected to produce clinical findings that would exclude a diagnosis of FHC.

The demonstration that FHC is caused by defects of the sarcomere raises two important questions: What types of sarcomeric mutations produce FHC? How do defects in the structure and function of the sarcomere result in myocyte disarray and hypertrophy? An analysis of the different mutation types found in FHC may provide insights into the mechanisms by which these mutations produce a dominant phenotype. That is, most of the FHC mutations in three sarcomeric genes are missense. These missense mutations may produce so-called poison polypeptides, mutant polypeptides that are incorporated into the growing sarcomere but disrupt function. Alternatively, these mutations may produce unstable polypeptides that could alter the stoichiometry of sarcomeric components and could prevent proper syn-

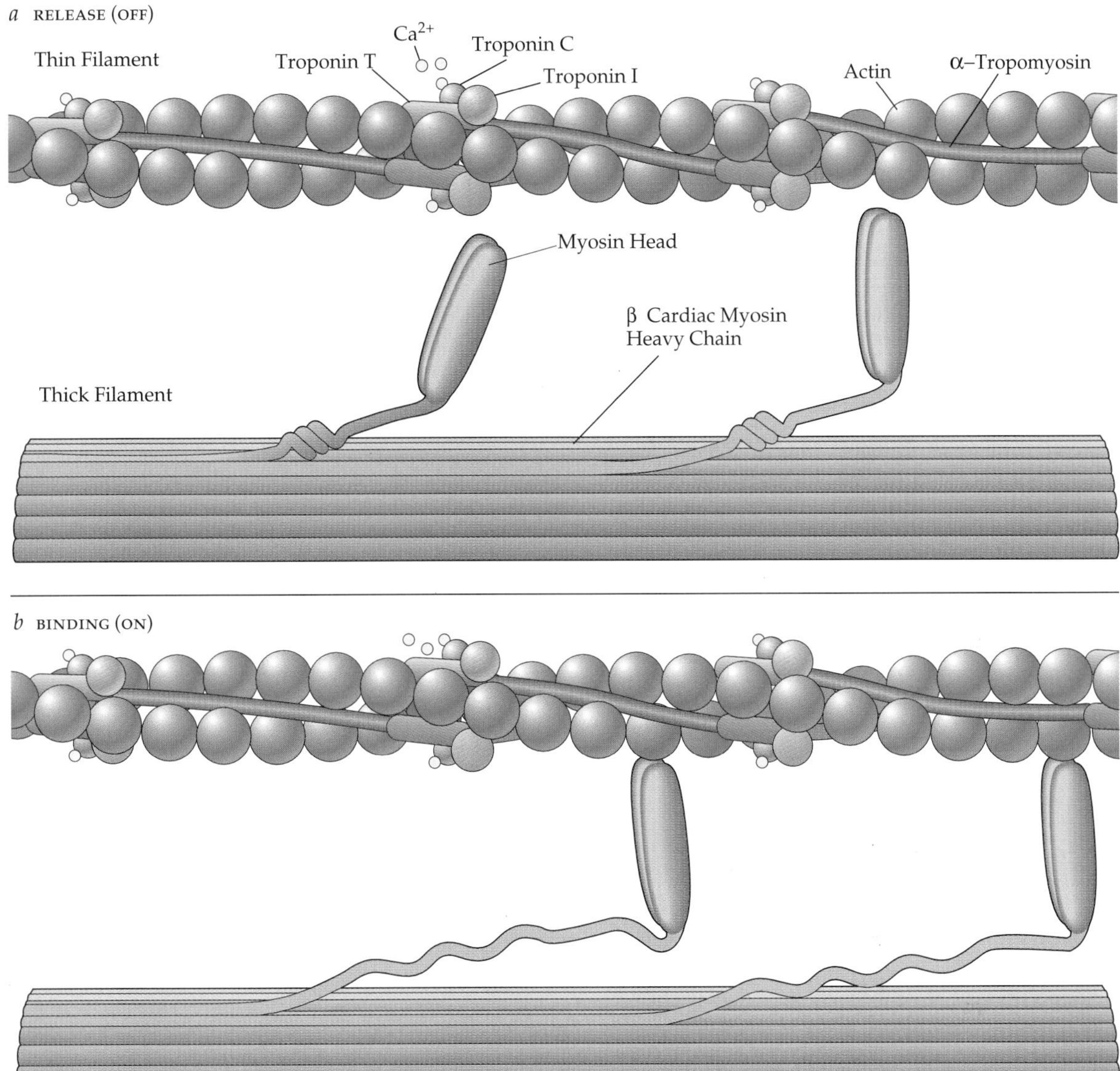

Figure 4 *The structure of the sarcomere, which is the basic contractile unit in striated muscle, is illustrated with myosin head "off" (a) and "on" (b). Contraction requires alternate binding to and releasing of actin by the myosin heavy-chain region, as mediated by* Ca^{2+} *concentration. Calcium binding further involves a shift in troponin I binding with actin and troponin C. Mutations thus far shown to be associated with FHC occur in the myosin head, α-tropomyosin, and troponin T. Two strands of α-tropomyosin that coil around actin are represented by a single strand.*

thesis of this structure. Expression of mutant β cardiac myosin heavy-chain polypeptides suggests that these act as poison peptides because they are stable in mammalian cells,[34] and when incorporated into reconstituted thick filaments, they have reduced motility as assessed by in vitro assays.[35]

Although mutant β cardiac myosin heavy-chain polypeptides appear to function as poison polypeptides, at least one cardiac troponin T mutation appears to function as a null mutation. The predicted effects of a mutation in the highly conserved 5′ splice donor sequence of intron 15 would be either the skipping of exons with the resultant transcript encoding a frame shift and premature termination, or use of a downstream cryptic splice signal, also resulting in premature termination. An analogous troponin T mutation has been described[36] in *Drosophila* (*upheld*^{2}), in which homozygous *upheld*^{2} flies lack troponin T polypeptide in flight muscle tissue.[37] Because the *upheld*^{2} appears to function as a null allele, the analogous human 5′ splice mutation may also be functionally a null allele. A null allele in cardiac troponin T would then be expected to cause FHC by altering the stoichiometry of sarcomeric components.

Whether by poison polypeptides or by altered ratio among the chains that make up the sarcomeric components, FHC mutations appear to cause cardiac hypertrophy by disrupting the sarcomere. What, then, is the mechanism by which disrupted sarcomeres lead to aberrant myocyte growth? Elucidating the steps in this pathway may identify new targets for therapeutics to treat FHC.

Clinical Implications of Molecular Diagnoses in Familial Hypertrophic Cardiomyopathy

Genetic studies have demonstrated that β cardiac myosin heavy-chain, cardiac troponin T, and α-tropomyosin mutations can cause FHC. In fact, mutations in these genes may cause as many as 70 percent of cases of FHC. Assuming that the remaining FHC genes encode sarcomeric proteins, we can anticipate that these genes will be identified in the near future. Knowledge of the full complement of disease genes will permit the genetic diagnosis of FHC. Although this task may still require analyses of several different genes, the identification of a disease-causing mutation in one individual will enable precise diagnosis of all family members, even before clinical findings of disease are present. Gene-based diagnosis also has the potential for improving the recognition of those individuals at risk for the serious sequelae of FHC.

The natural history and pathophysiology of FHC vary considerably in affected individuals from unrelated families. An early challenge for genetic studies of FHC was to determine if clinical or anatomic features of the disease could discriminate between the distinct genetic causes of the condition. Even before the cardiac troponin T and α-tropomyosin genes were demonstrated to cause FHC, clinical manifestations (symptoms and electrocardiographic and echocardiographic findings) of FHC caused by β cardiac myosin heavy-chain mutations were not distinct from disease features found in individuals with other gene defects.[38] In contrast, there may be differences in phenotype that are mutation-specific rather than allele-specific. Two unrelated families with FHC caused by α-tropomyosin mutations on chromosome 15 had significantly different degrees of cardiac hypertrophy.[29] Whether these differences reflect the unique effects of two different mutations within the same gene or the genetic and environmental background in which these mutations are expressed remains an area of active investigation.

Clinical outcome in individuals with FHC varies considerably. Physicians have recognized for many years that FHC in some families portends poor survival,[39] whereas in other families it may lead to a benign clinical course and a near-normal life expectancy.[8] Premature death in patients with FHC commonly results from either intractable heart failure (disease-related death) or sudden death. Neither the degree nor the distribution of hypertrophy correlates with clinical outcome, and unfortunately, the most common predictor of risk for premature mortality is the occurrence of sudden death in affected family members. Identification of the genetic causes of FHC may provide a better method for assessing prognosis.

Several groups have identified the same β cardiac myosin heavy-chain mutation in unrelated families with FHC. Comparison of life expectancies in individuals with different environmental, social, and genetic backgrounds, but who share an FHC gene defect, provides an indication of the effect that a particular mutation has on survival. Kaplan-Meier survival curves of life expectancy have been compiled for several different β cardiac myosin heavy-chain mutations [*see Figure 5*]. These studies demonstrate that some gene defects severely affect prognosis whereas others cause more benign disease.[24,25] For example, approximately half of all individuals with the Arg403Gln or Arg453Cys mutation (family A, [*see Figure 2*]) die by 40 years of age, whereas those with other mutation (e.g., Val606Met) have near-normal survival. It is intriguing that nonconservative mutations (or those that alter the charge of the encoded amino acid) appear to have a more significant effect on life expectancy than do conservative mutations, suggesting that changes in charge may contribute to the effects that a mutation has on myosin function.

Survival analysis in patients with cardiac troponin T mutation has also been revealing. Recent studies have demonstrated that life expectancy in four different cardiac troponin T mutations is comparable to that seen with malignant β cardiac myosin heavy-chain mutations, such as Arg403Gln[33] [*see Figure 5*]. This finding is particularly important because the cardiac hypertrophy produced by these mutations was typically mild and sometimes sub-clinical. The particularly poor prognosis associated with an inherited cardiomyopathy that presents with a subtle phenotype underscores the relevance of genetic diagnosis in patient management.

To date, many fewer mutations have been identified in the α-tropomyosin gene than in the β cardiac myosin heavy-chain or cardiac troponin T gene. However, because the hypertrophic responses in two different α-tropomyosin mutations are significantly different, different mutations in these genes will also likely produce a range in disease severity and hence will variably affect prognosis. As survival data are accumulated for a large number of mutations in the full complement of FHC genes, knowledge of genotype will likely enable a rigorous assessment of prognosis in affected individuals. Such data will provide important information to physicians and families and will allow aggressive therapies to be directed to those at risk for premature death.

Diagnosis of children at risk for developing FHC can be difficult and can require longitudinal studies. In many instances, disease phenotype does not manifest until puberty.[8,40] Because FHC is a dominant condition, each child of an affected individual has a 50 percent chance of developing the disease. Genetic diagnosis of children at risk will definitively identify those who have inherited an FHC mutation and will require repeated cardiovascular monitoring and counseling, particularly with regard to competitive sports. Gene-based preclinical diagnosis also makes early intervention possible, which may improve patients' survival and quality of life. Of equal im-

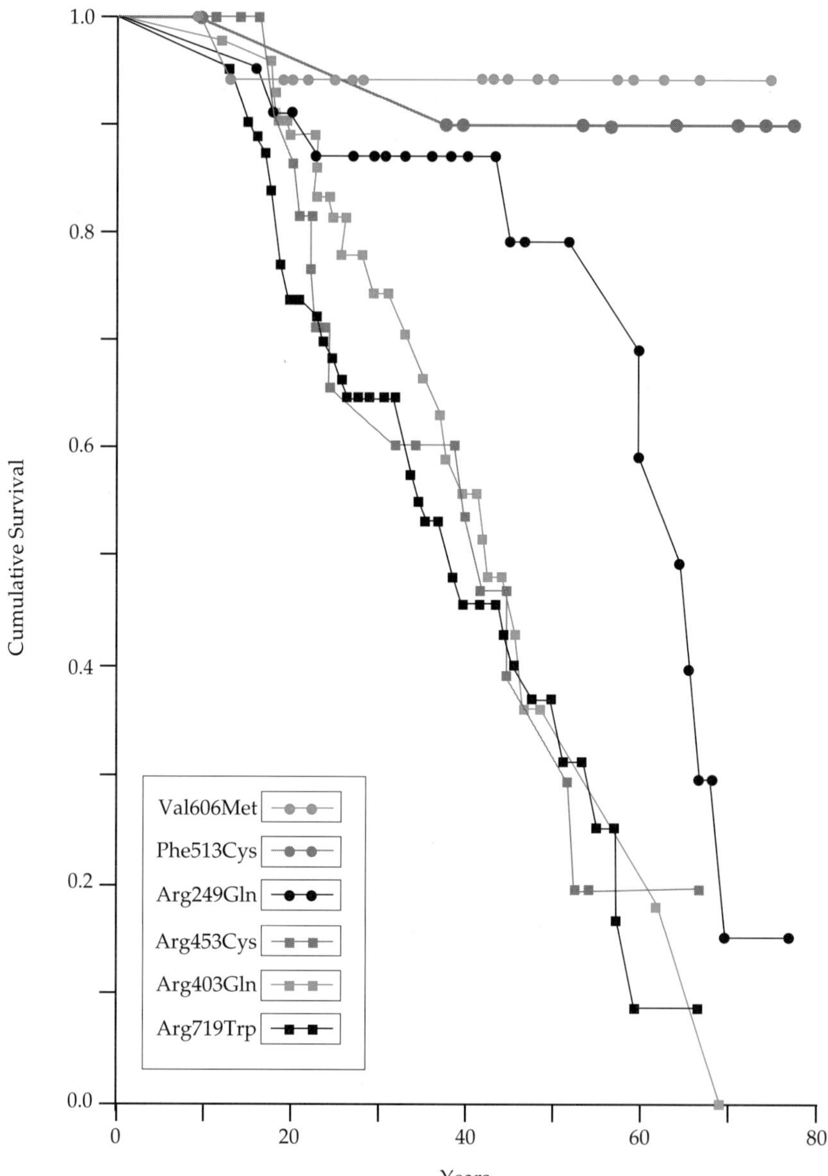

Figure 5 *Kaplan-Meier survival curves comparing the effects of different β cardiac myosin heavy-chain missense mutations on survival. Each point represents the current age or age of death of an affected individual with FHC caused by the corresponding mutation. Cumulative survival data has been compiled from affected individuals with the same β cardiac myosin heavy-chain mutation who are members of several unrelated families. The Phe513Cys survival data is derived from one large kindred.*

portance is the recognition of offspring who are unaffected. Gene-based recognition of unaffected offspring of individuals with FHC should prevent inappropriate restrictions and the psychological burdens that accompany a potentially inherited disease.

At present, genetic diagnosis of FHC genes is limited to families with mutations in the cardiac troponin T, α-tropomyosin, or β cardiac myosin heavy-chain gene. Because of the labor and expense involved in the identification of a precise mutation, linkage studies to define which gene is mutated are often performed first. However, as mutation screening technology improves, genetic diagnosis will certainly be possible in a single affected individual and in individuals whose clinical study results are equivocal for FHC. Inevitably, this will expand our knowledge of the repertoire of disease-causing mutations and will further define the relationship between phenotype and genotype.

Is Secondary Cardiac Hypertrophy a Disease of the Sarcomere?

The histopathology that typifies FHC can also be found in cardiac hypertrophy that results from such conditions as hypertension and valvular heart disease. The finding that FHC is a disease of the sarcomere has potential implications for the definition of the causes of noninherited forms of cardiac hypertrophy. In particular, one FHC mutation has been identified in a 5′ splice sequence of cardiac troponin T. This mutation appears comparable to a *Drosophila* 5′ splice sequence mutation that functions as a null allele[37]; that is, the transcripts resulting from the *Drosophila* mutation produce peptides that are not incorporated into the sarcomere. If the human cardiac troponin T gene mutation also functions as a null allele, the cardiac hypertrophy present in individuals with this mutation may result from altered stoichiometry of sarcomeric proteins. If confirmed, this finding would provide an intriguing model for secondary cardiac hypertrophy. Several studies have demonstrated that noninherited forms of cardiac hypertrophy are associated with changes in sarcomeric protein mRNA expression [*see also Chapter 12*].[41] Although these changes have been assumed to result from the development of hypertrophy, the troponin T null mutation that causes FHC suggests that changes in the stoichiometry of the sarcomeric components may be a fundamental event that triggers cardiac hypertrophy. Identification of the intracellular signals by which mutated sarcomeric proteins cause cardiac hypertrophy in FHC should provide new targets for the development of therapeutics for inherited and secondary cardiac hypertrophy.

Conclusions

The autosomal dominant condition FHC is a genetically heterogeneous condition that can be caused by mutations in genes that encode the sarcomeric components β cardiac myosin heavy chain, α-tropomyosin, and cardiac troponin T. Mutations in genes that encode other components of the thick and thin filaments will probably account for FHC that maps to other loci. These data classify FHC as a disease of the sarcomere. The ability to make genetic diagnoses of FHC has important consequences for patients, families, and physicians, partly because the severity of FHC appears to be related to the specific mutation that causes the disease. Thus, we anticipate that genetic diagnosis will become an additional tool for the cardiologist. We hope that by understanding the molecular basis of FHC, we will eventually be able to understand the molecular basis of cardiac hypertrophy that results from noninherited causes.

References

1. Hallopeau M: Retrecissement ventriculo-aortique. *Gazette Med Paris* 24:683, 1869
2. Codd MB, Sugrue DD, Gersh BJ, et al: Epidemiology of idiopathic dilated and hypertrophic cardiomyopathy. *Circulation* 67:1227, 1989
3. Maron BJ, Epstein SE, Roberts WC: Causes of sudden death in young athletes. *J Am Coll Cardiol* 7:204, 1986
4. Davies K: Diagnosing the heart of the problem. *Nat Genet* 4:211, 1993

5. Wynne J, Braunwald E: The cardiomyopathies and myocarditides: toxic, chemical, and physical damage to the heart. *Heart Disease: A Textbook of Cardiovascular Medicine*, 4th ed. Braunwald E, Ed. W.B. Saunders, Philadelphia, 1991, p 139
6. *Cardiomyopathies, Realisations and Expectations*. Goodwin J, Olsen E, Eds. Springer-Verlag, Berlin, 1993
7. McKenna W, Deanfield J, Faruqui A, et al: Prognosis in hypertrophic cardiomyopathy: role of age and clinical, electrocardiographic and hemodynamic features. *Am J Cardiol* 47:532, 1981
8. Spirito P, Chiarella F, Carratino L, et al: Clinical course and prognosis of hypertrophic cardiomyopathy in an outpatient population. *N Engl J Med* 320:749, 1989
9. van Dorp WG, ten Cate FJ, Vletter WB, et al: Familial prevalence of asymmetric septal hypertrophy. *Eur J Cardiol* 4/3:349, 1976
10. Maron BJ, Gottdiener JS, Epstein SE: Patterns and significance of distribution of left ventricular hypertrophy in hypertrophic cardiomyopathy: a wide angle, two dimensional echocardiographic study of 125 patients. *Am J Cardiol* 48:418, 1981
11. Maron BJ, Spirito P, Wesley Y, et al: Development and progression of left ventricular hypertrophy in children with hypertrophic cardiomyopathy. *N Engl J Med* 315:610, 1986
12. Chandrasekaran K, Aylward PE, Feegle SR, et al: Feasibility of identifying amyloid and hypertrophic cardiomyopathy with the use of computerized quantitative texture analysis of clinical echocardiographic data. *J Am Col Cardiol* 13:832, 1989
13. Solomon SD, Jarcho JA, McKenna W, et al: Familial hypertrophic cardiomyopathy is a genetically heterogeneous disease. *J Clin Invest* 86:993, 1990
14. Watkins H, Thierfelder L, Hwang D-S, et al: Sporadic hypertrophic cardiomyopathy due to de novo myosin mutations. *J Clin Invest* 90:1666, 1992
15. Greaves SC, Roche AH, Neutze JM, et al: Inheritance of hypertrophic cardiomyopathy: a cross sectional and M mode echocardiographic study of 50 families. *Br Heart J* 58:259, 1987
16. Jarcho JA, McKenna W, Pare JAP, et al: Mapping a gene for familial hypertrophic cardiomyopathy to chromosome 14q1. *N Engl J Med* 321:1372, 1989
17. Watkins H, MacRae C, Thierfelder L, et al: A disease locus for familial hypertrophic cardiomyopathy maps to chromosome 1q3. *Nat Genet* 3:333, 1993
18. Thierfelder L, MacRae C, Watkins H, et al: A familial hypertrophic cardiomyopathy locus maps to chromosome 15q2. *Proc Natl Acad Sci USA* 90:6270, 1993
19. Carrier L, Hengstenberg C, Beckmann JS, et al: Mapping of a novel gene for familial hypertrophic cardiomyopathy to chromosome 11. *Nat Genet* 4:311, 1993
20. Saez LJ, Gianola KM, McNally EM, et al: Human cardiac myosin heavy chain genes and their linkage in the genome. *Nucleic Acids Res* 15:5443, 1987
21. Nadal-Ginard B, Mahdavi V: Molecular basis of cardiac performance. *J Clin Invest* 84:1693, 1989
22. Marian AJ, Yu A-T, Mares A, et al: Detection of a new mutation in the β myosin heavychain gene in an individual with hypertrophic cardiomyopathy. *J Clin Invest* 90:2156, 1992
23. Tanigawa G, Jarcho JA, Kass S, et al: A molecular basis for familial hypertrophic cardiomyopathy: an α/β cardiac myosin heavy chain hybrid gene. *Cell* 62:991, 1990
24. Watkins H, Rosenzweig A, Hwang D-S, et al: Characteristics and prognostic implications of myosin missense mutations in familial hypertrophic cardiomyopathy. *N Engl J Med* 326:1108, 1992
25. Anan R, Greve G, Thierfelder L, et al: Prognostic implications of novel β myosin heavy chain gene mutations that cause familial hypertrophic cardiomyopathy. *J Clin Invest* 93:280, 1994
26. Fananapazir L, Epstein ND: Genotype-phenotype correlations in hypertrophic cardiomyopathy. *Circulation* 89:22, 1994
27. Geisterfer-Lowrance AAT, Kass S, Tanigawa G, et al: A molecular basis for familial hypertrophic cardiomyopathy: a β cardiac myosin heavy chain gene missense mutation. *Cell* 62:999, 1990
28. Watkins H, Thierfelder L, Anan R, et al: Independent origin of identical β myosin heavy chain gene mutations in hypertrophic cardiomyopathy. *Am J Hum Genet* 53:1180, 1993
29. Thierfelder T, Watkins H, MacRae C, et al: α Tropomyosin and cardiac troponin T mutations cause familial hypertrophic cardiomyopathy, a disease of the sarcomere. *Cell* 77:701, 1994
30. White SP, Cohen C, Phillips GN Jr: Structure of co-crystals of tropomyosin and troponin. *Nature* 325: 826, 1987
31. Zot AS, Potter JD: Structural aspects of troponin-tropomyosin regulation of skeletal muscle contraction. *Annu Rev Biophys Biomol Struct* 16: 535, 1987

32. Pan B-S, Gordon AM, Potter JD: Deletion of the first 45 NH_2-terminal residues of rabbit skeletal troponin T strengthens binding of troponin to immobilized tropomyosin. *J Biol Chem* 266:12432, 1991

33. Watkins H, McKenna W, Thierfelder L, et al: The role of cardiac troponin T and α-tropomyosin mutations in hypertrophic cardiomyopathy. *N Engl J Med* 332:1058, 1995

34. Straceski AJ, Geisterfer-Lowrance A, Seidman CE, et al: Functional analysis of myosin missense mutations in familial hypertrophic cardiomyopathy. *Proc Natl Acad Sci USA* 91:589, 1994

35. Sweeney HL, Straceski AJ, Leinwand LA, et al: Heterologous expression of a cardiomyopathic myosin that is defective in its actin interaction. *J Biol Chem.* 269:1603, 1994

36. Fyrberg E, Fyrberg C, Beall C, et al: *Drosophila melanogaster* troponin-T mutations engender three distinct syndromes of myofibrillar abnormalities. *J Mol Biol* 216:657, 1990

37. Mogami K, Nonomura Y, Hotta Y: Electron microscopic and electrophoretic studies of a *Drosophila* muscle mutant *wings-up* B. *Jpn J Genet* 56:51, 1981

38. Solomon SD, Wolff S, Watkins H, et al: Left ventricular hypertrophy and morphology in familial hypertrophic cardiomyopathy associated with mutations in the β myosin heavy chain gene. *J Am Coll Cardiol* 22:498, 1993

39. Maron BJ, Lipson LC, Roberts WC, et al: "Malignant" hypertrophic cardiomyopathy: identification of a subgroup of families with unusually frequent premature death. *Am J Cardiol* 41:1133, 1978

40. Rosenzweig A, Watkins H, Hwang D-S, et al: Preclinical diagnosis of familial hypertrophic cardiomyopathy by genetic analysis of blood lymphocytes. *N Engl J Med* 325:1753, 1991

41. Parker TG, Schneider MD: Growth factors, proto-oncogenes, and plasticity of the cardiac phenotype. *Annu Rev Physiol* 53:179, 1991

Acknowledgments

This work was supported by grants from the Howard Hughes Medical Institute, National Institutes of Health, American Heart Association, and Bristol-Myers Squibb Company.

Figure 2 Talar Agasyan.

Figure 3 Laura Brown.

Figure 3*c* Data from "Complete Nucleotide Sequence and Structural Organization of Rat Cardiac Troponin T Gene," by J. P. Jin, Q.Q. Huang, H. I.Yeh, J. S. Lin, in *Journal of Molecular Biology* 227:1269, 1992.

Figure 4 Tom Moore.

Figure 5 Laura Brown.

CHAPTER 14

Ion Channels and Cardiac Function

Harry A. Fozzard, M.D.

The heart is a large muscle that forms a four-chambered pump. Its electrical properties are specialized to its complex pump function. The right and left atria collect blood for the pulmonary and peripheral circulations, respectively, and they contract to propel the blood into the right and left ventricles through the atrioventricular valves. After a brief delay for filling, the ventricles contract in a synchronized way to close the atrioventricular valves, open the pulmonary and aortic valves to eject blood into the pulmonary and systemic circulations, and then relax to permit refilling. This sequence of compartmental synchronized contraction and relaxation allows the heart muscle to add potential (pressure) and kinetic (flow) energy efficiently to the blood to produce the circulation essential to deliver oxygen and nutrients to the body. How does this unusual muscle accomplish such a complex task 60 to 100 times per minute for the life of the organism?

Heart cells combine the properties of nerves to coordinate rapid events with the properties of muscle to contract and generate force, or shorten. Excitability, the nervelike function of heart cells, is found in their action potential, which is a propagated depolarization-repolarization process that provides an orchestrating signal to the muscle. A second complex process couples excitation to contraction. Depolarization of the membrane during the action potential secondarily causes a release of calcium from membrane-bound stores within the cells to initiate contraction. The contraction itself is a coordinated molecular interaction that causes one set of macromolecular filaments to march along another set. The stores then take up the calcium, allowing relaxation. These four processes are the key to normal cardiac cell function—excitation, excitation-contraction coupling, contraction, and relaxation.

The molecules critical to these four processes are proteins that regulate ion movement across membranes—ion channels and pumps—and proteins that form the sliding filaments for contraction. Many of these proteins have been cloned, and their primary sequences have been determined, allowing inference about their three-dimensional structures. The function of ion channels has been characterized biophysically in exquisite detail by the patch clamp method of studying simple molecular events. Similar biophysical studies of individual contractile proteins are also possible through optical methods. Because of the need for a delicate balance among the components of the cardiac electrical system, many genetic abnormalities of ion channels are lethal. However, subtler ion channel abnormalities are now being found that predispose to dysfunction. Commonly, ion channels and pumps are targets for environmental changes or disease. Ion channels play a significant role in normal morphogenesis, indicating that their abnormality may be found to be one mechanism for developmental dysfunction.

Membrane Proteins

Membranes form water and ion-impermeable barriers that allow isolated compartments to form. The most basic function of the surface membrane is to isolate the cytoplasm of the cell from the external environment, so that it can accomplish the many metabolic processes that require special conditions. This membrane is also depolarized during excitation through changes in its permeability properties. The cell is divided by membranes into many compartments, such as the nucleus, the mitochondria, and the endoplasmic reticulum, and variable structures, such as endosomes and transport vesicles. Membranes are composed of phospholipid and other lipids to form a hydrophobic barrier that is typically 30 to 40 Å thick. Although the impermeability of the basic membrane is essential, some means must exist for the entry and exit of solutes and for the regulation of cell volume. These functions are achieved by the intrinsic membrane proteins. Ion channels are intrinsic membrane proteins that are the structures responsible for excitation and excitation-contraction coupling. Pumps are also intrinsic membrane proteins that regulate ion concentrations, through such functions as pumping calcium into intracellular membrane-bound stores, so that the calcium may be released to initiate contraction. Membrane proteins differ from the better-studied soluble proteins, and the structures of membrane proteins have been harder to determine.

Synthesis

Proteins are strips of amino acids that are attached by amino-carboxy covalent linkages to form an –N–C–C–O– backbone. The rich variety of proteins is derived from the side chains of the 20 different amino acids that interact with one another and the environment. Although each amino acid is unique, amino acids can be divided into hydrophobic, polar, and charged types. The primary structure of a protein is a string of amino acids, and the protein may be formed from a handful to as many as 4,000 amino acids. In the past, the only way to determine the primary structure was to purify the protein, separate the terminal amino acid residues one by one, and identify them. The methods of molecular biology now allow the use of only a few such amino acids as templates for the extraction of mRNA, which can be used to isolate the full-length DNA sequence coding for the protein. The full protein primary structure can then be inferred from the nucleotide code for amino acids.

Self-association within the protein strand results in the formation of secondary structures, the most common of which are α helices, β strands, and random coils. α Helices are springlike coils of amino acids that are stabilized by hydrogen bonding into a fixed structure that typically has 3.6 amino acids per turn. These α helices, which are composed of about 18 to 25 mostly hydrophobic amino acids, are typical structures that cross the membrane hydrophobic barrier. β Strands are linear alignments of amino acids with bulky side chains on alternate sides of the strand. Strands are typically 8 to 16 residues long. They may terminate in a helix, or they may turn back on themselves to form a β hairpin with hydrogen bonds to the adjacent antiparallel strand. Random coils are less ordered structures. The helices, strands, and random coils arrange themselves into a tertiary structure. For a globular protein tertiary structure, this arrangement is influenced by the need for a hydrophobic interior and a hydrophilic surface. Membrane proteins have various patterns, with hydrophobic surfaces for interaction with membrane lipids and hydrophilic extracellular and intracellular domains. Many functional proteins, such as ion channels, are composed of several such tertiary units, forming a multidomain quaternary structure that is often symmetric or nearly so.

The complex structure of membrane proteins requires an equally complex process of synthesis. As the string of amino acids is formed by processing through the assembly line of the ribosome, some of the secondary structures are formed, and transmembrane crossings are accomplished. The amino end of the protein may contain a signal sequence that allows it to cross the endoplasmic reticulum membrane. This membrane crossing is the critical step for a transmembrane protein because the inside face of the endoplasmic reticulum membrane will eventually become the outside face of the surface membrane. This membrane polarity is preserved as the membrane and its embedded protein travel in the form of vesicles from the endoplasmic reticulum to the Golgi apparatus and eventually to the surface. In the Golgi apparatus, the partially folded protein receives further processing, such as glycosylation. Subunits may be associated at this processing stage or later. Finally, a vesicle containing the folded and assembled channel will travel to the membrane for fusion and insertion of the protein in its functional location. Proteins are not randomly distributed in the membrane; they may be clustered or even restricted to one side of a polar cell. The mechanism of such targeting and anchoring is not yet completely understood, but one component may be association with specific cytoskeletal proteins.

Structural Motifs

Five arbitrary categories of membrane proteins are (1) surface proteins that require only anchoring, (2) growth receptor, cell recognition, and cell adhesion proteins, (3) adrenergic receptors coupled to G-proteins, (4) pumps, and (5) channels. Proteins can be anchored on the surface of a cell simply by surface association with another membrane protein or lipid; this association is usually mediated by amphipathic helices or β structures (in which one face is hydrophobic and the other is hydrophilic). This process is used by enzyme systems that have circulating substrates. Other proteins are anchored to the membrane by the presence of one transmembrane (helical) segment and a small intracellular tail, with the principal part of the protein in the extracellular domain. This group includes the large family of cell-adhesion molecules, such as the integrins, the selectins, and the addressins. The transmembrane segment appears to function as an anchor for these molecules, but it may also mediate interaction with other transmembrane proteins. The cytoplasmic domain probably interacts with the cytoskeleton for localization. Some of these single-transmembrane segment proteins are receptors, such as the epidermal growth factor receptor. They have an outside N-terminal domain for binding of the ligand and a C-terminal intracellular signal-transduction domain that activates or functions as a protein kinase [*see Figure 1a*]. The transmembrane segment may also participate in signal transduction through dimerization of the receptors.

Adrenergic receptors characteristically have seven transmembrane helices, with the N-terminal outside and the C-terminal inside [*see Figure 1c*]. The extracellular domain and several of the hydrophobic helices make up the hormone-binding pocket, and the inside domain activates the intracellular messengers. Transmission of the signal from agonist binding to the effector element on the inside domain is by an unknown mechanism, but typically, the agonist causes the receptor to dissociate G-proteins, which then act as the receptor's intracellular effector molecules.

Pumps typically appear to have 10 to 14 transmembrane segments, often with two homologous domains, as shown in Figure 1e for a 12-transmembrane protein. The inside regions may contain regulatory or catalytic nucleotide binding sites. Presumably, the transmembrane components form the pathway for the transported substrates, such as ions or small molecules. This motif is also seen for some channels and for the enzyme system adenylyl cyclase.

Heart muscle has sodium and calcium channels, potassium channels, and chloride channels that generate its action potential. Ion channels have four essential components: an ion pore, a selectivity function, gates, and a gating sensor. Voltage-gated channels have voltage sensors and open and shut in response to membrane voltage. Ligand-gated channels have binding sites for hormones or neurotransmitters, and they open or close as a consequence of binding of the ligand. Voltage-gated channels are typically composed of a more-or-less symmetric four-subunit structure. Several kinds of potassium channels of the "Shaker" type[1] have six transmembrane α helices with N- and C-terminals on the cytoplasmic side [*see Figure 1d*]. The potassium channel is formed by noncovalent association of four of these molecules, which are either identical (homotetrameric) or different (heterotetrameric). The principal molecules for sodium and calcium channels, the α and α_1 subunits, respectively, contain four highly homologous sets of six α helices that are covalently linked to form the functional channel [*see Figure 1f*].

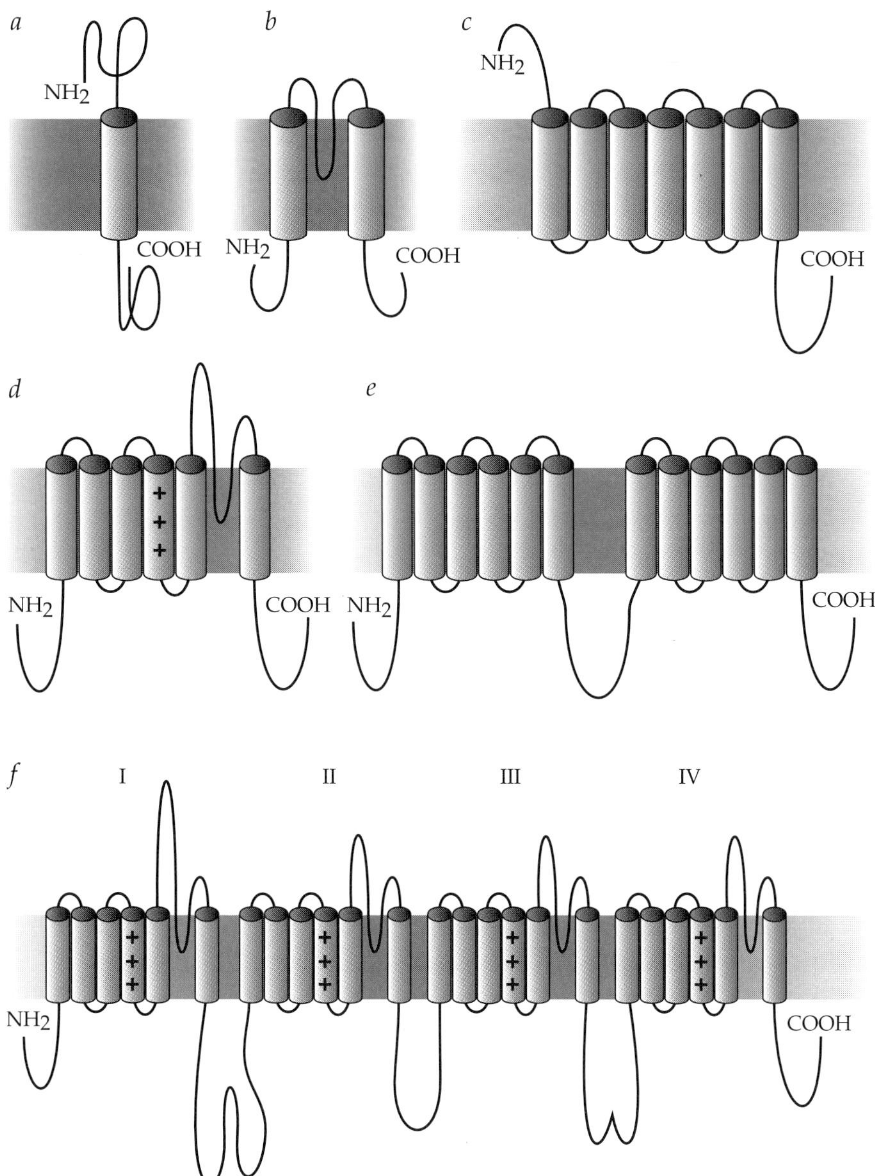

Figure 1 *Topology of various intrinsic membrane proteins functioning as ion channels or transporters. The N-terminals (NH_2) and C-terminals (COOH) are identified. The top of each membrane is extracellular. The barrels represent predicted α-helical structures spanning the membrane bilayer. (a) Single-transmembrane-segment proteins, including growth factor receptors and adhesion molecules. They often function as homodimers or heterodimers. (b) Two-transmembrane-segment proteins include a frequently occurring type of potassium channel. Functional channels are multimers that require at least four polypeptide monomers, but the exact number is unknown. (c) Seven-transmembrane-segment proteins are typical of the adrenergic receptors, which release a G-protein second messenger during ligand binding. (d) Six-transmembrane-segment proteins are characteristic of the voltage-gated potassium channel family. These protein channels form by the association of four similar molecules. (e) Two-domain proteins, each with six transmembrane segments. This pattern is seen in pumps as well as in ion channels. Alternative patterns for pumps are molecules with 10 or 14 transmembrane segments, and the N- and C-terminals may be extracellular. (f) Four-domain molecules, with each domain having six transmembrane segments. This structure is typical of voltage-gated sodium and calcium channels. (d and f) Some of the transmembrane structures are identified as having positively charged residues at every third position in the helix.*

The fourth α helix of each molecule or each homologous domain of the voltage-gated channels has a charged residue at each third position, so that four to six charges span the membrane electric field. This structure functions as the channel's voltage sensor. Some of the sodium and calcium channels also have additional subunits that modify the principal α subunit function. For further description, see W.A. Catterall.[2]

Typical ligand-gated channels contain five subunits that are arranged circumferentially to form a pore in the center. Each subunit is usually represented as having four transmembrane α helices, but considerable controversy now exists over the topology and secondary structures of these proteins. The prototype ligand-gated channel is the acetylcholine receptor in the neuromuscular junction, but glycine and glutamate receptors seem to be similar. Because these channels are composed of five circumferential subunits, their pore is larger than for the voltage-gated channels, and they are generally not very selective. This type of ion channel is not found in heart muscle.

A new class of cloned potassium-selective channels is not very voltage sensitive. These channels have two transmembrane segments that resemble the fifth and sixth transmembrane segments of the Shaker-type potassium channel, thereby omitting the pattern of charges in the fourth transmembrane segment that appears to function as the voltage sensor for Shaker-type potassium channels, sodium channels, and calcium channels [*see Figure 1b*]. These relatively voltage-insensitive potassium channels are usually gated by such ligands as G-protein, cyclic adenosine monophosphate (cAMP), or adenosine triphosphate (ATP). The number of subunits that form this type of potassium channel is not known. Finally, a small single-transmembrane segment protein called min-K can also form a channel when it is expressed in *Xenopus* oocytes, although some evidence suggests that its normal physiologic role may be partly as a regulator of other channels.

Ion Channels and Excitation

Channel Biophysics

Ion movement through channels can be rapid. For example, a single open sodium channel may allow a picoampere of current to flow, representing 10^7 ions/sec, compared with the rate of transport of the ATP-dependent sodium-potassium pump, which can achieve a maximum of only 200 to 300 cycles/sec. This very high ionic flow rate in channels requires that very little friction be encountered during the passage of the ion past the walls of the channel pore. However, channels must be capable of being selective, discriminating not only between anions and cations but even between such similar monovalent cations as Na^+ and K^+. Such discrimination requires that the ion interact with the channel protein closely during its transit. Channel selectivity does not simply mean that the channel acts as a sieve, because some channels allow passage of larger ions while rejecting smaller ones. Although the molecular mechanism of selectivity is not fully understood, the important variables include atomic size, valence, and energy of hydration.

Simple open ionic pores would permit ionic movement that is proportional to the difference in electrochemical energy between the two sides of the membrane. This property can be considered to be an application of Ohm's law to ion channels. In this application, the force causing ions to move is the transmembrane electrochemical gradient, which is a sum of the chemical concentration difference and the electric field acting on the ion's charge. The resistance of the channel is the friction of ion movement, and the current is the net transfer of charge per unit of time. However, many channels have more complicated permeation that favors ion movement in one direction more than the other, a process called rectification. This rectification is a prominent property of the family of potassium channels that are formed by two transmembrane segment proteins [*see Figure 1b*]. One example of the rectification process is the tendency of intracellular Mg^{2+} to block this type of rectifying potassium channel when the electrical field favors Mg^{2+} entry into the mouth of the pore. In this way, potassium may enter the cell from the outside without block but may have difficulty leaving the cell because of magnesium block.

Channels have the capability of opening or shutting in response to ligands, such as neurotransmitters or second messengers (ligand gating), or in response to membrane electric field (voltage gating). Ligand gating is most comparable to allosteric modulation of enzyme function. Voltage gating requires that some portion of the channel sense the electric field across the membrane and that there be a means of connecting the sensor to the gate itself. In both cases, the gating represents a conformational change in the membrane protein that could be as subtle as a loss of flexibility in the side chain of an amino acid in the selectivity filter or as dramatic as the movement of a large peptide segment into a blocking position in the pore. Generally, gates can change position quickly; a change in status from fully closed to fully open may occur in microseconds. However, some channels have subconductances, in which stepwise changes in current flow may result from partially open gates.

Gating can be studied by single-channel recording using a patch-clamp technique. A glass pipette with a small opening of approximately 1 μm in diameter seals to the cell membrane, electrically isolating the patch of membrane beneath the pipette tip. An amplifier can control voltage within the pipette, which is sealed to the outside surface of the membrane. If, for example, the pipette potential is set to be at the same level as the intracellular potential, no electric gradient exists across the patch. If a channel opens, the amplifier must supply amounts of current that are equal (and opposite in sign) to that of the current through the channel so that voltage is kept constant. Using this method, one can directly record the opening and closing of single channels as a function of ligand concentration or membrane potential. The opening and closing processes behave according to the predictions of first-order reactions, which are stochastic at the single-molecule level. Consequently, the individual behavior of the single channel is random and is described in terms of probabilities—much like radioactive decay, which is a random process that is analyzed statistically. For further discussion of channel biophysics, see B. Hille.[3]

Excitability and the Action Potential

All cells have a transmembrane potential that is typically 40 to 90 mV, with the interior being negative with respect to the exterior. This status is the consequence of the difference in ionic concentrations between the cytoplasm and the outside solution and of the selectively permeable nature of the membrane. A membrane pump, in all but a very few cell types, transfers Na^+ out of the cell and K^+ into it, splitting ATP in the process. K^+ is the predominant cytoplasmic cation. The resting membrane has a cation permeability primarily to K^+, so that some K^+ leaks out of the cell along its electrochemical gradient until a large-enough negative potential builds up in the cell to balance K^+ influx and efflux. In excitable cells, there is also a small inward leak of Na^+, and this leak is balanced by the sodium-potassium pump. If the inward Na^+ leak increases or the outward K^+ leak is reduced by changes in the distribution of open channels, the cell will lose part of its resting potential.

Excitable cells have a transient depolarization-repolarization event called the action potential. If the membrane depolarizes to a threshold voltage, it shifts its permeability so that it is primarily permeable to Na^+ or Ca^{2+}, which allows large numbers of positive charges into the cell, causing it to depolarize. This system has a positive-feedback property because depolarization increases the chance that sodium and calcium channels will open, and the current through the channels causes further depolarization, increasing even more the probability that the channels will open. The rapid local depolarization at the original site of the action potential produces currents that flow to adjacent parts of cells. Cardiac cells are coupled by low-resistance gap junction channels, which are large nonselective ion channels that permit current to flow easily from cell to cell, thereby propagating the action potential into the next cell. These currents, if large enough, can be recorded on the body surface, making electrocardiographic study possible. Sodium channels have a second gate that closes relatively slowly during depolarization, so that the sodium current turns itself off. Like sodium channels, calcium channels are voltage gated.

Depolarization opens several types of potassium channels in addition to the sodium and calcium channels. Both the opening of potassium channels and the closing of sodium or calcium channels favor repolarization back to the resting potential. In contrast to the one- to two-millisecond-long nerve action potentials, cardiac action potentials are 100 to 300 milliseconds long. This prolonged depolarization permits a substantial Ca^{2+} current to flow and to activate contraction. Prolonged depolarization also prevents premature reactivation, so that the muscle has time to complete its contraction and relax before the next activation. This mechanism of the long action potential is some mix of a prolonged small inward current from sodium and calcium channels and a transient fall in K^+ current that results from inward rectification. Repolarization results both from the eventual shutting of sodium and calcium channels and from the slow opening of potassium channels.

Additional factors that alter the resting and action potentials over long periods of time relative to the action potential are special potassium channels [*see Figure 1b*], which are opened secondarily by acetylcholine released from the vagal nerve, and chloride channels of several types, which are opened by voltage or by phosphorylation via the cAMP pathway. These potassium channels are gated by G-proteins that are released from a receptor of the seven-membrane spanning type [*see Figure 1c*], which is activated by acetylcholine. The phosphorylation-gated chloride channels can be activated by any stimulus that increases cellular cAMP. The topology of chloride channels is not yet clear, but they are most like pumps, as illustrated in Figure 1e. Some pumps and exchangers can have electrogenic effects, contributing small but occasionally important currents. In addition, other channels may become active in disease states. One such surface membrane channel is activated by intracellular calcium and allows entry of cations that can then depolarize the cell and trigger an action potential. This current is noted as [I_{NS}] in Figure 2. It is one cause of ventricular tachycardia in ischemia and in digitalis toxicity. Another channel that has an important role in ischemic heart disease is the K(ATP) channel, which is a potassium-selective channel that is kept closed in the presence of normal cellular levels of ATP but that opens during ischemia when ATP levels fall to the range of 1 mmol/L. When open, this channel causes the cardiac action potential to be shortened, and it may be responsible for the T-wave changes seen electrocardiographically during ischemia. Current through this channel is identified in Figure 2 by the symbol [$I_{K(ATP)}$]. Because different parts of the heart have different complements or densities of channels and pumps, the action potentials can differ substantially, and they can respond to pathological conditions or drugs differently. Overall, more than 10 channel types that contribute to the cardiac electrical system interact with voltage and with each other to produce the resting and action potentials [*see Figure 2; see also Task Force of the Working Group on Arrhythmias of the European Society of Cardiology*].[4]

Excitation-Contraction Coupling and Contraction

Excitation-Contraction Coupling

Excitation-contraction coupling is the process by which membrane depolarization is translated into mechanical action. The process occurs in three stages. First, calcium must be explosively increased to permit the initiation of a series of steps, beginning with the binding of calcium to troponin, which then allows myosin to interact with actin, resulting in contraction. Second, calcium must be reduced to its resting level to stop the actin-myosin interaction and permit relaxation. Finally, the calcium release process must recover before the next contraction occurs. Figure 3 shows the path that calcium traverses during excitation, contraction, and recovery. When calcium is bound to troponin, contraction is initiated.

The first stage of excitation-contraction coupling is initiated by membrane depolarization, which activates voltage-gated calcium channels in the surface membrane. Ca^{2+} enters and binds to ryanodine receptors (so named for the high-affinity chemical used for their isolation biochemically) of the sarcoplasmic reticulum. This action triggers release of Ca^{2+} from the terminal cisternae of the sarcoplasmic reticulum via the ryanodine receptor, which is a calcium-sensitive, nonselective channel. Ca^{2+} entering the cell through the surface-membrane calcium channel combines with Ca^{2+} released from the sarcoplasmic reticulum to interact with troponin C; this interaction results in the initiation of contraction. The delay between depolarization and onset of contraction is typically two to four milliseconds. The magnitude of the rise in

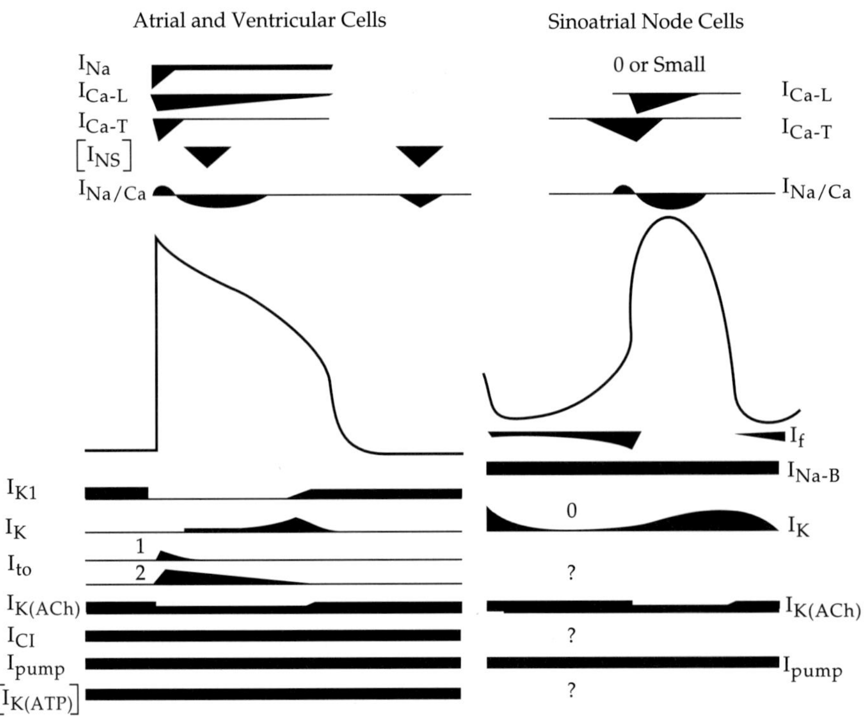

Figure 2 *Currents and channels involved in generating the resting and action potentials. The time course of stylized action potential of atrial and ventricular cells is shown on the left, and that of sinoatrial cells, on the right. Above the action potentials are the various channels and pumps that contribute inward (depolarizing) currents, and below are the channels and pumps for outward (repolarizing) currents. Associated with each current (I) is a subscript identifying the channel type.* $I_{Ca\text{-}L}$ *is the L-type calcium channel current, and* $I_{Ca\text{-}T}$ *is the T-type calcium channel current.* I_{K1} *is the* K^+ *current responsible for maintaining the resting potential near the* K^+ *equilibrium potential in atrial and ventricular cells.* $I_{Na\text{-}B}$ *is the proposed background* Na^+ *current through a voltage-independent channel in sinoatrial cells.* I_f *is the inward current carried by* Na^+ *through a relatively nonspecific cationic channel.* I_{to} *is the* K^+ *current that turns on rapidly after depolarization and then inactivates. The approximate time courses of the currents associated with the channels or pumps are symbolized by the variation in line weight. No effort is made to represent their magnitudes relative to each other. The heavy bars for* I_{CI}, I_{pump}, *and* $I_{K(ATP)}$ *indicate only the presence of these channels or pumps. The cationic nonselective channel and the potassium-selective adenosine triphosphate channel [*I_{NS} *and* $I_{K(ATP)}$*] are active only under pathological conditions. In sinoatrial cells,* I_{Na} *and* I_{K1} *are small or absent (0). Question marks indicate that experimental evidence is insufficient to decide the roles of these currents. Other channels and currents exist under nonphysiologic conditions, but their roles are not yet resolved.*

Ca^{2+} is determined by the size of the membrane Ca^{2+} current, the quantity of Ca^{2+} in the sarcoplasmic reticulum, the sensitivity of the sarcoplasmic reticulum release system, and the Ca^{2+}-buffering capacity of the cytoplasm. The principal Ca^{2+} buffer in heart cells, other than troponin C itself, is calmodulin.

The Relaxation Process

Although Ca^{2+} binds quickly to troponin C, the dissociation of Ca^{2+} from troponin is relatively slow, so free cytoplasmic Ca_i declines before contraction peaks. The time course of normal relaxation is controlled mainly by the Ca^{2+} dissociation process. Ca^{2+} released from troponin C is reaccumulated into the sarcoplasmic reticulum by an ATP-dependent Ca^{2+} pump, or it is transferred to the outside by a surface membrane sodium-calcium antiporter and a second ATP-dependent Ca^{2+} pump.

The Ca^{2+} release process must recover before another normal contraction can occur. This recovery process lags behind recovery of the surface membrane calcium channels and the Ca^{2+} pump of the sarcoplasmic reticulum. The process probably depends on recovery of the ryanodine receptor, which is the release channel of the sarcoplasmic reticulum.

The Roles of Calcium Channels

Essential to the contraction system are the surface-membrane calcium channels.[5] Two kinds of sarcolemmal calcium channels are found in heart cells: L type and T type. T-type calcium channels may be important for pacemaker behavior, but their role in normal excitation-contraction coupling is usually minor. The L-type calcium channels, however, are essential in regulating the electrical activity of the heart. They are activated by depolarization to between -40 and zero millivolts. The rapid influx of calcium from its relatively high extracellular level raises Ca^{2+} just beneath the surface membrane to high levels. These channels are inactivated partly by a voltage-dependent process, but the main process is by binding of Ca^{2+} at a site on the inside surface of the channel. After inactivation, channel recov-

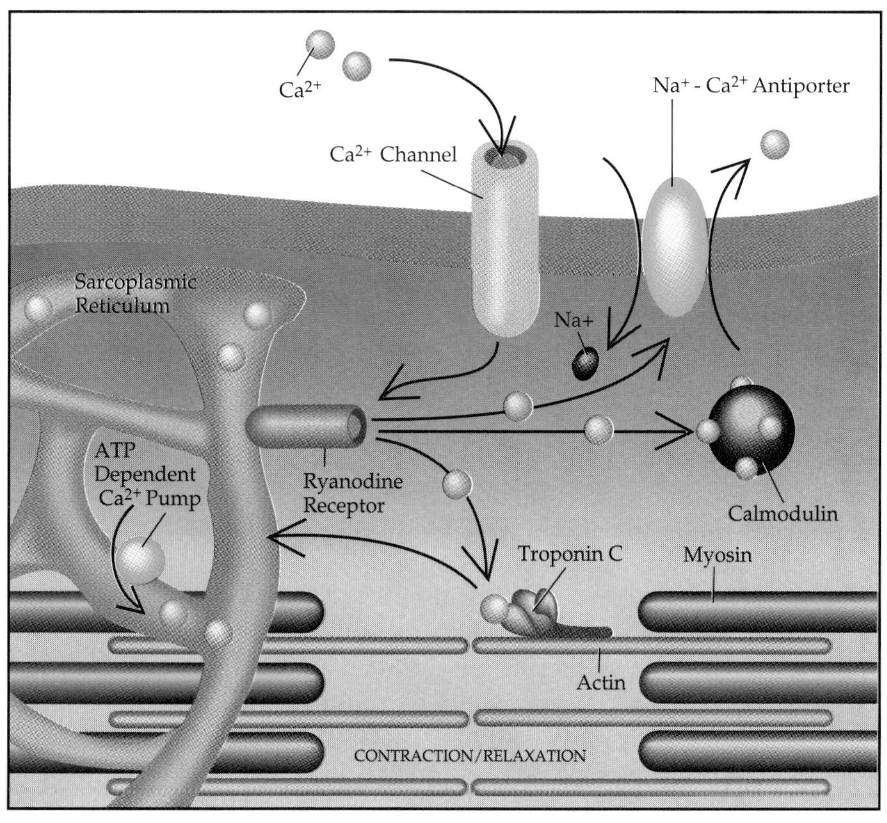

Figure 3 *Illustration of cardiac cellular calcium cycling. The surface-membrane calcium channel allows Ca^{2+} entry when the channel is opened by depolarization during the action potential. The entering Ca^{2+} diffuses to the calcium-release channel (the ryanodine receptor) of the terminal cisternae of the sarcoplasmic reticulum. Ca^{2+} released from this store is transported out of the cell by the sodium-calcium antiporter, and it binds to intracellular buffers, represented here by calmodulin, and to troponin C to initiate contraction. Ca^{2+} is also pumped back into the sarcoplasmic reticulum by an ATP-dependent Ca^{2+} pump, thereby lowering intracellular Ca^{2+} and producing relaxation.*

ery requires both reduction of Ca_i and repolarization, and it is usually complete in several hundred milliseconds.

The L-type calcium channel is the target for most of the clinically used calcium channel–active drugs. The current is reduced by verapamil and diltiazem and the dihydropyridine family of molecules, although some molecules related in structure to calcium channel drugs can increase the Ca^{2+} current. These drugs act at three separate but cooperative sites on the channel. The dihydropyridine site has been located on the α_1 subunit, and the others are probably there also. The L-type calcium channel is also modulated by various hormones and biologically active molecules. The best-studied mode of modulation is calcium-channel enhancement by beta-adrenergic stimulation. This process results from channel phosphorylation by protein kinase A, which is activated by cAMP that is derived from the stimulated adenylyl cyclase. Phosphorylation alters single-channel kinetics to increase the probability that the channel will open on depolarization and to prolong openings as well. Examples of agents that reduce the L-type Ca^{2+} current are acetylcholine, which reduces cAMP via its muscarinic receptor, G-proteins that inhibit adenylyl cyclase or directly inhibit the channel, and adenosine, which acts by a yet unresolved second messenger system. This topic is thoroughly reviewed by McDonald et al.[5]

L-type calcium channels are large proteins that contain probably five subunits. The α_1 subunit is structurally similar to the voltage-gated sodium channel in that it has four homologous domains of six transmembrane segments each [*see Figure 1f*]. When the RNA coding for the subunit is expressed in heterologous cells, it possesses the principal pore properties and some of the pharmacological properties of the native channel, but it shows abnormal kinetics. Coexpression of the α_1 subunit with the α_2 and β subunits tends to restore normal kinetics and perhaps adrenergic modulation. The roles of the two other subunits are not yet clear.

The Sarcoplasmic Reticulum and Ca^{2+} Release

The sarcoplasmic reticulum is a highly structured intracellular membrane compartment that incorporates the Ca^{2+} uptake system and terminal cisternae near the Z line. It has long been known to sequester Ca^{2+} by action of an ATP-dependent Ca^{2+} pump. The pump affinity for Ca^{2+} transport is sufficiently high that it can lower Ca_i to subthreshold levels for contraction. In the heart, this pump is suppressed by an associated protein called phospholamban. When phospholamban is phosphorylated by protein kinase A, it is partially inhibited, and Ca^{2+} uptake into the sarcoplasmic reticulum is enhanced. The quantity of Ca^{2+} in the sarcoplasmic reticulum is large, and most of it is bound by calsequestrin, an effective Ca^{2+} buffer.

The terminal cisternae membranes release Ca^{2+} via the ryanodine receptor, which is a channel composed of four homologous proteins with a molecular weight of about 500 kilodaltons each.[6] The ryanodine receptor binds the alkaloid ryanodine, which opens the channel. The structure of this channel appears to be quite special, with one opening on the inside of the terminal cisterna and four openings on the outside. This complex from animal tissue has been reconstituted in lipid bilayers, where its properties can be studied directly. The reconstituted cardiac channel is triggered to open by Ca^{2+}, in a manner similar to that observed in animal tissues. This behavior is a positive-feedback system, in which a little trigger Ca^{2+} entering from the outside results in release of more Ca^{2+}. A major problem in understanding the function of this Ca^{2+}-release system is its graded behavior. In intact cells, a small Ca^{2+} current triggers a partial release, producing a graded contraction rather than the all-or-nothing release that would be expected from its positive-feedback property. The ryanodine receptor channel may also have a Ca^{2+}-inhibitory site that can turn the channel off.

Regulation of Intracellular Ca^+ and Relaxation

Contractile relaxation and recovery require restoration of normal cytoplasmic levels of Ca_i of 50 to 200 nmol/L. The major part of relaxation is the steady-state reuptake of Ca^+ by the ATP-dependent Ca^+ pump of the sarcoplasmic reticulum. However, Ca^{2+} is also added to the cell by entry through the calcium channel, typically in five to 10 percent of the amount used in the contraction. If steady state is to be maintained, this increment must be ejected from the cell during each contraction-relaxation cycle. The surface membrane contains a powerful system for the transport of Ca^{2+} to the outside, the sodium-calcium exchange protein, which is an antiporter that transports three Na^+ into the cell while transporting one Ca^{2+} out of the cell. It does not consume ATP in this process but uses the large electrochemical gradient for Na^+ as its energy source for calcium efflux. Note that the sodium-calcium exchange protein is electrogenic, allowing three positive charges into the cell in exchange for two positive charges out, so it acts as a depolarizing current when in its Ca^{2+}-efflux mode. Under the right circumstances, it can reverse its direction and transport Ca^{2+} into the cell in exchange for Na^+. For normal Na^+ gradients that are maintained by the sodium-potassium pump, the equilibrium for the sodium-calcium antiporter will take Ca_i to submicromolar levels. The sodium-calcium antiporter system has a high transport rate, so it begins to operate as soon as Ca^{2+} is released from the sarcoplasmic reticulum, thereby contributing to the Ca_i decline during systole and continuing at a lower rate in diastole. An ATP-dependent Ca^{2+} pump, also found in the surface membrane, has a low transport rate, but its K_D for inside Ca^{2+} is lower, and it may be important in setting the final diastolic level of Ca_i.

Regulation of Ca_i is obviously complex and involves numerous ion channels, transporters, and buffers. Some aspects of their interrelationship and relative importance in activation and relaxation of contraction remain controversial, and the feedback processes necessary for the stability of the system remain to be identified. Under pathological conditions, such as ischemia or excessive hypertrophy, or under the influence of drugs, this very sensitive Ca^{2+}-regulation process can be disrupted, resulting in poor contraction or relaxation or in lethal arrhythmias.

Conclusions

Ion channels play important roles in cardiac electrogenesis and contraction. The normal resting potential results from high membrane permeability to K^+ by potassium channels and from the ion gradient generated by the sodium-potassium pump. The action potential is a transient depolarization lasting 200 to 300 milliseconds. The depolarization in ventricular, atrial, and His-Purkinje cells is the result of transient openings of voltage-dependent sodium channels, which allow a large positive inward current that propagates the action potential throughout the heart. Depolarization of sinoatrial node and atrioventricular node cells is caused by opening of the calcium channels. The depolarization is maintained by a balance between Na^+ and Ca^{2+} currents, which carry a positive inward current, and K^+ currents, which carry a positive outward current. Repolarization occurs because the K^+ currents eventually dominate.

Calcium channels in the surface membrane admit a relatively small Ca^{2+} current that triggers release from intracellular stores of Ca^{2+} located in the terminal cisternae of the sarcoplasmic reticulum. These Ca^{2+} stores are released through a different calcium channel called the ryanodine receptor. After it is released, the Ca^{2+} is taken back into the sarcoplasmic reticulum by a Ca^{2+} pump. After contraction occurs, there is a partial refractory period caused by a slow recovery of this Ca^{2+}-release system.

The surface membrane and terminal cisterna ion channels are intrinsic membrane proteins, some of which are highly selective for permeating ions and others less selective. They may be opened or shut by membrane voltage (sodium and calcium channels and some potassium channels), by intracellular messengers (some potassium channels), or by intracellular Ca^{2+} (calcium channels and ryanodine receptor channels). Many of the channels have now been cloned and expressed in heterologous cells, and rapid progress is being made in the resolution of their structure and function.

References

1. Roberds SL, Knoth KM, Po S, et al: Molecular biology of the voltage-gated potassium channels of the cardiovascular system. *J Cardiovasc Electrophysiol* 4:68, 1993
2. Catterall WA: Cellular and molecular biology of voltage-gated sodium channels. *Physiol Rev* 72(suppl):S15, 1992
3. Hille B: *Ionic Channels of Excitable Membranes*. Sinauer Associates, Sunderland, MA, 1992
4. Task Force of the Working Group on Arrhythmias of the European Society of Cardiology: The Sicilian gambit. A new approach to the classification of antiarrhythmic drugs based on their actions on arrhythmogenic mechanisms. *Circulation* 84:1831, 1991
5. McDonald TF, Pelzer S, Trautwein W, et al: Regulation and modulation of calcium channels in cardiac, skeletal, and smooth muscle cells. *Physiol Rev* 74:365, 1994
6. Meissner G: Ryanodine receptor/Ca^{2+} release channels and their regulation by endogenous effectors. *Annu Rev Physiol* 56:485, 1994

Acknowledgments

Figure 1 Laura Brown.

Figure 2 Laura Brown. Adapted from "The Sicilian Gambit. A New Approach to the Classification of Antiarrhythmic Drugs Based on Their Action on Arrhythmogenic Mechanisms" by the Task Force of the Working Group on Arrhythmias of the European Society of Cardiology, in *Circulation* 84:1831, 1991.

Figure 3 Dana Burns-Pizer.

CHAPTER 15

Molecular Mechanisms in Hypertension

Victor J. Dzau, M.D., Jose E. Krieger, M.D., Ph.D., Howard Hutchinson, M.D.

Hypertension is a polygenetic disease that is characterized by dysfunction of vascular, cardiogenic, renal, neurogenic, and endocrine mechanisms, which interact in a complex but integrated manner to regulate blood pressure. Evidence suggests that altered genetic and environmental interactions play a key role in the genesis of primary hypertension. Molecular biology research has improved our understanding of the mediators of blood pressure control, such as angiotensin II, atrial natriuretic peptide, endothelin, and nitric oxide, and their potential roles in hypertension. Once initiated, hypertension tends to self-amplify via structural changes in the blood vessels, heart, and kidneys. These changes increase both systemic vascular resistance and cardiac output and impair sodium handling. Thus, the cellular and molecular processes of cardiovascular remodeling are important mechanisms in hypertension. Finally, our understanding of the molecular mechanisms of hypertension has been facilitated by genetic manipulations in vivo, such as transgenic models, homologous recombination, and in vivo gene transfer. The genetics of hypertension is reviewed in Chapters 16 and 17 of this book. This chapter focuses on the molecular biology of the systems that control hypertension.

Molecular Biology of the Hypertension Control Systems

Blood pressure homeostasis is maintained by a balance of countervailing forces that affect blood flow, vascular resistance, electrolyte and water handling, and cell growth. Complex interactions of endogenous biologically ac-

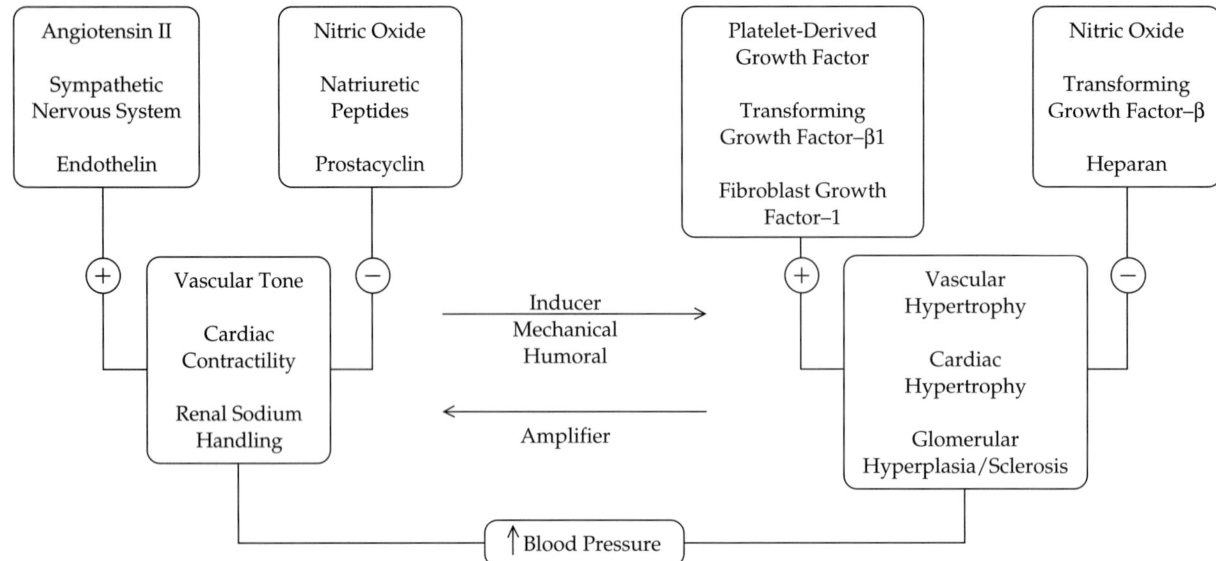

Figure 1 *The complex interaction among the biological substances and processes that regulate blood pressure. An imbalance in favor of vasoconstriction or sodium retention or of cardiovascular hypertrophy and hyperplasia can result in sustained hypertension.*

tive substances maintain fluid and electrolyte homeostasis, proper cellular growth, and a normal hemodynamic state. An imbalance of these forces in favor of sodium and water retention, cardiovascular hypertrophy and hyperplasia, or vasoconstriction can lead to sustained hypertension [*see Figure 1*]. Renal, endocrine, neurogenic, cardiogenic, and vascular mechanisms have been demonstrated to participate in the pathophysiology of hypertension. Molecular and cellular biologic research has contributed significantly to our understanding of the basic mechanisms underlying the control process and their potential roles in the pathogenesis of hypertension. In particular, major strides have been made in elucidating the molecular biology of substances that are involved with blood pressure regulation. These substances include the components of the renin-angiotensin system, the natriuretic peptide system, endothelins and their receptors, and nitric oxide synthase, which is responsible for endogenous nitric oxide production. The complementary and genomic DNAs for many of these factors have been cloned, sequenced, expressed in vitro, mutated, and tested as candidate genes for hypertension.

Renin-Angiotensin System

The importance of the renin-angiotensin system (RAS) for maintenance of normal cardiovascular homeostasis and its participation in hypertension and cardiovascular diseases is well established. A detailed review of this system is presented in Chapter 17. The classic endocrine view of the RAS has evolved to include the novel concept of tissue angiotensin systems directing the production of angiotensin at local tissue sites with paracrine and autocrine functions. Indeed, recent data have demonstrated that all, or at least part, of the components of the RAS are present in several tissues important for maintaining cardiovascular homeostasis. In particular, at local tissue sites, angiotensin-converting enzyme (ACE) can also play an important rate-limiting role and regulate the rate of local angiotensin II production. The peptide angiotensin II, of circulatory or tissue origin, activates specific receptors in multiple target organs. Several isoforms of angiotensin II receptors have been reported to exist, and so far, two isoforms, the type 1 (AT1) and type 2 (AT2) have been cloned. Because ACE and angiotensinogen are reviewed in detail elsewhere in this book, this chapter concentrates on the molecular biology of the tissue angiotensin system and angiotensin receptors.

Endocrine and Tissue Angiotensin System

In addition to the angiotensin II formed in the circulation as a hormone, local synthesis of angiotensin II occurs in multiple tissues.[1,2] The production of local angiotensin II occurs because of the existence and action of one or more components of the RAS in these target tissues. The presence of these components is due to their uptake from plasma or local gene expression. In particular, ACE is widely expressed in the endothelium of all blood vessels (arteries to capillaries), and this endothelial membrane-bound enzyme can potentially control local angiotensin II synthesis in specific vascular beds. Local angiotensin II can exert autocrine-paracrine effects on local tissue functions and participates in the pathophysiology of cardiovascular diseases.

Among the various components of the RAS, ACE appears to be particularly important as a regulator of angiotensin II production in tissues. Many studies have shown that chronic increases in tissue ACE expression and activity within the physiologic range (two- to threefold) result in parallel increases in tissue angiotensin II production.[3,4] We observed that an increased cardiac ACE expression due to a pressure overloading of the ventricle resulted in an increased intramyocardial conversion of angiotensin I to angiotensin II.[3] In the microvasculature of the heart, which is characterized by a significant capillary surface area containing ACE, angiotensin I is converted to angiotensin II. The microvasculature-derived angiotensin II translocates into the interstitium, with subsequent binding to myocyte and fibroblast receptors. The activation of myocyte receptors can increase contractility and stimulate cellular hypertrophy.[5,6] These effects are amplified by angiotensin's ability to stimulate catecholamine release from sympathetic nerve endings, leading to additional positive inotropic and hypertrophic effects.[7] Recent evidence suggests the presence of ACE within cells of the myocardium in addition to its location in the microvasculature. The existence of a second myocardial enzyme, angiotensin I convertase (or human chymase), which can convert angiotensin I to angiotensin II, has also been described.[8,9] This enzyme is found to be abundant and confirms the ability of the myocardium to produce angiotensin II independent of that delivered by the circulation. Local ACE gene expression appears to be triggered in response to ventricular wall tension, leading to increases in tissue angiotensin. The increased angiotensin can lead to subsequent alterations in myocardial structure (cardiac remodeling) by activating myocytes and nonmyocytes, promoting expression of autocrine-paracrine growth factors, and favoring the formation of connective tissue by fibroblasts and mesenchymal cells. The highly organized collagen network present in the normal myocardium becomes disrupted in hypertensive heart disease, leading to hypertrophy, increased myocardial stiffness, and abnormalities in diastolic and/or systolic function. Inhibition of the myocardial RAS leads to regression of left ventricular hypertrophy, reduced diastolic stiffness, and reduced interstitial fibrosis.[10]

In the vessel wall, ACE is primarily localized in the endothelium, although recent evidence also suggests the existence of ACE-like enzymes in the media and adventitia. Vascular ACE is activated in hypertension and vascular diseases. Okamura and colleagues[4] reported that during the chronic (non–renin-dependent) phase of two-kidney, one-clip renovascular hypertension in the rat, vascular ACE activity increased threefold secondary to the increase in blood pressure. The increased vascular ACE led to a parallel increase in vascular angiotensin I to angiotensin II conversion.[4] In intimal lesions of rat carotid arteries produced by angioplasty injury, ACE can be detected in vascular smooth muscle cells. In human atherosclerotic lesions, ACE immunohistochemical staining is present in macrophages and vascular smooth muscle cells. Vascular ACE is important not only for vascular smooth muscle contractility but also for growth of vascular smooth muscle cells that contributes to the development of intimal hyperplasia or medial hypertrophy. The role of local ACE in vascular structural abnormalities has been shown by in vivo gene transfer of ACE into intact blood vessels. ACE complementary DNA (cDNA) was transfected in vivo into an intact, injured common carotid artery of a rat, and the consequences were studied two weeks later. We observed a threefold increase in vascular ACE as well as local angiotensin-mediated hypertrophy in the transfected segment of the common carotid artery but not in the nontransfected control vessel or in the vessel transfected with the control vector (not containing ACE cDNA).[9] These results are strong evidence for a local ACE effect on angiotensin II production, affecting structural changes (i.e., hypertrophy) in the arterial media.

Taken together, these data suggest that in addition to the circulating RAS, local angiotensin production is an important modulator of tissue function and structure. Whereas circulating compounds of the RAS may be taken up by various tissues, local compartments within these tissues may generate angiotensin II with different enzyme substrate concentration and kinetics. Thus, the circulating RAS is important not only for systemic cardiovascular regulation but also in individual tissues, where local activation of this system can alter functions, such as cardiac and vascular remodeling and atherosclerosis, and have no effect on blood pressure.

Molecular Biology of Angiotensin Receptors

Ligand binding studies and molecular cloning efforts have shown the existence of a family of angiotensin II receptors.[11] The receptor that exists in the blood vessels, kidneys, heart, adrenal glands, and brain belongs to the AT1 subtype and mediates the known actions of angiotensin II, such as vasoconstriction and aldosterone release. This receptor is a member of the superfamily of seven-transmembrane, G-protein–coupled receptors. Angiotensin II binds to specific sites on the extracellular and membrane-spanning portions of the receptor, resulting in the coupling of a specific G protein to the receptor and the subsequent stimulation of intracellular events that lead to specific cellular responses. In vascular smooth muscle cells, stimulation of the AT1 receptor results in coupling with the protein Gq and the activation of phospholipase C, thereby increasing production of inositol trisphosphate and metabolites, leading to calcium influx, and in the generation of diacylglycerol, leading to protein kinase C activation. In the liver, angiotensin II receptor couples with the protein Gi, with subsequent inhibition of adenylate cyclase and a reduction of cyclic adenosine monophosphate. The AT1 antagonist losartan binds specifically to the AT1 receptor and inhibits the action of angiotensin II.

In the rat and mouse, the AT1 receptor has been shown to consist of two isoforms, AT1a and AT1b.[12,13] Most of the amino acid differences between these two isoforms are in the C-terminal region of the peptide. However, when comparing AT1a to AT1b sequences, the replaced amino acids are not the same in the rat and mouse. We and others have compared the ligand-binding, signal-transduction, desensitization, and internalization characteristics between rat AT1a and AT1b receptor isoforms, and thus far, no significant pharmacological or functional differences can be shown. Of note, recently, is that a second AT1 receptor subtype was cloned from a human placental cDNA library.[14] Once again, no significant pharmacological or functional difference from the previously characterized human AT1 receptor has been found.

A growing body of evidence suggests that angiotensin II exerts some of its actions via the activation of proto-oncogenes such as c-*fos* and c-*myc,* but the detailed signal-transduction pathways involved as well as the final events underlying the protein–DNA interactions, which finally determine the level of gene transcription, remain poorly understood. The results of the studies by Takeuchi and colleagues[15] and Naftilan and colleagues[16] suggest that at least some of the effects of angiotensin II may be associated with activation of a well-known enhancer element AP-1. AP-1 consists of two groups of proteins, Fos-related antigens (fra) and Jun proteins, and has been found to be important in controlling transcription of several other genes. Activation of AP-1 is dependent on a protein kinase C pathway. These findings may help to explain the molecular events by which angiotensin II exerts its mitogenic effects on vascular smooth muscle cells. Similarly, angiotensin II has recently been shown to induce hypertrophy and hyperplasia in neonatal mammalian cardiac myocytes and nonmyocytes (mainly fibroblasts), respectively, independent of hemodynamic and neurohumoral effects.[6] This response includes the activation of several so-called immediate early genes (c-*fos*, c-*jun*, *junB*, *egr*1, and c-*myc*), late markers of cardiac hypertrophy (skeletal α-actin and atrial natriuretic peptide), and also increased expression of angiotensinogen and transforming growth factor–β1 genes. Although neonatal cardiac cells contain both AT1 and AT2 receptor subtypes, this response is primarily mediated by the AT1 receptor.

Extensive pharmacological evidence indicates that almost all of the known effects of angiotensin II in human adult tissues are attributable to the AT1 receptor.[12,17] Much less is known about the second subtype of angiotensin II receptor, the AT2 receptor. It is abundantly and widely expressed in fetal and immature brain tissues,[18] but its presence in adults is limited to low quantities in the adrenal gland, brain, uterine myometrium, and atretic ovarian follicles.[19,20] Its expression is activated in skin wounds and in the neointima following vascular injury.[21] Recently, we and others have cloned the cDNA encoding the AT2 receptor subtype.[22,23] The AT2 receptor also has a seven-transmembrane structure. It is only 34 percent identical in primary amino acid sequence to the AT1 receptor, and the intracellular signaling pathway has not been defined. Preliminary experiments suggest that the AT2 receptor may participate in cell development and growth-related mechanisms and may actually activate pathways that oppose the actions mediated by the AT1 receptor.[24] At present, studies are under way to determine its physiologic role.

Natriuretic Peptides

As discussed earlier, blood pressure is controlled by a balance between vasoconstrictive/antinatriuretic and vasodilatory/natriuretic forces. The natriuretic peptides are a family of hormones that oppose the actions of the renin-angiotensin system. Within this family are three major hormones, atrial natriuretic peptide (ANP), brain natriuretic peptide (BNP), and C-type natriuretic peptide (CNP). These hormones induce natriuresis and vasodilation and have antimitogenic properties. ANP and BNP are the major circulating forms, of which ANP predominates.

Gene Structure and Regulation

ANP is a hormone produced mainly in the atria of the heart.[25] This peptide exhibits diuretic, natriuretic, and vasorelaxant properties and inhibits the secretion of renin, aldosterone, and vasopressin. Recently, it has been shown to exert antimitogenic properties also. Atrial distention is probably the most powerful stimulus for ANP release, yet other stimuli appear to modulate its rate of synthesis and secretion. Stimuli such as thyroid hormones and glucocorticoids have been demonstrated to influence the rate of transcription of the ANP gene. Prostaglandins increase the rate of transcription of the ANP gene, and it appears that a 2.5-kilobase region on the 5′ side of the gene contains the regulatory sequences necessary for this response.

Alpha-adrenergic stimulation increases ANP gene expression in cardiac myocytes. The signal-transduction pathway for this response appears to involve at least two routes, one that requires activation of protein kinase C and one that involves the activation of calmodulin-regulated kinases. Because protein kinase C activates AP-1 protein expression, at least one of the pathways is mediated by the activation of an AP-1–like binding site protein in the proximal regulatory domains of the ANP gene. This observation is consistent with the identification of an AP-1 recognition site within 640 base pairs from the initiation of transcription, which is important for the expression of ANP.

A second natriuretic peptide, BNP, has been identified and proposed as a novel human cardiac hormone.[26] BNP has patterns of synthesis, secretion, and clearance distinct from those of ANP. BNP has been shown to be secreted mainly from human ventricles and attains a lower circulating level relative to ANP (secreted from the atria) under basal conditions. In pathological states such as heart failure, BNP levels increase by a significantly higher percentage than the percentage increase in ANP levels.[27] The increase in BNP is secondary to an increased BNP synthesis-secretion from heart ventricles and also to a slower rate of clearance of the peptide. The physiologic importance of these findings deserves further investigation.

Recently, a third natriuretic peptide, CNP, was isolated from porcine brain.[28,29] As opposed to ANP and BNP, this peptide is not found in the circulation. The diuretic and natriuretic properties of CNP are 100 times less potent than those of ANP or BNP; however, the vasorelaxant and antimitogenic properties of CNP are far more potent.[28] The physiologic importance of this peptide is unclear at present. Recent studies from our laboratory indicate that CNP expression may increase locally in states of pathological cellular growth, such as occur with vascular injury.

Messenger RNA Localization and Regulation

In contrast to the adult heart ventricles, the fetal and neonatal ventricles highly express the ANP gene and its encoded protein, suggesting the possibility that ANP may play a greater role in control of the cardiovascular system at early stages of life.[30,31] In experimental models of pressure or volume overload in the adult, the pattern of expression of ANP in the ventricles resembles the fetal pattern. This high expression of ANP messenger RNA (mRNA) in the ventricles has been demonstrated in a variety of pathological conditions, including human congestive heart failure,[32] as well as in rats with myocardial infarction and failure,[33] rats subjected to pressure overload,[34] and spontaneously hypertensive rats.[35,36]

Molecular Action

The cellular actions of the natriuretic peptides are believed to be mediated through the production of cyclic guanosine monophosphate by the activation of guanylate cyclase–linked receptors. To date, three major receptors have been cloned, ANP-A, ANP-B, and ANP-C. ANP-A and ANP-B are guanylate cyclase–coupled receptors with molecular weights of approximately 130,000, an amino acid sequence homology of 62 percent, and four distinct domains (ligand-binding, transmembrane, protein kinase, and catalytic).[37,38] The presence of both a protein kinase domain and a guanylate cyclase domain raises the fascinating possibility that the natriuretic peptides could participate in two very diverse intracellular signal transduction pathways. In contrast to ANP-A and ANP-B, ANP-C is a low-molecular-weight receptor (MW 60,000), lacking both the kinase and cyclase domains.[39] At present, the role of this receptor is controversial. Data from Maack and colleagues[40] suggest that the ANP-C receptor acts as a clearance receptor capable of buffering excess circulating ANP. However, other studies suggest that ANP-C may play a role in regulating cyclic adenosine monophosphate levels and phosphoinositol metabolism through G-protein–coupled mechanisms.[41] Of note is that a recent report by Mizuno and colleagues[42] suggests that ANP-C may exist in more than one form through alternate RNA splicing. The presence of other yet-unidentified natriuretic peptide receptors that differ in distribution, regulation, and function cannot be ruled out.

The contribution of the natriuretic peptide system to the control of blood pressure and the pathophysiology of hypertension depends not only on circulating levels of hormone but also on the distribution of receptors in various tissues. Receptor selectivity has been noted within the natriuretic peptide family.[43] The rank order of potency for cyclic guanosine monophosphate production for ANP-A after ligand binding appears to be ANP > BNP > CNP, and for ANP-B, CNP > ANP > BNP. The receptor binding affinity for ANP-C appears to be ANP > CNP > BNP. Receptor distribution differs not only with cell type but also with the phenotypic state of the cell.[43] The physiologic significance of these differences is unclear. Several lines of evidence suggest that the natriuretic peptides are important in cardiovascular regulation and disease. It is intriguing to hypothesize that an aberrance in natriuretic gene expression or an alteration in receptor distribution or function may result in hypertension.

Endothelin

In addition to the roles of circulating hormones such as ANP, renin, angiotensin, and vasopressin, recent research has demonstrated the importance of local autocrine-paracrine mechanisms in the control of blood pressure. The endothelium produces potent vasoconstrictive and vasodilatory substances. Endothelin, a potent vasoconstrictive peptide, has been isolated from cultured porcine endothelial cells.[44] The molecular biologic characteristics of endothelin have been a subject of active investigation.

Gene Structure and Regulation

Three distinct loci in the human genome encode for three related but unique sequences of the endothelin peptide, ET1, ET2, and ET3.[45] A number of additional functions have been associated with endothelin, including stimulation of growth of mesenchymal cells, release of vasoactive substances (eicosanoids, endothelium-derived relaxing factor, and ANP), and inhibition of renin release from glomeruli. The molecular mechanisms of endothelin gene expression remain poorly understood. Lee and colleagues[46] and Wilson and colleagues[47] demonstrated that a sequence spanning positions –143 (–141) to –129 (–127) from the human *ET1* gene contains the regulatory sequences necessary for endothelin promoter function and transcriptional control. In addition, posttranscriptional regulation of endothelin mRNA appears to be important because endothelin mRNA has an intracellular half-life of only about 15 minutes.[48] Indeed, the endothelin gene contains in the 3′ untranslated region several AUUUA motifs that have been associated with selective mRNA destabilization of short-lived transcripts. These findings are fundamental to our understanding of the control of endothelin gene expression.

Messenger RNA Localization and Regulation

Endothelin mRNA levels in cultured endothelial cells have been shown to increase in response to physical stimuli such as shear stress[49] and chemical stimuli including thrombin, calcium ionophore A23187, and transforming growth factor–β1.[50] However, until recently, the demonstration of endothelin mRNA expression in vivo was restricted to endothelial cells of the aorta and umbilical vein. The results reported by Nunez,[51] MacCumber,[52] and Koseki[53] and their colleagues demonstrate that endothelin mRNA is not restricted to endothelial cells but has a broad tissue and cell distribution. These findings are consistent with the role of endothelin as a local hormone, with its synthesis and release being locally controlled. This model is further supported by the results of Yoshizawa and colleagues,[54] who identified endothelin mRNA expression in the hypothalamus and the neurohypophysis, suggesting that endothelin may participate in important physiologic activities at these neuronal centers. In addition, these investigators observed that after dehydration, endothelin immunoreactivity decreased in the posterior pituitary, suggesting the release of endothelin or decreased synthesis.

Molecular Action

The identification of three related isopeptides from the same endothelin family that express diverse functional and pharmacological profiles suggested the existence of different receptor subtypes. In agreement with these conjectures, two groups simultaneously reported the cloning of the cDNAs encoding two endothelin receptor subtypes.[55,56] The deduced amino acid sequences of both cDNAs resemble those of G-protein–coupled receptors. The ET-A receptor, which displays highest selectivity to ET1, has wide tissue distribution but is expressed mainly in the heart and lungs. The ET-B is nonselective, expressed in several tissues, and not found in vascular smooth muscle cells. Current data obtained from different cell lines suggest that the activation of the endothelin receptors by the three isopeptides results in phospholipase C activation and high levels of intracellular calcium. This increase in intracellular calcium has been ascribed either to calcium mobilization from intracellular pools subsequent to phospholipase C activation or to extracelluar calcium entry related to the activation of a voltage-dependent calcium channel.[57] Further studies will be necessary to identify the specific signal-transduction pathway involved with each of the several endothelin receptors and the relationship to physiologic and pathological conditions. For instance, Muldoon and colleagues[58] demonstrated that endothelin is a potent stimulus for phosphatidylinositol turnover and subsequent activation of gene transcription in rat fibroblast and smooth muscle cells. This effect may underlie a potential role of endothelin as a modulator of gene expression in hypertension. The colocalization of endothelin receptor mRNA and specific binding sites for ligand in all endothelin-producing tissues suggests that the endothelin system is a local rather than a circulating system.

To understand the developmental and physiologic significance of endothelin, Kurihara and colleagues[59] disrupted mouse embryonic stem cells by homologous recombination to generate mice deficient in ET1 (knockout technology). Homozygous mice died of respiratory failure at birth. Heterozygous mice, which produced lower levels of endothelin than wild-type mice, developed elevated blood pressure, suggesting a physiologic role of endothelin in cardiovascular homeostasis.

Nitric Oxide Synthase

Nitric oxide (NO) synthesized by the endothelium is a powerful vasodilator. Inhibition of its production systemically with N^G-monomethyl-L-arginine results in an increase in blood pressure in the intact animal. In experimental and human hypertension, there is no evidence for an impairment of vasorelaxation that depends on endothelial NO.

Gene Structure and Regulation

The understanding of the physiologic and pharmacological properties of the NO system is advancing rapidly after the cloning and sequencing of the cDNAs that encode the enzyme nitric oxide synthase (NOS). NO and its redox-activated forms are simple molecules that exert a variety of effects important for the control of vascular function,[60] neuronal transmission,[61] and immune targeting.[62] They are generated by the recently identified NOS family of proteins that convert L-arginine to NO and L-citrulline. To date, at least three isoforms have been identified, and their genes cloned and sequenced. They include two constitutive calcium/calmodulin-dependent NOSs—brain NOS (bNOS) and endothelial NOS (ENOS)—and an inducible calcium-independent NOS (iNOS) isoform. The constitutive ENOS found in vascular endothelium shares common biochemical and pharmacological properties with bNOS, but whereas bNOS is primarily a cytosolic protein, the former is membrane associated. NO produced by endothelial cells is an important vascular relaxant and inhibitor of vascular smooth muscle cell growth,[63] whereas the NO synthesized by neuronal cells appears to be a novel type of neurotransmitter that acts by activation of guanylate cyclase in specific areas of the peripheral, autonomic, and central nervous systems. The molecular mechanisms underlying the regulation of NOS genes remain largely unknown. However, there appear to be putative AP-1, AP-2, NF-1, heavy metal, shear stress, and acute-phase responses and sterol-regulatory *cis*-elements that may be involved in mediating different signal-transduction pathways responsible for proper control of the gene in several physiologic conditions. The three isoforms show protein kinase recognition sequence motifs, and in vitro phosphorylation of bNOS has been demonstrated,[64] suggesting that phosphorylation may participate in the activation of the enzyme.

Messenger RNA Localization and Regulation

ENOS mRNA has a broad tissue distribution and is more abundant in aorta, heart, lung, kidney, adrenal gland, spinal cord, and urogenital tissues, whereas bNOS is localized mainly in organs containing neural elements, such as brain regions, intestine, stomach, spinal cord, adrenal gland, and aorta.[65] The tissue distribution of bNOS is consistent with the proposed role for NO as a nonadrenergic, noncholinergic neurotransmitter responsible for smooth muscle relaxation.[66] iNOS, previously isolated from murine macrophages, has recently been cloned in vascular smooth muscle cells.[67,68] In normal vessels, ENOS production helps to modulate vascular tone. However, iNOS production is induced in vascular smooth muscle cells by the cytokines interferon gamma, tumor necrosis factor, and interleukin-1 and in pathological states such as vascular injury. The endogenous production of NO at the site of injury and in response to cyokines may contribute to control of blood flow, vascular tone, and blood fluidity.[69] A recent report by von der Leyen and associates[70] suggests that iNOS may also regulate growth of vascular smooth muscle cells at sites of vascular injury and therefore may also participate in remodeling of the injured blood vessel wall. Further studies are under way to elucidate the factors that regulate NOS mRNA expression.

In summary, much is known about the molecular biology of the major control systems that regulate blood pressure. The application of the powerful tools of molecular biology should provide an improved understanding of the molecular and genetic mechanisms of hypertension. The subsequent sections of this chapter review the roles of these systems in the pathogenesis of hypertension and the secondary structural adaptations observed during the course of this disease.

Structural Adaptation

The development and maintenance of hypertension are associated with structural changes in the cardiovascular system characterized by vascular smooth muscle cell hypertrophy, replication, or both and by myocardial hypertrophy [*see Figure 1*]. In general, these hypertrophic changes are believed to be the consequence of an elevated blood pressurc; however, genetic abnormalities that predispose vascular smooth muscle cells or myocardium to hypertrophy cannot be excluded. The molecular mechanisms by which an increase in blood pressure induces cell hypertrophy and replication are not well known but must involve an activation of the transcription of genes encoding the proteins responsible for growth. Therefore, identification of the factors controlling the expression of these genes is paramount. A growing body of evidence suggests that the cardiovascular remodeling observed in pathological states such as hypertension occurs in response to mechanical and hormonal stimulation.

Mechanical Factors

The development of myocardial hypertrophy in response to pressure-volume overload is associated with the reexpression of the fetal contractile proteins β cardiac myosin heavy-chain isoform[71] and α-skeletal actin.[72] The molecular mechanisms underlying the mechanical activation of cardiac hypertrophy are discussed in detail in Chapter 12.

The increase in blood vessel wall mass in chronic hypertension can be seen in vessels of all sizes, ranging from large conduit arteries to resistance arterioles. The thickening of the vessel wall is a result of increased cell mass within the subintimal space and the media, as well as an expansion of the extracellular matrix. The enhanced muscle mass may be due to an increase in cell size (hypertrophy) or an increase in cell number (hyperplasia). In animal studies, smooth muscle cell hypertrophy appears to predominate in the large conduit vessels, whereas hyperplasia is observed in the small arteries and arterioles.[73,74] Many investigators have also reported an increase in cellular DNA content associated with the increase in cell mass (polyploidy).[75]

The arterial wall in hypertensive animals is also characterized by changes within the extracellular matrix. The extracellular matrix expands by an increase in collagen, elastin, and glycosaminoglycans.[76] There is an invasion of inflammatory cells, which may modulate the remodeling process by the secretion of growth factors, proteases, and cytokines. In addition to extracellular matrix alterations, intimal and subintimal changes are also observed. The endothelium in hypertensive vessels loses much of its vasodilator capacity and some of its ability to inhibit platelet aggregation and to retard leukocyte adhesion.[77] Moreover, there is intimal thickening. Vascular smooth muscle–like cells have been observed to migrate into the subintimal space. These functional and structural alterations combine to reduce lumen area, limit vasodilation, and promote thrombosis.

Hemodynamic and humoral factors have been proposed as stimuli responsible for the initiation of vascular smooth muscle cell growth in hypertension. The autoregulatory response is a well-known phenomenon that shows the tendency of blood flow to remain constant in response to variations in blood perfusion pressure to several tissue beds. The basic mechanisms underlying autoregulation are not well understood, but mechanical as well as humoral/metabolic factors have been proposed to explain this response. An intriguing possibility is that this same phenomenon may also initiate some of the structural changes observed in hypertension, such as vessel wall growth, which may underlie a chronic adaptive response to high blood pressure, blood flow, or both.

The contribution of the mechanical stimulus of hypertension to vessel wall growth is implied by the effects of various pharmacological and nonpharmacological antihypertensive treatments in attenuating or reversing the vessel wall growth noted in animal models of hypertension.[73,78] Mechanical stretch of skeletal muscle induces muscle hypertrophy, indicating a direct effect of a mechanical stimulus on muscle growth. In fact, growth-promoting factors have been extracted from skeletal muscle with stretch-induced hypertrophy as well as from the hypertrophied cardiac muscle.[79,80] Similarly, it has been observed that mechanical stretch of vascular myocytes in vitro enhances protein synthesis and induces hypertrophy.[81] These studies support the postulate that increased wall tension produced by elevations in blood pressure may induce vascular myocyte growth. Moreover, it has been previously documented that a decrease in flow can trigger a remodeling of the blood vessel so that the luminal diameter is reduced.[82] As noted previously, the hypertensive vessel has a reduced luminal diameter and a higher resistance during maximal vasodilation. This alteration in vessel structure could represent a similar process of remodeling produced by a mechanical stimulus.

The results of several studies suggest that in the blood vessels, the mechanotransduction process could be initiated at the level of endothelial cells. Lansman and colleagues[83] proposed that stretch-activated ion channels in endothelial cells mediate the transduction of hemodynamic stresses. More recently, Olesen and colleagues[84] demonstrated that shear stress activates a potassium current in vascular endothelial cells. Transduction of events to underlying smooth muscle cells may take place by electrical signaling mechanisms via gap junction or by the release of effector molecules, such as growth factors. Taken together, these findings are consistent with the concept that the hemodynamic forces can directly initiate intracellular events controlling vascular tone and cell growth. The exact involvement of the different ion channels in mechanical transduction and its relevance to cardiovascular remodeling remain to be determined.

Humoral Factors

A variety of vasoactive agents appear to modulate vascular growth. Current data suggest that endogenous vasoconstrictors (such as angiotensin) are promoters of vascular smooth muscle cell growth, whereas endogenous vasodilators (such as NO or prostacyclin) possess growth-inhibiting properties. Thus, it is tempting to speculate that vasoactive substances may be involved with short-term regulation of vascular tone as well as long-term regulation of vascular structure. Additionally, vascular smooth muscle cell mitogens, such as platelet-derived growth factor and epidermal growth factor, have been shown to be vasoconstrictors. These findings indicate that factors regulating vascular function exhibit common properties with factors that regulate vascular structure. Thus, it appears that cellular signals that initiate a short-term increase in vascular resistance may mediate long-term remodeling of blood vessels. The latter process may then promote the maintenance of increased vascular resistance and thereby perpetuate hypertension.

The hypertrophic effect of angiotensin II in vitro has been associated with activation of proto-oncogenes, such as c-*fos* and c-*jun,* and growth factors, such as platelet-derived growth factor, basic fibroblast growth factor, and transforming growth factor–β1.[85,86] Additionally, Taubman and colleagues[87] have suggested that induction of c-*fos* is dependent on mobilization of intracellular calcium and protein kinase C activation. Tsuda and Alexander[88] provided evidence that nuclear lamins can be phosphorylated in vascular smooth muscle cells exposed to angiotensin II, suggesting that phosphorylation of nuclear proteins via protein kinase C activation may be an important mechanism by which angiotensin II controls intracellular processes that modify gene expression and cell growth. As discussed earlier, endothelin is a potent constrictor of vascular smooth muscle cells that is derived from endothelial cells. Recently, endothelin has been shown to induce hypertrophy of cultured rat cardiac and vascular myocytes.[89] Moreover, these responses were associated with intracellular accumulation of diacylglycerol and calcium, suggesting that the growth effects on the endothelium involve the activation of the phosphoinositide signal-transduction pathway. The sympathetic nervous system and catecholamines are believed to exert a trophic influence on smooth muscle cells, in addition to their well-established effects on the control of vascular tone. Majesky and colleagues[90] provided data suggesting that the trophic effects of catecholamines may involve the induction of growth-related genes via the alpha$_1$-adrenergic receptors.

In contrast, vasorelaxant substances, such as ANP and NO, have an antigrowth effect on vascular smooth muscle cells.[63,91] These findings suggest that ANP and NO may play an important counterregulatory role in hypertension via a long-term influence on vascular structure by inhibiting vascular hypertrophy. In short, the modulation of vascular tone and vascular growth involves a complex interaction between vasodilatory (growth-inhibitory) and vasoconstrictive (growth-promoting) factors. An understanding of the molecular biology of these processes may result in novel therapeutic strategies for the prevention and treatment of the complications of hypertension.

References

1. Dzau VJ: Circulating versus local renin-angiotensin system in cardiovascular homeostasis. *Circulation* 77(suppl 19):1, 1988
2. Paul M, Bachman J, Ganten D: The tissue renin-angiotensin systems in cardiovascuar disease. *Trends Cardiovasc Med* 2:94, 1992
3. Schunkert H, Dzau VJ, Tang SS, et al: Increased rat cardiac angiotensin converting enzyme activity and mRNA expression in pressure overload left ventricular hypertrophy: effects on coronary resistance, contractility, and relaxation. *J Clin Invest* 86:1913, 1990
4. Okamura T, Miyazaki M, Inagami T, et al: Vascular renin-angiotensin system in two-kidney, one clip hypertensive rats. *Hypertension* 8:560, 1986
5. Baker KM, Aceto JF: Angiotensin II stimulation of protein synthesis and cell growth in chick heart cells. *Am J Physiol* 259:H610, 1990
6. Sadoshima J, Izumo S: Molecular characterization of angiotensin II-induced hypertrophy of cardiac myocytes and hyperplasia of cardiac fibroblasts: critical role of the AT1 receptor subtype. *Circ Res* 73:413, 1993
7. Xiang J, Linz W, Becker H, et al: Effects of converting enzyme inhibitors ramipril and enalapril on peptide action and sympathetic neurotransmission in the isolated rat heart. *Eur J Pharmacol* 113:215, 1984
8. Urata H, Kinoshita A, Misono KS, et al: Identification of a highly specific chymase as the major angiotensin II forming enzyme in the human heart. *J Biol Chem* 265:22348, 1990
9. Morishita R, Gibbons GH, Zhang L, et al: Novel and effective gene transfer technique for study of vascular renin angiotensin system. *J Clin Invest* 91:2580, 1993
10. Dzau VJ: Local expression and pathophysiologic role of renin-angiotensin in the blood vessels and heart. *Basic Res Cardiol* 88(suppl):1, 1993
11. Chiu AT, Herblin WF, McCall DE, et al: Identification of angiotensin II receptor subtypes. *Biochem Biophys Res Commun* 165:196, 1989
12. Sasamura H, Hein L, Krieger JE, et al: Cloning, characterization, and expression of two angiotensin receptor (AT-1) isoforms from the mouse genome. *Biochem Biophys Res Commun* 185:253, 1992
13. Kitami Y, Okura T, Marumoto K, et al: Differential gene expression and regulation of type-1 angiotensin II receptor subtypes in the rat. *Biochem Biophys Res Commun* 188:446, 1992
14. Konishi H, Kuroda S, Inada Y, et al: Novel subtype of human angiotensin II type 1 receptor: cDNA cloning and expression. *Biochem Biophys Res Commun* 199:467, 1994
15. Takeuchi K, Nakamura N, Cook NS, et al: Angiotensin II can regulate gene expression by the AP-1 binding sequence via a protein kinase C-dependent pathway. *Biochem Biophys Res Commun* 172:1189, 1990
16. Naftilan AJ, Gilliland GK, Eldridge CS, et al: Induction of the protooncogene c-*jun* by angiotensin II. *Mol Cell Biol* 10:5536, 1990
17. Sasaki K, Yamano Y, Bardhan S, et al: Cloning and expression of a complementary DNA encoding a bovine adrenal angiotensin II type-1 receptor. *Nature* 351:230, 1991
18. Grady EF, Sechi LA, Griffin CA, et al: Expression of AT2 receptors in the developing rat fetus. *J Clin Invest* 88:921, 1991
19. Pucell AG, Hodges JC, Sen I, et al: Biochemical properties of the ovarian granulosa cell type 2-angiotensin II receptor. *Endocrinology* 128:1947, 1991
20. Millan MA, Jacobowitz DM, Aguilera G, et al: Differential distribution of AT1 and AT2 angiotensin II receptor subtypes in the rat brain during development. *Proc Natl Acad Sci USA* 88:11440, 1991
21. Hutchinson HG, Kim DK, Hein L, et al: Quantitative RT/PCR analysis of AT2 expression during vascular development and vascular injury. *Circulation* 90:I-463, 1994
22. Mukoyama M, Nakajima M, Horiuchi M, et al: Expression cloning of type 2 angiotensin II receptor reveals a unique class of seven-transmembrane receptors. *J Biol Chem* 268: 24539, 1993
23. Ichiki T, Herold CL, Kambayasi Y, et al: Cloning of the cDNA and the genomic DNA of the mouse angiotensin II type 2 receptor. *Biochim Biophys Acta* 1189:247, 1994

24. Nakajima M, Horiuchi M, Morishita R, et al: Growth inhibitory function of type 2 angiotensin II receptor: gain of function study by in vivo gene transfer. *Hypertension* 24:379, 1994

25. Brandt RR, Wright RS, Redfield MM, et al: Atria natriuretic peptide in heart failure. *J Am Coll Cardiol* 22:86A, 1993

26. Imura H, Nakao K, Itoh H: The natriuretic peptide system in the brain: implications in the central control of cardiovascular and neuroendocrine functions. *Front Neuroendocrinol* 13:217, 1992

27. Yasue H, Yoshimura M, Sumida H, et al: Localization and mechanism of secretion of B-type natriuretic peptide in comparison with those of A-type natriuretic peptide in normal subjects and patients with heart failure. *Circulation* 90:195, 1994

28. Sudoh T, Minamino N, Kangawa K, et al: C-type natriuretic peptide (CNP): a new member of natriuretic peptide family identified in porcine brain. *Biochem Biophys Res Commun* 168:863, 1990

29. Minamino N, Kangawa K, Matsuo H: N-terminally extended form of C-type natriuretic peptide (CNP-53) identified in porcine brain. *Biochem Biophys Res Commun* 170:973, 1990

30. Bloch KD, Seidman JG, Naftilan JD, et al: Neonatal atria and ventricles secrete atrial natriuretic factor via tissue-specific secretory pathways. *Cell* 47:695, 1986

31. Gardner DG, Hedges BK, Wu J, et al: Expression of the atrial natriuretic peptide gene in human fetal heart. *J Clin Endocrinol Metab* 69:729, 1989

32. Saito Y, Nakao K, Arai H, et al: Augmented expression of atrial natriuretic polypeptide gene in ventricle of human failing heart. *J Clin Invest* 83:298, 1989

33. Drexler H, Hanze J, Finckh M, et al: Atrial natriuretic peptide in a rat model of cardiac failure. *Circulation* 79:620, 1989

34. Izumo S, Nadal-Ginard B, Mahdavi V: Protooncogene induction and reprogramming of cardiac gene expression produced by pressure overload. *Proc Natl Acad Sci USA* 85:339, 1988

35. Matsubara H, Mori Y, Yamamoto J, et al: Diabetes-induced alterations in atrial natriuretic peptide gene expression in Wistar-Kyoto and spontaneously hypertensive rats. *Circ Res* 67:803, 1990

36. Arai H, Nakao K, Saito Y, et al: Augmented expression of atrial natriuretic polypeptide gene in ventricles of spontaneously hypertensive rats (SHR) and SHR-stroke prone. *Circ Res* 62:926, 1988

37. Chinkers M, Garbers DL, Chang M-S, et al: Molecular cloning of a new type of cell surface receptor: a membrane form of guanylate cyclase is an atrial natriuretic peptide receptor. *Nature* 338:78, 1989

38. Schulz S, Singh S, Bellet RA, et al: The primary structure of a plasma membrane guanylate cyclase demonstrates diversity within this new receptor family. *Cell* 58:1155, 1989

39. Fuller F, Porter JG, Arfsten AE, et al: Atrial natriuretic peptide clearance receptor. *J Biol Chem* 263:9395, 1988

40. Maack T, Suzuki M, Almeida FA, et al: Physiologic role of silent receptors of atrial natriuretic factor. *Science* 238:675, 1987

41. Anand-Srivastava MB, Sairam MR, et al: Ring-deleted analogs of atrial natriuretic factor inhibit adenylate cyclase/cAMP system. *J Biol Chem* 265:8566, 1990

42. Mizuno T, Iwashina M, Itakura M, et al: A variant form of the type C atrial natriuretic peptide receptor generated by alternative RNA splicing. *J Biol Chem* 268:5162, 1993

43. Suga S, Nakao K, Hosoda K, et al: Receptor selectivity of natriuretic peptide family, atrial natriuretic peptide, brain natriuretic peptide, and C-type natriuretic peptide. *Endocrinology* 130:229, 1992

44. Yanagisawa M, Kurihara H, Kimura S, et al: A novel potent vasoconstrictor peptide produced by vascular endothelial cells. *Nature* 332:411, 1988.

45. Inoue A, Yanagisawa M, Kimura S, et al: The human endothelin family: three structurally and pharmacologically distinct isopeptides predicted by three separate genes. *Proc Natl Acad Sci USA* 86:2863, 1989

46. Lee ME, Bloch KD, Clifford JA, et al: Functional analysis of the endothelin-1 gene promoter. *J Biol Chem* 265:10446, 1990

47. Wilson DB, Dorfman DM, Orkin SH: A nonerythroid GATA-binding protein is required for function of the human preproendothelin-1 promoter in endothelial cells. *Mol Cell Biol* 10:4854, 1990

48. Yanagisawa M, Inoue A, Takuwa Y, et al: The human preproendothelin-1 gene: possible regulation by endothelial phosphoinositide turnover signaling. *J Cardiovasc Pharmacol* 13:S13-S17, 1989

49. Yoshizumi M, Hurihara H, Sugiyama T, et al: Hemodynamic shear stress stimulates endothelin production by cultured endothelial cells. *Biochem Biophys Res Commun* 161:859, 1989

50. Kurihara H, Yoshizumi M, Sugiyama T, et al: Transforming growth factor-β stimulates the expression of endothelin mRNA by vascular endothelial cells. *Biochem Biophys Res Commun* 159:1435, 1989

51. Nunez DJR, Brown MJ, Davenport AP, et al: Endothelin-1 mRNA is widely expressed in porcine and human tissues. *J Clin Invest* 85:1537, 1990

52. MacCumber MW, Ross CA, Glaser BM, et al: Endothelin: visualization of mRNAs by in situ hybridization provides evidence for local action. *Proc Natl Acad Sci USA* 86:7285, 1989

53. Koseki C, Imai M, Hirata Y, et al: Autoradiographic distribution in rat tissues of binding sites for endothelin: a neuropeptide? *Am J Physiol* 256:R858, 1989

54. Yoshizawa T, Shinmi O, Giaid A, et al: Endothelin: a novel peptide in the posterior pituitary system. *Science* 247:462, 1990

55. Arai H, Hori S, Aramori I, et al: Cloning and expression of a cDNA encoding an endothelin receptor. *Nature* 348:730, 1990

56. Sakurai T, Yanagisawa M, Takuwa Y: Cloning of a cDNA encoding a non-isopeptide-selective subtype of the endothelin receptor. *Nature* 348:732, 1990

57. Yanagisawa M, Masaki T: Molecular biology and biochemisity of the endothelins. *Trends Pharmacol Sci* 10:374, 1989

58. Muldoon LL, Rodland KD, Forsythe ML, et al: Stimulation of phosphatidylinositol hydrolysis, diacylglycerol release, and gene expression in response to endothelin, a potent new agonist for fibroblasts and smooth muscle cells. *J Biol Chem* 264:8529, 1989

59. Kurihara Y, Kurihara H, Suzuki H, et al: Elevated blood pressure and craniofacial abnormalities in mice deficient in endothelin-1. *Nature* 368:703, 1994

60. Moncada S, Palmer RMJ, Higgs EA: Nitric oxide: physiology, pathophysiology, and pharmacology. *Pharmacol Rev* 43:109, 1991

61. Bredt DS, Snyder SH: Nitric oxide mediates glutamate-linked enhancement of cGMP levels in the cerebellum. *Proc Natl Acad Sci USA* 86:9030, 1989

62. Stuehr DJ, Nathan CF: Nitric oxide: a macrophage product responsible for cytostasis and respiratory inhibition in tumor target cells. *J Exp Med* 169:1543, 1989

63. Garg UC, Hassid A: Nitric oxide-generating vasodilators and 8-bromo-cyclic guanosine monophosphate inhibit mitogenesis and proliferation of cultured rat vascular smooth muscle cells. *J Clin Invest* 83:1774, 1989

64. Bredt DS, Ferris CD, Snyder SH: Nitric oxide synthase regulatory sites: phosphorylation by cyclic AMP-dependent protein kinase, protein kinase C, and calcium/calmodulin protein kinase; identification of flavin and calmodulin binding sites. *J Biol Chem* 267: 10976, 1992

65. Sessa WC, Harrison JK, Luthin DR, et al: Genomic analysis and expression patterns reveal distinct genes for endothelial and brain nitric oxide synthase. *Hypertension* 21:934, 1993

66. Desai KM, Sessa WC, Vane JR: Involvement of nitric oxide in the reflex relaxation of the stomach to accommodate food or fluid. *Nature* 351:477, 1991

67. Geng YJ, Almqvist M, Hansson GK: cDNA cloning and expression of inducible nitric oxide synthase from rat vascular smooth muscle cells. *Biochim Biophys Acta* 1218:421, 1994

68. Nunokawa Y, Ishida N, Tanaka S: Cloning of inducible nitric oxide synthase in rat vascular smooth muscle cells. *Biochem Biophys Res Commun* 191:89, 1993

69. Hansson GK, Geng YJ, Holm J, et al: Arterial smooth muscle cells express nitric oxide synthase in response to endothelial injury. *J Exp Med* 180:733, 1994

70. Von der Leyen H, Gibbons GH, Morishita R, et al: Successful gene therapy for blocking vascular neointimal lesion: in vivo transfer of ec-nitric oxide synthase. *Proc Natl Acad Sci USA* (in press)

71. Izumo S, Lompré A-M, Matsuoka R, et al: Myosin heavy chain messenger RNA and protein isoform transitions during cardiac hypertrophy. *J Clin Invest* 79:970, 1987

72. Schiaffino S, Samuel JL, Sassoon D, et al: Nonsynchronous accumulation of α-skeletal actin and β-myosin heavy chain mRNAs during early stages of pressure-overload-induced cardiac hypertrophy demonstrated by in situ hybridization. *Circ Res* 64:937, 1989

73. Mulvany MJ, Hansen PK, Aalkjaer C: Direct evidence that the greater contractility of resistance vessels in spontaneously hypertensive rats is associated with a narrowed lumen, a thickened media, and an increased number of smooth muscle cell layers. *Circ Res* 43:854, 1978

74. Owens GK: Influence of blood pressure on development of aortic medial smooth muscle hypertrophy in spontaneously hypertensive rats. *Hypertension* 9:178, 1987

75. Barrett TB, Sampson P, Owens GK, et al: Polyploid nuclei in human artery wall smooth muscle cells. *Proc Natl Acad Sci USA* 80:882, 1983

76. Udenfriend S, Cardinale G, Spector S: Hypertension induced vascular fibrosis and its reversal by antihypertensive drugs. *Frontiers in Hypertension Research*. Laragh JH, Buhler FR, Seldin OW, Eds. Springer-Verlag, New York, 1981, p 404

77. Lockette W, Otsuka Y, Carretero O: The loss of endothelium-dependent vascular relaxation in hypertension. *Hypertension* 8(suppl II):II-161, 1986

78. Sano T, Tarazi RC: Differential structural responses of small resistance vessels to antihypertensive therapy. *Circulation* 75:618, 1987

79. Hammond GL, Lai YK, Markert CL: The molecules that initiate cardiac hypertrophy are not species-specific. *Science* 216:529, 1982

80. Sadoshima J, Xu Y, Slayer HS, et al: Autocrine release of angiotensin II mediates stretch-induced hypertrophy of cardiac myocytes in vitro. *Cell* 75:977, 1993

81. Leung DYM, Glagov S, Mathews MB: Cyclic stretching stimulates synthesis of matrix components by arterial smooth muscle cells in vitro. *Science* 191:475, 1976

82. Langille BL, O'Donnell F: Reductions in arterial diameter produced by chronic decreases in blood flow are endothelium dependent. *Science* 231:405, 1986

83. Lansman JB, Hallam TJ, Rink TJ: Single stretch-activated ion channels in vascular endothelial cells as mechanotransducers? *Nature* 325:811, 1987

84. Olesen S-P, Clapham DE, Davies PT: Haemodynamic shear stress activates a K^+ current in vascular endothelial cells. *Nature* 331:168, 1988

85. Naftilan AJ, Pratt RE, Dzau VJ: Induction of platelet-derived growth factor A-chain and c-*myc* gene expressions by angiotensin II in cultured rat vascular smooth muscle cells. *J Clin Invest* 83:1419, 1989

86. Itoh H, Mukoyama M, Pratt RE, et al: Multiple autocrine growth factors modulate vascular smooth muscle cell growth response to angiotensin II. *J Clin Invest* 91:2268, 1993

87. Taubman MB, Marmur JD, Rosenfield CL, et al: Agonist-mediated tissue factor expression in cultured vascular smooth muscle cells: role of Ca^{2+} mobilization and protein kinase C activation. *J Clin Invest* 91:547, 1993

88. Tsuda T, Alexander RW: Angiotensin II stimulates phosphorylation of nuclear lamins via a protein kinase C-dependent mechanism in cultured vascular smooth muscle cells. *J Biol Chem* 265:1165, 1990

89. Shubeita HE, McDonough PM, Harris AN, et al: Endothelin induction of inositol phospholipid hydrolysis, sarcomere assembly, and cardiac gene expression in ventricular myocytes: a paracrine mechanism for myocardial cell hypertrophy. *J Biol Chem* 265: 20555, 1990

90. Majesky MW, Daemen MJAP, Schwartz SM: Alpha 1-adrenergic stimulation of platelet-derived growth factor A-chain gene expression in rat aorta. *J Biol Chem* 265:1082, 1990

91. Itoh H, Pratt RE, Dzau VJ: Atrial natriuretic polypeptide inhibits hypertrophy of vascular smooth muscle cells. *J Clin Invest* 86:1690, 1990

Acknowledgments

This work is supported by NIH grants HL46631, HL35252, HL35610, HL48638, and HL07708 and the American Heart Association–Bugher Foundation Centers for Molecular Biology in the Cardiovascular System. Dr. Krieger is supported by grants from FINEP/Brazil (66.93.0023.00) and Fundacão EJ Zerbinin.

Figure 1 Talar Agasyan.

CHAPTER 16

Genetics of Hypertension

Klaus Lindpaintner, M.D., Reinhold Kreutz, M.D., Detlev Ganten, M.D., Ph.D.

Hypertension has been recognized over the past half century as one of the most important risk factors for the development of cardiovascular and related ailments, including cardiac hypertrophy; coronary, cerebrovascular, and peripheral vascular disease; nephrosclerosis; and retinopathy. Despite hypertension's high prevalence and great impact on public health, little is still known about its causes, owing to the great complexity of its pathogenesis but perhaps also to certain traditional perceptions and classifications concerning its etiology. We find ourselves today at the brink of significant advances in the understanding of hypertension, made possible through recombinant DNA technology and advances in molecular genetics. This progress will require an open mind; already, we are seeing familiar concepts and tenets being called into question.

The Challenge of Hypertension Genetics

In the vast majority of patients with hypertension, no discernible anatomic, metabolic, or endocrine derangement can be found, and hypertension in these cases is regarded as a primary, genetically determined illness; hence the term primary or essential hypertension. This view is strongly influenced and supported by data from epidemiological and twin studies that demonstrate familial aggregation of the disease. The absence of simple patterns of monogenetic mendelian inheritance indicates that hypertension is a polygenic disease in which more than one gene, perhaps even several genes interacting, control the level of blood pressure. As is well appreciated by physicians treating patients with hypertension, the degree of blood pressure elevation varies widely depending on environmental factors, such as dietary or psychosocial variables, identifying hypertension as a multifactorial disease. Moreover, identical environmental perturbations, acting on a particular gene, may have markedly different effects in different individuals, suggesting that certain environmentally responsive genes may be altered in a way that modulates this response quantitatively or qualitatively. It also appears certain that hypertension is not a single homogeneous disease, but that the set of genes responsible for blood pressure elevations is heterogeneous, differing among individuals and kindreds. Lastly, unlike the case with some monogenetic diseases, the phenotype parameter measured in hypertension—blood pressure itself—is a not a discrete or qualitative variable but a continuous, quantitative one; aside from considerations of how best and most representatively to determine blood pressure, we are still faced with an empirically chosen cutoff value for the diagnosis of the disorder. It is easy to see that the combination of properties listed here, all of which operate concomitantly, makes primary hypertension an exceedingly complicated disorder or, perhaps truer to the facts, array of disorders.

It is therefore not surprising that despite many years of dedicated research, we have so far failed to uncover any of the causative principles underlying hypertension. Recently, however, with the advent of recombinant DNA technology and its application to molecular genetic analyses, and with the parallel development of sophisticated statistical genetic tools, the discovery of genes contributing to complex disease such as hypertension has come within reach.

Analytic Tools and Conceptual Framework

Genetic Markers

Genetic markers, the principal tool of molecular genetic investigation, represent tags, based on unique DNA sequence characteristics, that identify particular genes or loci within the genome. If they are polymorphic, they exist as different alleles (based on sequence differences), allowing the distinction of one individual from another.

The first widely available method to visualize such polymorphic markers relied on restriction fragment length polymorphisms (RFLPs),[1] which are based on the variable presence of certain restriction endonuclease recognition sites in a gene of interest or the presence or absence of sequence domains located between two constant sites [*see Figure 1*]. The basic method of RFLP analysis has remained one of the mainstays of candidate gene analysis, and the application of the polymerase chain reaction (PCR) to this technique has greatly enhanced its practicability.

Currently, use of random markers represents the most common method for genotyping. Its application is based on the existence of repeated sequence elements that are present in multiple copies and widely dispersed throughout the genome. At any given localization, these sequence elements show a high degree of interindividual (or interstrain) variability that is attributed to differences in length (i.e., the number of repeats) or differences in their loca-

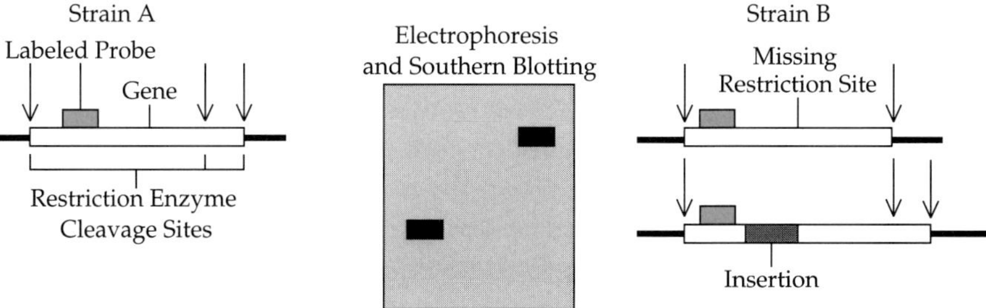

Figure 1 *In this representation of restriction fragment length polymorphism (RFLP) analysis, small segments of genomic DNA from two different strains (or two different, noninbred individuals) are shown, along with the location of specific restriction endonuclease sites (arrows). It should be recognized that the restriction enzyme will cut the genomic DNA used for this experiment in many different locations, resulting in a multitude of smaller and larger fragments that will be fractionated by size during electrophoresis (center panel). However, from this smear of different-sized fragments, only those complementary to the specific genetic probe used will trap (anneal to) this radiolabeled probe (light-gray rectangles) and thus be visualized as a band. Depending on the size of the probe and location of the specific restriction sites, one may see more than one band: in this case, restriction enzyme recognition sites lie within the area complementary to the probe, and the probe molecule then binds to more than one fragment of genomic DNA. Loss of a restriction site (top, strain B), insertion of genetic material between two restriction sites (dark-gray region, strain B), or deletion of genetic material between two restriction sites can result in banding patterns different from the original situation because annealing to the same probe now occurs on different-sized (and migrating) pieces of cut genomic DNA.*

tion relative to particular restriction endonuclease sites. These differences constitute an abundant source of polymorphic markers that literally cover the mammalian genome. Two broad classes of such tandem repeat elements can be distinguished: so-called minisatellites,[2] or variable number tandem repeats, and microsatellites,[3] or simple sequence length polymorphisms. The minisatellites usually have a single unit length of about 10 to 100 base pairs and are visualized by hybridization against specific radiolabeled complementary probes after genomic DNA digestion by restriction endonucleases, electrophoretic size fractionation, and Southern transfer to nitrocellulose or nylon membranes. The use of microsatellites, which represent very short (usually di-, tri-, or tetranucleotide) repeat units, most commonly $[CA]_n$, as the source of polymorphic markers has the primary advantage of being PCR based [*see Figure 2*]; this technique requires very small amounts of DNA and allows the efficient screening of large numbers of these markers. Currently, large panels of microsatellite markers that will offer comprehensive coverage of the genome are being developed for the human[4] as well as other species.[5,6] Anonymous markers can be anchored to chromosomes by hybridization in somatic cell hybrid panels and then are ordered into linkage groups to map their respective position on the chromosome.

Candidate Gene Testing Versus Genome Screening

Two major, conceptually different schemes for genetic analysis are generally used in the study of hypertension; each has its advantages and limitations. One, termed the candidate gene approach, takes advantage of polymorphisms in genes that encode proteins of known or suspected importance in the regulation of blood pressure or of importance in developmental or structural aspects of the cardiovascular system. In association studies, for which the candidate gene approach represents the only legitimate strategy, a positive result is considered strong evidence for a pathogenetic role of a particular gene. If this approach is applied to pedigree systems, a positive linkage result is of course highly suggestive of the involvement of that gene in the disease process, but it is also compatible with a similar role for a nearby gene. Use of this approach, however, limits the search for a disease-relevant gene to the 3,000 to 4,000 genes presently known (of an estimated 100,000 genes in the human genome), leaving most of the gene pool beyond the method's scope.

Therefore, the candidate gene approach is complemented, and increasingly overshadowed, by the alternative approach of genome screening. These reverse genetic and positional cloning approaches use large numbers of randomly distributed polymorphic markers that can be applied to interval mapping strategies. Note that these markers have no inherent relationship to the trait being studied. Reverse genetics refers to the direction of scientific detection: first, a gene is cloned, and subsequently, the function of the encoded protein is studied. Positional cloning[7] denotes that in contrast to conventional random or shotgun cloning, a specific region of the genome, previously identified by linkage analysis as carrying a disease-relevant gene, is targeted for cloning and physical mapping. Rather than assuming that the gene of interest is identified directly by the marker used, the working hypothesis for this approach assumes that the gene of interest is located somewhere between two of the markers (in the interval) tested. Successful interval mapping leads to the identification of a region of several hundred thousand base pairs that can be physically isolated, using yeast artificial chromosomes or similar techniques for the cloning of large fragments of genomic DNA, and subsequently analyzed by several different algorithms, including usually a large sequencing effort, for the presence of transcribable domains or open reading frames (i.e., genes). Eventually, the gene itself is identified and then further characterized by functional evaluation for its potential role in the pathogenesis of the disease under investigation.

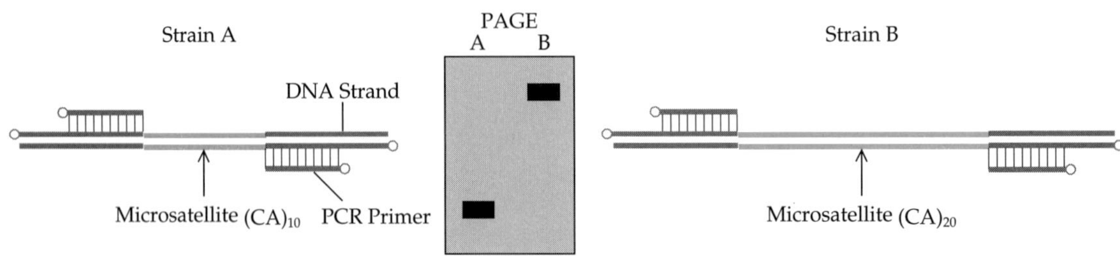

Figure 2 *Microsatellite mapping methodology. If individuals are to be typed for a microsatellite, knowledge of the flanking, unique DNA sequence is needed. With this information, specific polymerase chain reaction (PCR) primers may be designed and synthesized and then used to amplify the region of interest (the microsatellite) many millionfold. From minute amounts of genomic DNA, one thus arrives at quantities of DNA from the specific region of interest that are large enough to be analyzed directly. If one of the two primers carries a detection signal, the fragments amplified from different individuals may be visualized by autoradiography or other staining methods as bands on a polyacrylamide gel electrophoretic (PAGE) column.*

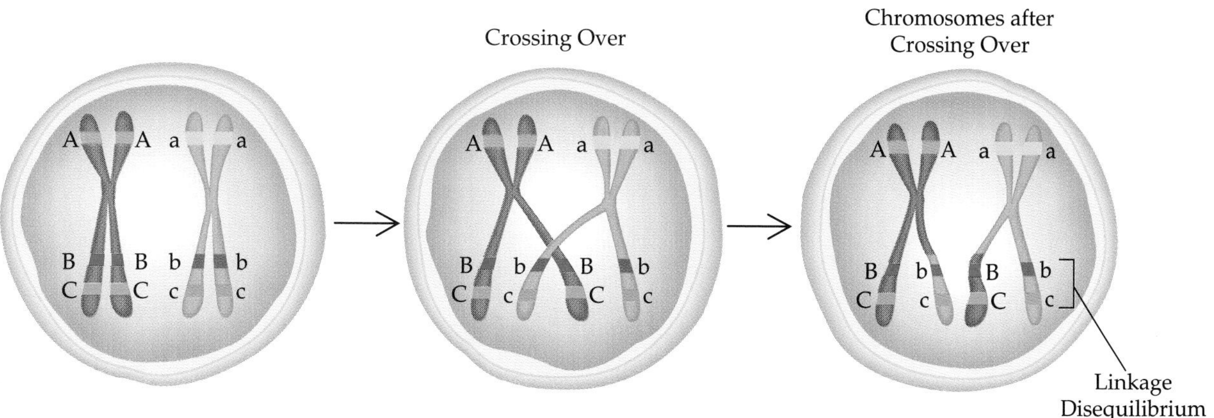

Figure 3 *Meiotic recombination (crossing over) is shown between homologous (carrying the same genes) but not identical (carrying specific alleles of the same genes) regions of two chromosomes. Two sets of sister chromatids are indicated by the blue and tan colors, respectively, and letters A, B, and C indicate three genes, with lowercase a, b, and c indicating different alleles of these same genes. As indicated, the close physical proximity between genes B and C results in linkage disequilibrium between the two loci, making a recombination event between genes B and C much less likely than between them and locus A. Thus, if gene C were unknown, using B and b as an indicator for the allele status at C would be practicable, as opposed to using A.*

Analytic Approaches: Linkage and Association

Classically, genetic investigations are based on studying the coinheritance of a putative marker allele with the disease among affected and unaffected members of a family. Because of the reshuffling of parental chromatids, and because of genetic recombination, allelic variants at any two genetic loci have a 50 percent chance of being inherited in one of two possible combinations (they are in linkage equilibrium). Only if they are located on the same chromosome and in relatively close proximity to each other is there a significant greater-than-chance likelihood of their being coinherited: they are said to be in linkage disequilibrium, or linked [*see Figure 3*]. Because the degree of linkage is directly proportional (in first approximation) to the physical distance of two loci, this information may be translated directly into the putative location of the disease gene. As a practical example, if in a large pedigree, 99 of 100 affected members carry a certain allele, *A*, and only one affected member carries a different allele, *a*, that is present in all unaffected members, then *A* is linked to the disease with a recombination frequency of one percent, or it is localized at a recombination distance of 1 centimorgan (equaling about one million base pairs). The statistic used to test the reliability of such investigative findings is based on likelihood methods that compare the odds of data arising from actual linkage to those of a chance occurrence, typically expressed as a logarithmic score (logarithm of odds, Lod). Conventionally, a Lod score of greater than 3, indicating 1,000:1 odds for the data to represent true linkage, is considered significant. In essence, such a result tells the investigator that the marker—usually well characterized with regard to its chromosomal localization—is close to the gene of interest, providing a critical way-point toward the identification of yet-unknown genes or a strong indication of the disease relevance of a candidate gene (in the case of candidate gene markers). Note, however, that linkage generally identifies a chromosomal region only as carrying the gene of interest and will pinpoint a particular gene only in the case of the fortuitous availability of very closely spaced markers and highly informative recombinant individuals.

Whereas among family members linkage analysis can be used successfully even with markers that map at some distance from the disease gene, linkage disequilibrium is rapidly lost among unrelated individuals, so that only markers that in essence represent the pathogenic mutation, or are at least localized within the same gene, can be used for association (case-control) studies among such populations. Statistical analysis of association studies is therefore based not on likelihood but on regression algorithms. Although it is important that proband samples in populations used for this approach do not contain blood relatives, these studies are highly sensitive to differences in the genetic background of cases and controls.

Genetic Analysis of Complex Disease

The two approaches to genetic analysis described here are well suited for the analysis of simple mendelian traits. In the case of a polygenic, complex genetic disease, they cannot discern any clear pattern of inheritance. However, we can conceptualize the phenotype as a composite that represents the net effect of additive (or multiplicative) influences of several genes, each of which segregates independently but according to classic mendelian doctrine. This allows, theoretically, the resolution or dissection of the remote phenotype into the intermediate phenotype effects of all of its contributing factors, in particular the genes involved. Each of them, segregating independently, will be found to confer a particular quantitative and qualitative effect (e.g., more or less blood pressure raising or lowering). Thus, the principles of classic linkage or association analysis can be applied to the investigation of a polymorphic marker's role in polygenic disease etiology, with the proviso that the concomitant effects of additional unknown genetic and other factors will increase noise and decrease statistical power, raising (often dramatically) the number of observations necessary to reach statistically meaningful results.

Because complex diseases such as hypertension are common yet genetically heterogeneous, have incomplete penetrance, and their onset is delayed, large informative pedigrees are usually not available nor are they necessarily desirable. For these traits, sibling-pair linkage approaches, based on the collection of data from many nuclear families with affected members, are the preferred way of investigation. Sophisticated mathematical and statistical algorithms have been developed[8,9] to analyze data from such populations. If through such studies a particular chromosomal region is found to have a high likelihood of containing a candidate gene (as always, linkage algorithms do not have the power to pinpoint a single gene), a second line of investigation, carried out among unrelated individuals as a case-control study, represents a very powerful means of testing for the role of a particular gene.

Paradoxically, the rapid development of molecular genetic methods and reagents over the past decade has by now created a situation where the tools of molecular analysis are no longer the limiting factor in genetic investigation. Rather, the collection of appropriate population or pedigree samples and the careful and precise determination of specific phenotype parameters represent the greatest challenges for this type of study, from both a logistical and a financial standpoint. Thus, it is the ascertainment and high-fidelity phenotyping of large proband samples, rather than the molecular genetic analysis, that make genetic epidemiological investigation a complex and costly undertaking.

Localization of Hypertension Genes in Experimental Animals

Use of fully inbred animal models expressing a genetically determined disease avoids the problem of genetic heterogeneity, which in humans reduces statistical power to a degree that may preclude detection of individual genetic factors. In an inbred strain, the same set of genes, with the same relative contribution from each gene, is responsible for blood pressure elevation in each animal (of the same sex and age, to be precise). In addition, animal experimentation allows a more precise control of environmental factors than is possible in clinical studies. Most important, the ability to produce specific cross-bred hybrid populations of predetermined genetic constellation and cohort size provides the investigator with a set of extremely powerful experimental tools for carrying out genetic linkage analyses far beyond the scope possible in even large human pedigrees, yet the data can be analyzed with very simple statistical tools.

Hypertensive Rat Models

Over the years, genetic models of hypertension have been developed in several animal species, including rats,[10] dogs,[11] rabbits,[12] turkeys,[13] and mice.[14] The rat model has been used most widely, as it combines several practical advantages, including feasibility of conducting sophisticated hemodynamic investigations, ease of breeding, relatively short generation times, and limited animal husbandry costs. In addition, the substantial number of rat models of genetic hypertension in existence today may be viewed as reflecting, in some ways, the heterogeneity of the hypertensive syndromes encountered in humans.

The characteristics of many of these rat strains have been reviewed.[10] This chapter focuses primarily on the spontaneously hypertensive rat (SHR) as a paradigm of genetic models of hypertension in the rat. This strain has been used more widely than any other in experiments into the nature and pathomechanism of hypertension. It was developed about 30 years ago by selective breeding from a colony of Wistar rats in which individual animals were observed to have elevated blood pressures.[15] SHRs show a steep rise of blood pressure early during postnatal development and a distinct sexual dimorphism, with higher blood pressures in males than females (a characteristic that is also commonly observed in humans). In the vast majority of studies directed at identifying the cause of hypertension in this strain, the investigators' strategy was to compare any of a large number of measurable physiologic, biochemical, pharmacological, and other parameters with similar measurements obtained in a normotensive reference strain, traditionally the Wistar-Kyoto (WKY) strain (which was developed in parallel with the SHR by selective inbreeding of Wistar rats with normal blood pressures).

Among other strains of genetically hypertensive rats, the Dahl rat[16] (later bred to homozygosity as SS/Jr and SR/Jr[17]) is paradigmatic for the multifactorial aspects of human hypertension, in which specific gene-environment (ecogenetic) interactions may play an important role. In the Dahl rat strains, the interaction with environmental factors, such as exposure to dietary salt loading, is critical for the development of hypertension in the salt-sensitive SS strain but has no effect in the salt resistant SR strain.

As a result of the breeding strategies, a large number of genetic (and therefore phenotypic) differences,[18,19] in addition to blood pressure, exist among pairs of strains, most of them fixed purely by chance and without any relevance to hypertension. Thus, the overwhelming majority of differences found by comparing two strains is expected to be either altogether unrelated to the hypertensive phenotype or secondary to it. Proof that any difference, be it phenotypic or genotypic, causally affects blood pressure must rely on the demonstration of cosegregation of the difference (i.e., the polymorphic marker) and blood pressure. Of all loci that differ among the parental strains and that segregate freely in hybrid progeny, only those truly relevant for expression of hypertension will remain associated with this phenotype.

The frequent question of which control strain to use becomes a moot issue for cosegregation studies; as long as both strains are inbred and differ in the phenotype of concern, they may be used in such an experiment to detect disease-relevant loci. However, it is important to realize that depending on the choice of nondiseased strain used for performing the cross, different loci may be detected as pathogenetically important in the same diseased model strain. This finding is characteristic for polygenic diseases: for example, of several genes that potentially raise blood pressure, all but one may differ between a hypertensive and a given normotensive strain, allowing the detection of all but this one locus. If the same hypertensive strain is crossed with a different normotensive strain, and the two strains differ at the previously undetectable locus but not at one of the others, a different set of hypertension-related genes will be detected in the same hypertensive strain, including now the previously undetectable locus.

Candidate Gene Studies in Rat Hypertension

Among the candidate genes for which cosegregation studies have been reported using various systems of polymorphism detection in a variety of intercross and backcross populations are the genes coding for renin,[20-22] atrial natriuretic peptide,[23] angiotensin-converting enzyme,[23] 11β-hydroxylase,[24] kallikrein,[25] the heat-shock protein Hsp70,[26] phospholipase C-δ1,[27] and the gene designated *SA*.[28-31]

Although the findings regarding most of these polymorphisms await independent experimental confirmation, more extensive information from the study of several independent experimental crosses is available in two of them. An RFLP from within the renin gene [*see Figure 1*] was the first DNA-based polymorphism reported to show linkage to blood pressure in a salt-stressed intercross of salt-sensitive and salt-resistant Dahl Jr rats.[20] A second investigation, performed in a hybrid cohort bred from SHR and Lewis rats, demonstrated elevated blood pressures in F_2 animals heterozygous for the renin allele but showed similarly low blood pressures in animals homozygous for either the SHR or the Lewis allele, a finding interpreted as being possibly attributable to the effects of a recessive hypotensive gene in linkage disequilibrium with the renin polymorphism[21] tested. A concomitant study in hybrids derived from WKY rats and a stroke-prone SHR (SHRSP) strain, in contrast, showed no cosegregation of the renin locus and baseline or sodium-stimulated blood pressure.[32] Lastly, a cosegregation study in a cross of the Lyon hypertensive and normotensive strains again found evidence for linkage between a polymorphic marker at the renin locus and diastolic blood pressure.[22] These data indicate that renin, or perhaps more likely a closely linked gene (no sequence differences have been found in the coding region and the 5′-untranslated region among Dahl SS/Jr and SR/Jr rats[33]), may indeed play a role in the pathogenesis of hypertension in selected rat strains. These data emphasize that depending on the presence or absence of divergent gene effects in a particular pair of strains at a particular locus, linkage between this locus and phenotype (such as hypertension) may or may not be apparent. This variable importance that a given gene (mutation) may have depending on the genetic reference to which it is compared is also illustrated by the finding of linkage between blood pressure and the angiotensin-converting enzyme (ACE) locus in a cross of the Dahl SS/Jr rat and the Milan normotensive rat, but not when the same hypertensive strain was crossed with the WKY rat or in several additional cross-bred cohorts involving various different strains.[23]

The *SA* gene represents an unusual candidate gene: whereas the nature and function of the encoded protein (the gene product) are still obscure, the gene (originally discovered through differential hybridization techniques applied to complementary DNA libraries prepared from the kidneys of hypertensive SHR and normotensive Sprague-Dawley animals) shows significantly enhanced levels of expression in the kidneys of SHR as compared with normotensive rats.[34] Its potential contribution to rat hypertension has been implied by demonstration of cosegregation of a genomic polymorphism at the *SA* locus with blood pressure in independent F_2 cohorts derived from SHR/WKY,[28,29,31] SHRSP/WKY,[30] and Dahl SS/Lewis[35] crosses. As with the previously cited examples, the makeup of the cross also affects the detectable biological role of the *SA* gene: in a Dahl SS/WKY cross, no effect could be shown.[35] The *SA* locus exhibits variable ecogenetic characteristics: in a SHRSP/WKY cross, blood pressure was shown to be linked to the *SA* locus (in this case tested by probes for the immediately neighboring leukosianine and myosin light-chain–2 loci on chromosome 1 [recombination distance to *SA* = 4 centimorgans[30]]) under basal conditions but not after sodium loading[36]; conversely, in another SHRSP/WKY cross, exactly the opposite was found.[30] As confusing as these discrepancies may appear, they most likely reflect genetic differences between strains that are nominally, but not biologically, identical, having been reared apart for years and often decades.[37-40]

Genome Screening in Rat Hypertension

The alternative approach to searching for disease-relevant genes, random marker linkage analysis (interval mapping), has been applied to SHRSP/WKY and Lyon hypertensive/normotensive crosses. In the experiment on the SHRSP/WKY cross, a total of 180 polymorphic mini- and microsatellite markers were typed in a cohort of 115 F_2 animals, resulting in the identification of a putative hypertension gene, *BP/SP-1*, on chromosome 10. Linkage was first detected between a microsatellite marker derived from sequence information for the growth hormone locus and systolic and diastolic blood pressure after dietary sodium loading.[41] The linkage group of markers to which this microsatellite belongs, and which also includes the gene encoding the fast nerve growth factor receptor, was known to be represented by synteny in humans on the long arm of chromosome 17, where the gene for ACE had previously been localized[42] [*see Figure 4*]. Because the ACE gene obviously represents a potential candidate gene, a polymorphic marker for the gene in the rat was developed based on homology to the mouse that was subsequently shown to be as closely linked to *BP/SP-1* as *GH* was. Although this finding was intriguing, it has since been improperly overinterpreted as evidence that the ACE gene causes hypertension in the SHRSP. Based on the spacing of markers and on the number of animals examined, the 100:1 odds interval for placing *BP/SP-1* still spans some 20 centimorgans, or 90 million base pairs (in the rat, 1 cM = 2×10^6 bp).

A second locus affecting blood pressure was found in this experiment to localize to the X chromosome.[41] The WKY allele at this locus tracked with higher blood pressures, and the SHRSP allele conferred lower blood pressures. This observation, seemingly paradoxical, highlights the principle that blood pressure phenotype is the net result of the effects of a number of genes that either raise or lower blood pressure; the fact that in the SHRSP, as compared with the WKY rat, blood pressure–elevating loci are more prevalent is certainly not incompatible with the finding that on some loci the WKY rat carries a gene that has a greater blood pressure–raising effect than

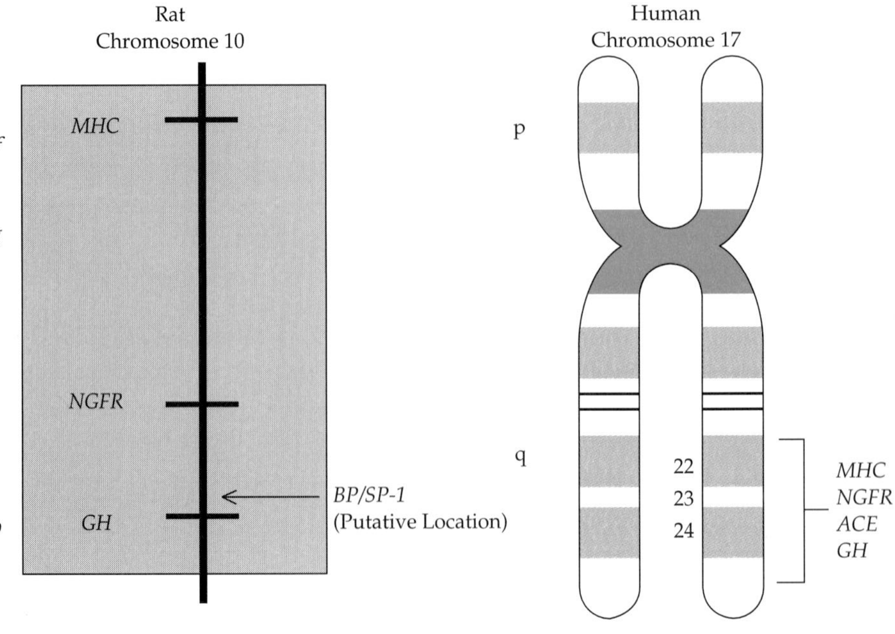

Figure 4 *The syntenic regions on rat chromosome 10 and human chromosome 17 are shown schematically. Because chromosome numbers in each species have been assigned somewhat arbitrarily, and because relatively large regions of contiguous DNA are often preserved undisrupted (syntenic) through evolution, corresponding homologous genome regions can be found on different chromosomes among different species. By comparison, one can often make inferences about the presence of additional genes in one species from the knowledge of their presence in another, as was done for the ACE gene in the rat, which turned out to map close to rat GH. GH, growth hormone; NGFR, nerve growth factor receptor.*

its homologue in the SHRSP. Alternatively, one could argue that the WKY allele at this X-chromosomal locus is associated with normal blood presure, whereas the SHRSP allele actually lowers blood pressure and thereby facilitates biological fitness and survival in the SHRSP strain. On a more general level, we may infer that for most polygenic disease phenotypes, one will find, depending on the genetic reference used, loci enhancing as well as attenuating the trait.

A second experiment that utilized a random marker approach demonstrated linkage between the carboxypeptidase B gene locus on rat chromosome 2 and pulse pressure (the differential of systolic and diastolic blood pressure, which may be a crude indicator of left ventricular performance or vascular compliance).[22] This experiment emphasizes the importance of determining perhaps somewhat esoteric-appearing phenotypes (sub- or intermediate phenotypes) that contribute specific elements to the remote, composite phenotype of actual interest.

Relevance of Studies in Experimental Hypertension to Human Disease

What can we learn from these studies in experimental animal strains about hypertension in humans? The lessons to be learned are likely to provide important conceptual and methodological guidance for the approach to human studies, as well as new insights into pathomechanisms that may result in the elevation of blood pressure. However, the hope that hypertensinogenic genes will be found in the rat that relate directly, by their human homologues, to the disease in humans—an argument often heard in support of animal experimentation—is likely to be naive, given the heterogeneity of both human hypertension and hypertensive rat strains. There is even a more disconcerting reason why research using various hypertensive rat strains may be leading us along a wrong path: although these strains provide very good model systems for hypertension with regard to blood pressure elevations, they show very little of the associated vascular and end-organ pathology that makes hypertension a clinically relevant and epidemiologically important issue in humans. In fact, coincidental with the selection for blood pressure–raising genes, an unrecognized selection against morbidity-susceptibility genes is likely to have occurred during the breeding of these rat strains to ensure their continued biologic fitness. This observation raises the conceptual issue of whether hypertension is to be regarded as a disease per se or as a sign (an epiphenomenon of a disease process that starts and strikes elsewhere). A notable exception is the SHRSP, which under appropriate environmental conditions shows a high incidence of cerebrovascular accidents.

Genetic Basis of Human Hypertension

Evidence for heritability of hypertension in humans comes primarily from large epidemiological surveys showing a pattern of familial aggregation[43-46] and from twin studies documenting excess disease concordance in monozygotic as compared with dizygotic twins.[47] The problems presented by this and similar complex diseases can now be addressed by the tools of molecular genetic epidemiology, which derives its resources from the successful interaction of molecular biology for data collection and sophisticated statistical genetic algorithms for data analysis.

Several studies have been conducted in human populations and pedigrees in the past using non–DNA-based indirect genetic markers. By far the most common of these markers were HLA antigens.[48] Whereas most of these studies have remained inconclusive and underpowered, an overall trend toward an association for certain antigens and hypertension was commonly seen, and a linkage study also supported localization of a hypertension-relevant gene to the major histocompatibility complex locus.[48] Likewise, haptoglobin isoforms have been shown to be associated with sodium-sensitive hypertension.[49] The purported role of the sodium-hydrogen antiporter as a determinant of blood pressure[50] serves as a case in point, demonstrating the unreliability and vagaries of linkage or association analyses using biochemical or physiologic markers: when the study was repeated in the same subjects using molecular probes to detect the genetic isoforms of the gene as well as linkage analysis with a panel of markers spanning the sodium-hydrogen antiporter locus, no linkage was detected.[51]

Among monogenetic forms of hypertension, the deployment of molecular genetic techniques has recently solved the riddle of glucocorticoid-remediable aldosteronism, a rare autosomal dominant disorder characterized by hypertension, occasional hyperaldosteronism, and the secretion of abnormal adrenal steroids, all suppressible by glucocorticoids or dexamethasone and under the control of adrenocorticotropic hormone.[52] This syndrome was traced to a fusion of the 11β-hydroxylase and aldosterone synthase genes by an unequal crossing-over event, rendering a chimeric enzyme with the actions that could explain all clinical features of the syndrome.

Very little is yet known about the genetic underpinnings of the more frequent polygenic forms of hypertension. Lacking large, well-characterized pedigrees (or the even larger affected sibling-pair registries that would be necessary), investigators have not yet applied interval mapping using anonymous markers to hypertension. Rather, several candidate genes, almost exclusively chosen from the renin-angiotensin system, have been examined. The most intriguing and promising of them so far is the gene coding for angiotensinogen, precursor of the vasoactive peptide angiotensin II. Chapter 17 describes the genes that code for the renin-angiotensin system and the evaluation of their potential role in human hypertension.

Sexual Dimorphism and Age of Onset

The presence of a sexual dimorphism affecting the incidence, age at onset, and severity of hypertension has long been appreciated in both human and experimental hypertension. In part, this dimorphism appears to represent a steroid hormone–related, sex-influenced trait—that is, the presence of male sex hormones affects certain genes or their gene products.[53,54] One of the candidate genes whose expression may be influenced by testosterone is renin,[55] although no specific hormone-responsive element has been characterized in the flanking region of the gene. Several elegant experimental studies[53,54,56] have provided evidence that the phenomenon is partially a holandric (Y chromosome–linked) effect, at least in certain strains of SHR. In addition, there is evidence for the existence of sex-linked (X chromosome–linked) inheritance of loci affecting blood pressure.[41] Very little is known about the origin of sexual dimorphism of blood pressure in humans, but we now have evidence that the angiotensinogen locus shows much less convincing linkage to hypertension in women than in men[57] (aside from the special case of preeclampsia[58]), suggesting that the effect of this locus may be influenced by gender. These observations have important implications on research in hypertension. In studies of human hypertension, it stands to reason that female and male subjects should be analyzed separately. Close attention also needs to be paid to proband age, as hypertension is a disease that shows delayed onset, and phenotype data need to be adjusted for the effects of age. For research with experimental animals, a careful study design is thus mandatory, involving duplication of the cross to incorporate Y chromosomes from both progenitor strains where appropriate.

Conclusion

With the availability and practical applicability of powerful new methods of molecular genetics, hypertension research, like many other areas of medicine, finds itself at the threshold of expanding into a new era of progress. We finally have the tools assembled that will make it possible to characterize the genetic basis of hypertension. It will not be a simple task, however, and mastering it will require a concerted, interdisciplinary effort of basic researchers and clinical investigators, of molecular biologists, clinicians, physiologists, geneticists, epidemiologists, pharmacologists, and statisticians, among others. A major burden will fall on the clinician to collect and characterize appropriate populations of afflicted patients. Whereas remarkable improvements in the prognosis for hypertensive patients have been achieved over the past decades by simple palliation, the ability to target specific disease mechanisms will truly revolutionize the therapy and, more important, prevention of hypertensive syndromes, a goal well worth our most intensive efforts.

References

1. Gusella JF, Wexler NS, Conneally PM, et al: A polymorphic DNA marker genetically linked to Huntington's disease. *Nature* 306:234, 1983
2. Jeffreys AJ, Wilson V, Thein SL: Hypervariable "minisatellite" regions in human DNA. *Nature* 314:67, 1985
3. Weber JL, May PE: Abundant class of human DNA polymorphisms which can be typed using the polymerase chain reaction. *Am J Hum Genet* 44:388, 1989
4. Weissenbach J, Gyapay G, Dib C, et al: A second-generation linkage map of the human genome. *Nature* 359:794, 1992
5. Dietrich W, Katz H, Lincoln SE, et al: A genetic map of the mouse suitable for typing intraspecific crosses. *Genetics* 131:423, 1992
6. Serikawa T, Kuramoto T, Hilbert P, et al: Rat gene mapping using PCR-analyzed microsatellites. *Genetics* 1992;131:701, 1992
7. Collins FS: Positional cloning: let's not call it reverse anymore [news]. *Nat Genet* 1:3, 1992
8. Lathrop GM, Lalouel JM, Julier C, et al: Strategies for multilocus linkage analysis in humans. *Proc Natl Acad Sci USA* 81:3443, 1984
9. Lander ES, Botstein D: Mapping mendelian factors underlying quantitative traits using RFLP linkage maps. *Genetics* 121:185, 1989

10. Lovenberg W, Horan M, Eds: Genetic rat models of hypertension: guidelines for breeding, care, use. *Hypertension* 9(suppl I):I-1, 1987
11. Katz JI, Skom JH, Wakerlin GE: Pathogenesis of spontaneous and pyelonephritic hypertension in the dog. *Circ Res* 5:137, 1957
12. Alexander N, Hinshaw LB, Drury DR: Development of a strain of spontaneously hypertensive rabbits. *Proc Natl Acad Sci USA* 86:855, 1954
13. El Halawani ME, Weibel PE, Appel JR, et al: Catecholamines and monoamine-oxidase activity in turkeys with high or low bood pressure. *Trans NY Acad Sci* 35:463, 1973
14. Schlager G, Weibust RS: Genetic control of blood pressure in mice. *Genetics* 55:497, 1968
15. Okamoto K, Aoki K: Development of a strain of spontaneously hypertensive rats. *Jpn Circ J* 27:282, 1963
16. Dahl LK, Heine M, Tassinari L: Role of genetic factors in susceptibility to experimental hypertension due to chronic excess salt ingestion. *Nature* 194:480, 1962
17. Rapp JP, Dene H: Development and characteristics of inbred strains of Dahl salt-sensitive and salt-resistant rats. *Hypertension* 7:340, 1985
18. Johnson ML, Ely DL, Turner ME: Genetic divergence between the Wistar-Kyoto and the spontaneously hypertensive rat. *Hypertension* 19:425, 1992
19. St. Lezin E, Simonet L, Pravenec M, et al: Hypertensive strains and normotensive "control" strains: how closely are they related? *Hypertension* 19:419, 1992
20. Rapp JP, Wang S-M, Dene H: A genetic polymorphism in the renin gene of Dahl rat cosegregates with blood pressure. *Science* 243:542, 1989
21. Kurtz TW, Simonet L, Kabra PM, et al: Cosegregation of the renin allele in the spontaneously hypertensive rat with an increase in blood pressure. *J Clin Invest* 85:1328, 1990
22. Dubay C, Vincent M, Samani NJ, et al: Genetic determinants of diastolic and pulse pressure map to different loci in Lyon hypertensive rats. *Nat Genet* 3:354, 1993
23. Deng Y, Rapp JP: Cosegregation of blood pressure with angiotensin converting enzyme and atrial natriuretic peptide receptor genes using Dahl salt-sensitive rats. *Nat Genet* 1:267, 1992
24. Cicila GT, Rapp JP, Wang JM, et al: Linkage of 11 beta-hydroxylase mutations with altered steroid biosynthesis and blood pressure in the Dahl rat. *Nat Genet* 3:346, 1993
25. Pravenec M, Kren V, Kunes J, et al: Cosegregation of blood pressure with a kallikrein gene family polymorphism. *Hypertension* 17:242, 1991
26. Hamet P, Kong D, Pravenec M, et al: Restriction fragment length polymorphism of hsp70 gene, localized in the RT1 complex, is associated with hypertension in spontaneously hypertensive rats. *Hypertension* 19:611, 1992
27. Katsuya T, Higaki J, Miki T, et al: Hypotensive effect associated with a phospholipase C-delta 1 gene mutation in the spontaneously hypertensive rat. *Biochem Biophys Res Commun* 187:1359, 1992
28. Iwai N, Inagami T: Identification of a candidate gene responsible for the high blood pressure of spontaneously hypertensive rats. *J Hypertens* 10:1155, 1992
29. Iwai N, Kurtz TW, Inagami T: Further evidence of the SA gene as a candidate gene contributing to the hypertension in spontaneously hypertensive rat. *Biochem Biophys Res Commun* 188:64, 1992
30. Lindpaintner K, Hilbert P, Ganten D, et al: Molecular genetics of the SA-gene: cosegregation with hypertension and mapping to rat chromosome 1. *J Hypertens* 11:19, 1993
31. Samani NJ, Lodwick D, Vincent M, et al: A gene differentially expressed in the kidney of spontaneously hypertensive rat cosegregates with increased blood pressure. *J Clin Invest* 92:1099, 1993
32. Lindpaintner K, Takahashi S, Ganten D: Structural alterations of the renin gene in stroke-prone spontaneously hypertensive rats: examination of genotype-phenotype correlations. *J Hypertens* 8:763, 1990
33. Alam KY, Wang Y, Dene H, et al: Renin gene nucleotide sequence of coding and regulatory regions in Dahl rats. *Clin Exp Hypertens* 15:599, 1993
34. Iwai N, Inagami T: Isolation of preferentially expressed genes in the kidneys of hypertensive rats. *Hypertension* 17:161, 1991
35. Harris EL, Dene H, Rapp JP: SA gene and blood pressure cosegregation using Dahl salt-sensitive rats. *Am J Hypertens* 6:330, 1993
36. Nara Y, Nabika T, Ikeda K, et al: Basal high blood pressure cosegregates with the loci on chromosome 1 in the F2 generation from crosses between normotensive Wistar Kyoto rats and stroke-prone spontaneously hypertensive rats. *Biochem Biophys Res Commun* 194:1344, 1993

37. Louis WJ, Howes LG: Genealogy of the spontaneously hypertensive rat and Wistar-Kyoto rat strains: implications for studies of inherited hypertension. *J Cardiovasc Pharmacol* 16(suppl 7):S1, 1990

38. Kurtz TW, Montano M, Chan L, et al: Molecular evidence of genetic heterogeneity in Wistar-Kyoto rats: implications for research with the spontaneously hypertensive rat. *Hypertension* 13:188, 1989

39. Kurtz TW, Morris RC Jr: Biological variability in Wistar-Kyoto rats: implications for research with the spontaneously hypertensive rat. *Hypertension* 10:127, 1987

40. Samani NJ, Swales JD, Jeffreys AJ, et al: DNA fingerprinting of spontaneously hypertensive and Wistar-Kyoto rat: implications for hypertension research. *J Hypertens* 7:809, 1990

41. Hilbert P, Lindpaintner K, Beckmann JS, et al: Chromosomal mapping of two genetic loci associated with blood-pressure regulation in hereditary hypertensive rats. *Nature* 353:521, 1991

42. Mattei MG, Hubert C, Alhenc-Gelas F, et al: Angiotensin I converting enzyme is on chromosome 17. *Cytogenet Cell Genet* 51:1041, 1989

43. Annest JL, Sing CF, Biron P, et al: Familial aggregation of blood pressure and weight in adoptive families: I. Comparisons of blood pressure and weight statistics among families with adopted, natural or both natural and adopted children. *Am J Epidemiol* 110:479, 1979

44. Higgins M, Keller J, Moore F, et al: Studies of blood pressure in Tecumseh, Michigan: I. Blood pressure in young people and its relationship to personal and familial characteristics and complications of pregnancy in mothers. *Am J Epidemiol* 111:142, 1980

45. Diaz JF, Hachinski VC, Pederson LL, et al: Aggregation of multiple risk factors for stroke in siblings of patients with brain infarction and transient ischemic attacks. *Stroke* 17:1239, 1986

46. Havlik RJ, Garrison RJ, Feinleib M, et al: Blood pressure aggregation in families. *Am J Epidemiol* 110:304, 1979

47. Levine RS, Hennekens CH, Perry A, et al: Genetic variance of blood pressure levels in infant twins. *Am J Epidemiol* 116:759, 1982

48. Gerbase-DeLima M, DeLima JJ, Persoli LB, et al: Essential hypertension and histocompatibility antigens: a linkage study. *Hypertension* 14:604, 1989

49. Weinberger MH, Miller JZ, Fineberg NS, et al: Association of haptoglobin with sodium sensitivity and resistance of blood pressure. *Hypertension* 10:443, 1987

50. Hasstedt SJ, Wu LL, Ash KO, et al: Hypertension and sodium-lithium countertransport in Utah pedigrees: evidence for major-locus inheritance. *Am J Hum Genet* 43:14, 1988

51. Lifton RP, Hunt SC, Williams RR, et al: Exclusion of the Na(+)-H+ antiporter as a candidate gene in human essential hypertension. *Hypertension* 17:8, 1991

52. Lifton RP, Dluhy RG, Powers M, et al: A chimaeric 11 beta-hydroxylase/aldosterone synthase gene causes glucocorticoid-remediable aldosteronism and human hypertension. *Nature* 355:262, 1992

53. Ely DL, Daneshvar H, Turner ME, et al: The hypertensive Y chromosome elevates blood pressure in F11 normotensive rats. *Hypertension* 21:1071, 1993

54. Turner ME, Johnson ML, Ely D: Separate sex-influenced and genetic components in spontaneously hypertensive rat hypertension. *Hypertension* 17:1097, 1991

55. Bachmann J, Feldmer M, Ganten U, et al: Sexual dimorphism of blood pressure: possible role of the renin-angiotensin system. *J Steroid Biochem Mol Biol* 40:511, 1991

56. Ely DL, Turner ME: Hypertension in the spontaneously hypertensive rat is linked to the Y chromosome. *Hypertension* 16:277, 1990

57. Jeunemaitre X, Soubrier F, Kotelevtsev YV, et al: Molecular basis of human hypertension: role of angiotensinogen. *Cell* 71:169, 1992

58. Arngrimsson R, Purandare S, Connor M, et al: Angiotensinogen: a candidate gene involved in preeclampsia [letter]? *Nat Genet* 4:114, 1993

Acknowledgments

Figures 1, 2, 4 Talar Agasyan.

Figures 3 Dimitry Schidlovsky. From "Medical Genetics," by R. W. Erbe, in *Scientific American Medicine,* edited by E. Rubenstein and D. D. Federman, Section 9, Subsection IV. Scientific American, Inc. New York, 1994.

CHAPTER 17

The Renin-Angiotensin System in Human Hypertension

Pierre Corvol, M.D., Xavier Jeunemaitre, M.D., Anne Charru, M.D., Florent Soubrier, M.D.

Blood pressure is a quantitative trait that varies continuously throughout the population and whose regulation is controlled by mechanisms that involve several genetic loci and environmental factors. However, little is known about the genes involved in human hypertension, their importance in determining blood pressure level, and their interaction with other genes and environmental components. Epidemiologic studies have shown that individual blood pressure levels are determined by both genetic predisposition and environmental factors; the evidence suggests that approximately 30 percent of the variance of blood pressure is attributable to genetic heritability and 50 percent to environmental influences.[1] The heritable component of blood pressure has been documented in familial and twin studies.

No data exist on the number of genetic loci involved in the regulation of blood pressure, the frequency of deleterious alleles, the mode of transmission, or the quantitative effects of any single allele on blood pressure. The unimodal distribution of blood pressure within each age group and in each sex strongly suggests that several loci are involved. Because of the probable etiologic heterogeneity of the disease, a single biochemical or DNA genetic marker is not likely to help the clinician in the treatment of most hypertensive patients. However, genetic markers are useful indicators for the genetic loci linked to high blood pressure. The genetic approach can discount the importance of a gene because it is not frequently implicated in blood pressure level or in hypertension. Conversely, the discovery of a positive linkage between a given locus and high blood pressure will promote new studies for improving or finding new intermediate phenotypes of the locus. In addition, molecular genetics can reveal an underestimated or even unexpected mechanism of blood pressure control.

Even though the genetic loci that control blood pressure are unknown, an initial logical approach is to study genes that are likely to contribute to the variance of blood pressure because of their well-known effects on the cardiovascular system. The genes of the renin-angiotensin system are good candidates for such an approach because this system is well known to be involved in the control of blood pressure. The renin-angiotensin system consists of four main proteins: renin, angiotensinogen, angiotensin-converting enzyme, and angiotensin II receptor. During the past 10 years, considerable progress has been achieved since the complementary DNAs (cDNAs) encoding these proteins and their corresponding genes were cloned [*see Table 1*]. Molecular cloning of the renin-angiotensin system genes has provided investigators with new tools for studying the structure and function of these proteins and for developing new inhibitors. It has also opened new avenues for the investigation of the expression and regulation of these genes in various tissues, and for seeking a possible relation between high blood pressure and abnormalities of one of these genes. This review discusses the recent progress made in the molecular genetics of the renin-angiotensin system genes in human hypertension.

The Renin Gene

The renin gene is important because the renin-angiotensinogen reaction is the first and rate-limiting step leading to angiotensin II production. Numerous studies have linked renin to experimental forms of hypertension and to human hypertension. A fulminant hypertension develops in transgenic rats harboring the mouse *ren*2 gene.[2] In humans, about 30 percent of subjects with essential hypertension have higher renin levels than do normotensive subjects of the same age when they are examined under the same metabolic conditions.[3] Recently, it was shown that the patients with higher renin levels are at higher risk for developing a cardiovascular complication than are those with normal renin levels.[4]

The first component of the renin-angiotensin system to be cloned was the mouse renin cDNA.[5] Comparison of the amino acid sequence deduced from

Table 1 Genes of the Renin-Angiotensin System

Gene	*Gene Family*	*Chromosomal Localization in Humans*	*Gene Polymorphism*
Renin	Aspartyl protease	1q32–1q42[10]	RFLP[13]
Angiotensinogen	Serine protease inhibitor	1q42[58]	Microsatellite[75] Mutations[76]
Angiotensin-converting enzyme	Zinc metallopeptidase	17q23[35]	Insertion/deletion[30]
Angiotensin II receptor	G-coupled receptor	3q21–3q25	Mutations

Table 2 Linkage or Association of the Renin-Angiotensin System Gene Variants with Human Hypertension

Gene	*Study Design*	*Results*
Renin	Linkage study in a Utah pedigree[11]	Negative
	Sib pair analysis[14]	Negative
	Association studies	Negative
	French hypertensive population[13]	Negative
	Australian hypertensive population[12]	Negative
Angiotensin-converting enzyme	Linkage study in French normotensive families[32]	Negative
	Sib pair analysis in Utah hypertensives[37]	Negative
	Association studies	Negative
	Dutch hypertensives and offspring study[41]	Negative
	Japanese hypertensive population[40]	Negative
	Four-corners study[38]	Negative
	Australian hypertensive population[36]	Positive
Angiotensinogen	Linkage and association studies in Utah and French hypertensives[76,78]	Positive
	Linkage study in pregnancy-induced hypertension[83]	Positive
	Association study in pregnancy-induced hypertension[82]	Positive

the cDNA sequence with that obtained from the mature protein itself allowed investigators to propose a model for the processing of prorenin into renin.[6] Renin cloning also confirmed that renin belonged to the aspartyl protease family, in which two aspartyl residues are present in the catalytic site. The human renin gene contains 10 exons and 9 introns and spans approximately 12 kilobases.[7-9] It is located on the short arm of chromosome 1 (1q32-1q42).[10]

Several studies have been conducted to seek an association or a linkage between renin genotype and hypertension [*see Table 2*]. These studies were facilitated by the identification of various polymorphisms located throughout the renin gene by several investigators: *Taq*I and *Bgl*I polymorphisms were located in the 5′ region; *Hin*dIII, in the 3′ region; and *Hin*fI, in the first intron. In a single large Utah human pedigree with high prevalence of coronary disease and hypertension, no significant association existed between renin restriction fragment length polymorphisms (RFLPs) and blood pressure or plasma renin activity.[11] Interpretation was, however, limited by the very low number of patients studied. In another preliminary report, Morris and Griffiths[12] compared the renin RFLPs of 29 subjects undergoing antihypertensive treatment with those of 202 adult white patients. No association was found between hypertension and the renin gene allele, but, again, no definite conclusion could be drawn because only a few hypertensive patients were studied, clinical data were not available, and the renin gene polymorphism was defined by a single and weakly informative RFLP.

Soubrier et al.[13] reported on a study comparing the frequency of renin gene polymorphisms in a large population of normotensive and hypertensive subjects. A group of 102 hypertensive patients was selected according to strict criteria of age (between 20 and 60 years), established diagnosis of essential hypertension, and familial history of hypertension (defined as occurring before the age of 65 years in at least one parent and one sibling). A group of 120 normotensive subjects without a personal history of high blood pressure or a family history of hypertension was matched for age, sex ratio, and body-mass index. In all cases, patients presenting with other hypertensive risk factors, such as elevated body mass index, excessive alcohol intake, oral contraceptive treatment, or diabetes mellitus, were excluded. Renin gene polymorphism was studied using three restriction enzymes (*Taq*I, *Hin*fI, and *Hin*dIII). For each restriction enzyme, the genotype frequencies satisfied the Hardy-Weinberg proportion, which ensures a random distribution of alleles for a given gene locus. Allele frequencies were similar in the hypertensive and the normotensive groups. In the absence of parental genotypes, the haplotype frequencies estimated by the likelihood method were found to be similar in the two groups. The results of this investigation do not support an association between the renin genotype and high blood pressure. A definite conclusion could not, however, be drawn, because the effect of the renin gene might be too weak to be revealed in this study.

To explore further the potential role of the renin gene as a genetic determinant of hypertension, another type of study was undertaken by Jeunemaitre et al.[14] in hypertensive sib pairs. This method has several advantages: (1) it does not assume any specific mode of inheritance at the test locus and looks only for a distortion of segregation between a genetic marker and the disease, (2) the use of a single adult generation decreases problems caused by the age-related increase in blood pressure, and (3) analysis of hypertensive sib pairs can partly resolve the problem of genetic heterogeneity generated by the analysis of extended multigenerational families. Using the same clinical criteria as Soubrier et al.[13] and the same renin genotypes, these authors found no linkage between the renin gene and hypertension, suggesting again that the renin gene does not have a frequent or important role in the pathogenesis of essential hypertension. However, the definitive exclusion of a contribution of the renin gene in the heritability of essential hypertension requires more powerful linkage studies, such as the use of a reliable renin intermediate phenotype and discovery of a more polymorphic marker of the renin locus. At present, it is not possible to exclude a minor role of this gene in blood pressure level in a large population of patients or a major effect of the gene in rare families.

The Angiotensin-Converting Enzyme

Angiotensin-converting enzyme (ACE) is a zinc metallopeptidase whose main function is to convert angiotensin I into angiotensin II and to inactivate bradykinin. This step of the renin-angiotensin system has been assumed to be not limiting, and indeed no evidence indicates that plasma ACE levels are related to blood pressure levels. However, the molecular genetics of ACE in humans open a new and fascinating area in the study of cardiovascular diseases.

Structure of Somatic and Testicular ACE and Organization of the ACE Gene

Molecular cloning of the human endothelial ACE cDNA[15] and of the mouse kidney ACE cDNA[16] revealed that the enzyme consists of two highly homologous domains, indicating a gene duplication event in the course of evolution [*see Figure 1*]. The human somatic ACE is a 170-kilodalton (kd) protein inserted in the plasma membrane by a hydrophobic α-helix located near the C-terminal.[17] ACE also circulates in a soluble form in plasma. Its solubilization is a posttranslational enzymatic process that has been elucidated in Chinese hamster ovary cells expressing recombinant ACE.[18] A series of site-directed mutageneses aimed to inactivate either the N- or the C-domain showed that both domains of ACE are catalytically active[19] and are able to bind ACE inhibitors.[20] Angiotensin I and bradykinin, the two main ACE substrates, are cleaved at the same rate by the two domains of ACE.

However, several functional differences exist between the two domains of ACE. First, the catalytic activity of the C-domain for some substrates strongly depends on chloride concentration, whereas the N-domain is much less dependent on chloride.[19] Second, some substrates are more favorably cleaved by the N-domain than by the C-domain. Luteinizing hormone–releasing hormone is hydrolyzed by both domains, but the amino terminal endoproteolytic cleavage of this peptide is performed 30 times faster by the N-domain than by the C-domain.[21] Last, the two domains exhibit differential binding affinities for various ACE inhibitors.[20] The physiologic and clinical relevance of the different behavior of the two ACE active catalytic sites is not known.

In the testis, in addition to the somatic ACE, a distinct 100-kd isoform occurs in germinal cells. It is specifically expressed in mature spermatids at the onset of puberty. Molecular cloning revealed that it corresponds to the C-domain of ACE and contains one of the two putative catalytic sites identified in endothelial ACE.[22-24] However, the amino terminal sequence is specific for the germinal ACE of the mature spermatids and results from the specific transcription of an exon not transcribed in somatic ACE.

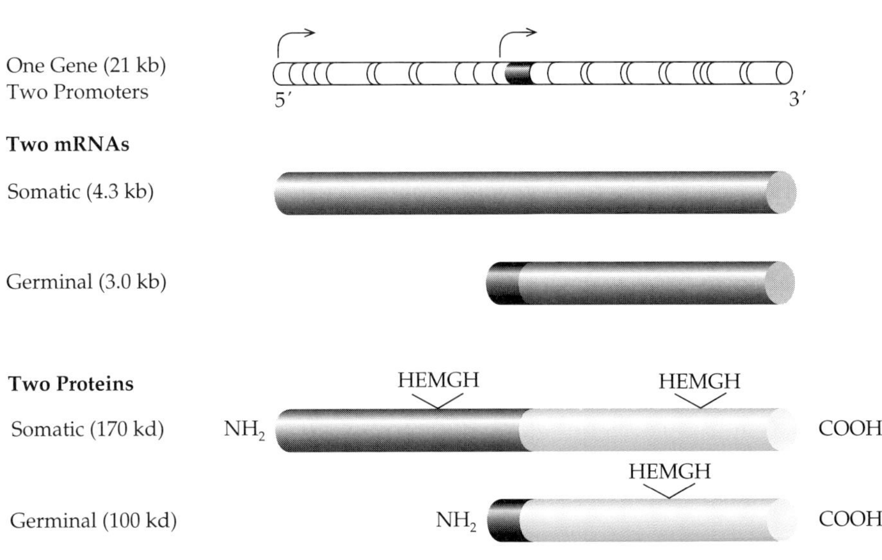

Figure 1 *Schematic structure of the human ACE gene, ACE somatic and germinal mRNAs, and the corresponding ACE proteins. Two alternative promoters direct the transcription of somatic ACE mRNA and germinal ACE mRNA. Exon 13 is specifically transcribed in germinal ACE. Somatic ACE consists of two homologous domains, each containing an active catalytic site with the Zn^{2+} metallopeptidase consensus sequence His-Glu-X-X-His. The zinc-binding site in ACE has the sequence His-Glu-Met-Gly-His. The germinal ACE contains a single functional domain.*

The human ACE gene contains 26 exons, and the organization of its structure provides further support for the duplication of an ancestral gene.[25] Two alternative promoters exist: a somatic promoter localized on the 5′ side of the first exon of the gene and a germinal, intragenic promoter located on the 5′ side of the specific 5′ end of germinal messenger RNA.[25,26] The two alternative promoters of the ACE gene exhibit highly contrasting cell specificities; the somatic promoter is active in endothelial, epithelial, and neuronal cell types, whereas the germinal promoter is active only in a stage-specific manner in male germinal cells.[27]

Relation Between ACE Phenotype and Genotype

In a large series of normal individuals, Alhenc-Gelas et al.[28] found that plasma ACE levels could differ markedly, as much as fivefold, from subject to subject; however, the levels remain remarkably constant when measured repeatedly in a given subject. This important variability primarily results from a major genetic effect, as shown by Cambien et al.[29] in a family population study: a genetic analysis conducted in a sample of 87 healthy families showed an intrafamilial resemblance between plasma ACE levels and suggested that a major gene accounted for approximately 30 and 75 percent of the variance of ACE in parents and in offspring, respectively.

The role of the ACE gene in the genetic control of plasma ACE concentration was assessed using ACE DNA polymorphism. A polymorphism consisting of the presence or the absence of a 287–base pair DNA fragment was detected and used as a marker genotype.[30] In 80 healthy subjects, allele frequencies were 0.6 and 0.4 for the shorter (D) and the longer (I) allele, respectively. Serum ACE levels were measured in every subject and were classified according to ACE genotypes. Patients who were homozygous for the shorter allele had an immunoreactive ACE level that was almost twice as high as that of patients homozygous for the longer allele, whereas heterozygous patients had an intermediate ACE level. This insertion/deletion polymorphism accounted for 47 percent of the total variance of serum ACE, indicating that the ACE gene locus plays an important role in determining serum ACE levels.

Human T cells also express ACE. ACE levels vary widely between individuals and are all influenced by the polymorphism of the ACE gene. As in serum ACE levels, T cell ACE levels are significantly higher in patients who are homozygous for the deletion than they are in the other patients.[31] Another study, combining segregation and linkage analysis in 98 healthy nuclear families, showed that the ACE long allele/short allele (I/D) polymorphism is in fact only a neutral marker that is in strong linkage disequilibrium with the putative variant.[32] Therefore, the I/D polymorphism is not directly involved in the genetic regulation of serum and tissue ACE, and the cause of variations in ACE levels has not been found. Altogether, these results suggest that the level of ACE expression in cells synthesizing the enzyme is genetically determined. In vascular endothelial cells present in kidney, brain, and heart, the presence of a local renin-angiotensin system has been described, and ACE could be a rate-limiting step in the generation of angiotensin I and in the degradation of bradykinin.

ACE Gene Polymorphism and Cardiovascular Diseases

ACE Gene and Hypertension

The observation that plasma ACE levels are under direct control of a variant of the ACE gene renders attractive the hypothesis that ACE is a possible candidate gene for high blood pressure. Two recent studies performed in genetically hypertensive rats made this hypothesis even more attractive. An F_2 rat population generated from stroke-prone spontaneously hypertensive rats (SHRSP) and normotensive Wistar-Kyoto crosses was studied by two laboratories, using a set of gene markers evenly spaced throughout the rat genome.[33,34] Both groups of investigators found a significant linkage between sodium chloride–loaded hypertension and a gene locus on rat chromosome 10. This locus contributed as much as 20 percent of blood pressure variance in rats that had high salt intake and contained the ACE gene. The ACE gene maps in a syntenic region of the human genome, at band 17q23.[35]

The finding that ACE was one of the many genes linked to blood pressure variance in rat genetic hypertension prompted studies to detect possible linkage or association of this locus in human hypertension, even though no relation was found between plasma ACE levels, ACE genotype, and blood pressure in a study of 98 healthly nuclear families.[32]

All reported studies, except one association study comparing a normotensive population with a hypertensive Australian population that had two hypertensive parents,[36] failed to detect an association or a linkage of hypertension to the ACE gene locus. The most conclusive study was that of Jeunemaitre et al.,[37] who, using a highly polymorphic marker locus, showed no evidence of linkage between blood pressure levels and the ACE locus in hypertensive sib pairs from Utah. Another study was performed by Harrap et al.,[38] who investigated the distribution of the ACE I/D gene polymorphism in young adults with contrasting genetic predisposition to high blood pressure ("four-corners approach").[39] Young adults with high blood pressure and two parents with high blood pressure did not show any significant difference in the I/D allele frequencies of the ACE gene when compared with adults of the same age but with low blood pressure and no genetic predisposition to high blood pressure. Other association studies also showed no association [*see Table 2*].[40,41] Taken together, these results suggest that the ACE gene does not play a major role in blood pressure variance in these populations.

ACE Gene and Myocardial Infarction

Although the ACE gene is not linked to high blood pressure, the ACE I/D polymorphism does seem to be a potent risk factor for coronary heart disease, especially in patients formerly considered at low risk according to commonly used criteria. A case control study was performed in different populations in France and Belfast to identify variants of candidate genes that predispose to myocardial infarction. Cambien et al.[42] found that the ACE DD genotype was associated with a higher incidence of myocardial infarction than occurred in the I/D and II genotypes. In addition, they made the important observation that in a low-risk group defined according to plasma apolipoprotein B levels and body mass index, the ACE I/D polymorphism was an independent risk factor, and the ACE DD genotype increased 2.7 times the relative risk (approximated by an odds ratio) of developing myocardial infarction. In a subsequent study, the same group showed that an association existed between ACE genotype and parental history of fatal myocardial infarction: a significant excess of both DD and ID genotypes existed among the patients with a parental history of myocardial infarction.[43] The deleterious effect of the DD genotype may result from an overexpression of ACE, giving rise to a local increase in angiotensin II in some vascular territories, like the coronary circulation. In a preliminary report, Otishi et al.[44] showed a higher incidence of coronary artery stenosis after coronary artery dilation in patients carrying the ACE DD genotype than in those carrying the II genotype. Other studies are in progress in several countries to test the hypothesis that the ACE I/D gene polymorphism could be a new and potent risk factor for coronary diseases.

Two recent studies indicate that the ACE DD genotype frequency is increased in patients with ischemic or idiopathic dilated cardiomyopathy[45] and in familial hypertrophic cardiomyopathy.[46] This finding suggests that the ACE gene variant may contribute to the pathogenesis of cardiomyopathy and that a gene-gene interaction might play a detrimental role in familial hypertrophic cardiomyopathy and sudden cardiac death. Finally, results of a population-based study performed in 141 women and 149 men with left ventricular hypertrophy suggest that the DD genotype of ACE is a genetic marker of left ventricular hypertrophy, especially in middle-aged men.[47]

The Angiotensinogen Gene

Angiotensinogen, the renin substrate, is mainly synthesized by the liver and is the unique substrate for renin. The K_m of renin for angiotensinogen is around 1.25±0.1 μM, and is more than 10 times lower than the K_m of renin for the homologous synthetic tetradecapeptide substrate (20.7±7 μM).[48] Because the concentration of angiotensinogen in rat and human plasma is around 1 μM, 10 times more angiotensinogen than is naturally present would be necessary to reach a zero-order enzymatic reaction. For this reason, although the concentration of angiotensinogen present in plasma seems large, it is actually in a range in which variations in concentration directly affect the activity of renin.

Direct evidence supporting the limiting role of plasma angiotensinogen in angiotensin I generation comes from the effect of injection of pure angiotensinogen in salt-depleted rats, which increases blood pressure,[49] and the passive transfer of antiangiotensinogen antibodies, which decreases blood pressure and plasma renin activity to an extent that depends on the state of sodium balance.[50] However, neither injection of angiotensinogen nor transfer of antiangiotensinogen antibodies affects the blood pressure of binephrectomized animals.

If one assumes that the rate of angiotensin I formation is half its maximum at the usual plasma angiotensinogen concentration, it is logical for one to suspect that the rise in angiotensinogen induced by administration of synthetic estrogens or glucocorticoids plays a role in the pathophysiology of some secondary forms of hypertension, such as oral contraceptive–induced hypertension or Cushing's syndrome.[51] Subtle changes in renal blood flow have been observed in women whose angiotensinogen levels were increased by oral treatment with synthetic estrogens.[52] In normal patients, an angiotensinogen increase results in an elevation of plasma angiotensin II concentration, which in turn decreases renin secretion to restore a normal plasma angiotensin II concentration. A chronic state of increased plasma angiotensinogen concentration might facilitate the development of hypertension in predisposed individuals through an abnormally short feedback loop between angiotensin II and renin release. An exclusively angiotensinogen-dependent hypertension is thus theoretically difficult to imagine, even though two exceptional cases of hypertension associated with hepatic cell tumors that produced large amounts of angiotensinogen have been reported.[53,54]

Structure of the Human Angiotensinogen Gene

The human angiotensinogen cDNA structure[55] shows the presence of a coding region that corresponds to 1,455 nucleotides and codes for 485 amino acids. The mature form consists of 452 amino acid residues; the first 10 amino acids correspond to angiotensin I and the other most important part constitutes des-angiotensin I–angiotensinogen, the part of the angiotensinogen molecule that remains after angiotensin I is released by renin. The genomic organization of rat and human angiotensinogen has also been elucidated.[56,57] The human angiotensinogen gene encompasses five exons and four introns spanning 13 kb of genomic sequence. The first exon is very short (37 nucleotides) and corresponds to the 5′ untranslated sequence of the mRNA. The second exon codes for 59 percent of the protein and contains the nucleotide sequences coding for the signal peptide and angiotensin I. Exons 3 and 4 code for 48 and 62 amino acids of the protein, respectively, whereas the last exon codes for the C-terminal part of the protein and the 3′ untranslated sequence of the mRNA.

A single human angiotensinogen gene has been localized to chromosome 1q42-3 by in situ hybridization.[58] The renin gene has also been assigned to the long arm of chromosome 1 in the q32 region. However, neither loci belongs to a syntenic region. In the mouse, the angiotensinogen gene is located on chromosome 8,[59] whereas the renin 1 and 2 genes are on chromosome 1.[60] In the rat, the angiotensinogen and renin genes are located on chromosomes 19 and 13, respectively.[61,62]

Sites of Expression of Angiotensinogen

Angiotensinogen is a widely expressed glycoprotein.[63,64] The liver is the major site of angiotensinogen synthesis, and plasma angiotensinogen level reflects mainly this synthesis. The brain, large arteries, heart, kidney, and adipose tissues are also established sites of angiotensinogen synthesis.

There is conflicting evidence as to whether angiotensinogen is expressed in the tunica media (smooth muscle layer) or the adventitia of the arterial wall.[65-68] Naftilan et al.[68] showed that expression of angiotensinogen in the tunica media was regulated by sodium intake. Increased angiotensinogen expression in the tunica media has also been induced by vascular injury, suggesting a role for angiotensinogen in myotimal proliferation.[69]

In the heart, angiotensinogen mRNA is expressed mostly in the atria and with less abundance in the ventricles.[65,70] The presence in heart tissue of mRNA of the different components of the renin-angiotensin system, including those of angiotensin II receptors, supports the hypothesis of a physiologic role of the renin-angiotensin system in this organ. Increased ACE activity and angiotensinogen expression have also been demonstrated after experimental left ventricular hypertrophy,[71] suggesting, as have other studies, that the cardiac renin-angiotensin system may have an important role in the modulation of growth and hypertrophy of the heart.

Angiotensinogen mRNA is detectable in the kidney at a much lower level than in the liver.[65] Alteration of renal hemodynamics caused by experimental heart failure has been shown to induce a specific increase of kidney angiotensinogen mRNA, suggesting its contribution to the activation of the intrarenal renin-angiotensin system.[72]

The investigation of local renin-angiotensin systems involves the cellular localization of the four main proteins of this system (angiotensinogen, renin, ACE, and angiotensin II receptors). Because regulation of angiotensinogen expression is tissue specific, local synthesis sites may play biologic roles independent of the circulating angiotensinogen. However, the biochemical or molecular evidence for the presence of the components of the renin-angiotensin system (mRNA or protein) should ideally be supported by the demonstration of a biologic effect of their stimulation or their blockade, such as has been obtained in the heart.

Angiotensinogen Gene and Human Hypertension

The contribution of the renin substrate to blood pressure regulation is still unclear. Plasma angiotensinogen concentration is easy to measure but reflects only the liver-derived substrate, not the role of local tissue angiotensinogen. Plasma angiotensinogen does not seem to play a major role in plasma angiotensin II production under normal conditions. However, different studies have indicated a relationship between plasma angiotensinogen level and blood pressure in humans. A strong correlation between plasma angiotensinogen level and blood pressure was reported in a large study involving 574 subjects.[73] Higher levels of plasma renin substrate have been observed in hypertensive subjects and in offspring of hypertensive parents than in normotensive subjects.[74] Finally, an increased plasma angiotensinogen concentration was associated with a blood pressure increase in offspring with contrasted parental predispostion to hypertension.[39] The similar results of all these studies favor the hypothesis that angiotensinogen is a determinant of blood pressure.

Essential Hypertension

The molecular genetic approach is another powerful way to estimate the role of angiotensinogen in hypertension. A very polymorphic dinucleotide GT repeat (80 percent heterozygosity) located in the 3′ region of the angiotensinogen gene has been described,[75] as have other diallelic single-strand conformation polymorphisms located in the 5′ regulatory region and in intronic sequences of the gene.[76]

An extensive study of the potential role of the angiotensinogen gene in human essential hypertension was recently performed in two large series (Salt Lake City, Utah and Paris, France) of hypertensive sibships that yielded a total of 379 sib pairs.[76] Using the highly polymorphic GT microsatellite, we obtained evidence of genetic linkage between the angiotensinogen gene and hypertension. This linkage (17 percent excess of allele sharing) was found in severely hypertensive patients (characterized by a diastolic blood pressure of greater than 100 mm Hg or a therapy consisting of administration of two or more antihypertensive medications). In both the Utah and the Paris groups, although a significant linkage was obtained in male pairs, no excess of shared angiotensinogen alleles was observed in female comparisons, suggesting the influence of an epistatic hormonal phenomenon.

The polymerase chain reaction was used to examine genomic sequences at the angiotensinogen locus.[77] Among the 15 observed variants, five were missense mutations, and three were observed in single families [*see Figure 2*]. In the white subjects of both groups, the M235T variant (Met→Thr in amino-acid position 235) was found more frequently in hypertensive probands, especially in the more severe index cases (0.50), than in control subjects (0.38). Finally, a significant increase in plasma angiotensinogen level was observed for patients bearing the M235T variant, with a 10 and a 20 percent increase in heterozygotes (MT) and homozygotes (TT), respectively, compared with wild-type homozygotes (MM). More recently, these results were confirmed in hypertensive patients regardless of family history of hypertension.[78] The corroboration and replication afforded by these results support the interpretation that molecular variants of angiotensinogen, of which M235T may be only one example, are associated with inherited predisposition to essential hypertension in humans.

Another recent study, in United Kingdom families, showed a strong association of the angiotensinogen gene locus with essential hypertension.[79] No association existed between hypertension and the M235T variant, which could be the result of population differences because the frequency of the wild-type allele at the 235 position was similar to that of the 235T allele in the Paris and Utah populations.[76]

Pregnancy-Induced Hypertension

The results of the aforementioned studies support the hypothesis of a susceptible allele of the angiotensinogen gene that is associated with an increase in both plasma angiotensinogen concentration and blood pressure,

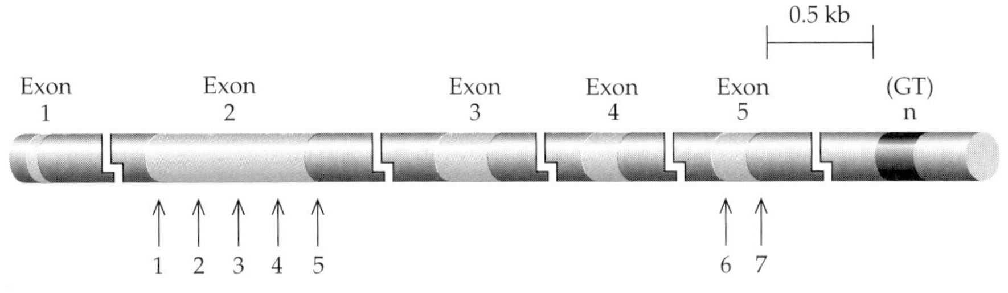

Figure 2 *Missense mutations at the human angiotensinogen gene: 1, L1OP; 2, T104M; 3, T174M; 4, M235T; 5, Y248C; 6, L359M; and 7, V388M. (GT)n is a microsatellite repeat 5 kilobases downstream from the 3′ region.*

an effect that could be more striking in conditions of stimulation of angiotensinogen expression, such as pregnancy or oral estrogen administration. Clinical studies have documented a familial tendency to develop preeclampsia, and familial studies have suggested both a genetic inheritance and the influence of environmental factors.[80,81]

Two recent reports indicate that the angiotensinogen locus could play an important role in the occurrence of pregnancy-induced hypertension. Ward et al.[82] found a significant association between the 235T variant and preeclampsia in white and Japanese samples. Using another strategy, analysis of the allelic inheritance of the GT repeat in 52 sibling pairs of preeclamptic sisters, Arngrimsson et al.[83] were able to demonstrate significant linkage between the angiotensinogen locus and preeclampsia in Icelandic and Scottish families. Thus, although different mechanisms have been proposed for preeclampsia and essential hypertension, these results suggest that some common variants of the angiotensinogen gene could predipose to both diseases.

From all these studies, the angiotensinogen gene appears to be involved in the determination of human familial hypertension and some forms of pregnancy-induced hypertension. However, as for all predisposing genes for a common disease, other clinical studies will have to be conducted in different populations and races to ascertain the role of the angiotensinogen gene in high blood pressure. Finally, several issues will have to be resolved: (1) at present, it is not possible to determine whether the observed molecular variants of angiotensinogen directly affect angiotensinogen function or whether they serve as markers for functional variants that have not been detected; (2) if, indeed, the mutation of a methionine into a threonine in the 235 position is directly affecting plasma angiotensinogen concentration, it will be necessary to look for a possible difference in clearance rate or K_m for renin between the two angiotensinogen isoforms; and (3) the response to antihypertensive agents, especially those blocking the renin system, will have to be evaluated in patients classified according to their angiotensinogen genotype.

Conclusion

Molecular genetic studies make possible the evaluation of the contributions of the renin-angiotensin system genes to blood pressure variance and hypertension in animals and humans. At present, neither the renin nor the ACE genes are likely to significantly contribute to genetic hypertension, at least in humans. However, they could be still involved in a subset of the human population that has yet to be defined. Molecular variants of the angiotensinogen gene are associated with inherited predispositions to essential hypertension in humans and are likely involved in some cases of pregnancy-induced hypertension. Finally, an ACE gene polymorphism associated with an increase in plasma and tissue ACE levels appears to be a strong marker of coronary and cardiac disease.

All these results show that some molecular variants of angiotensinogen (e.g., M235T) or of ACE (e.g., ACE DD genotype) are associated with increased plasma or tissue angiotensinogen and ACE levels, respectively. This relationship could result in a small increase in the formation rate of angiotensin II, especially in tissues in which these proteins are rate limiting for angiotensin II generation. This genetically chronic overstimulation of the renin system would then favor kidney sodium reabsorption and vascular hypertrophy and may also increase sympathetic nervous system activity and predispose to the development of common cardiovascular diseases.

References

1. Ward R: Familial aggregation and genetic epidemiology of blood pressure. *Hypertension: Pathophysiology, Diagnosis and Management.* Laragh JH, Brenner BM, Eds. Raven Press, New York, 1990, p 81
2. Mullins JJ, Peters J, Ganten D: Fulminant hypertension in rats harbouring the mouse *Ren 2* gene. *Nature* 344:541, 1990
3. Brunner HR, Laragh JH, Baer L: Essential hypertension: renin and aldosterone heart attack and stroke. *N Engl J Med* 286:441, 1972
4. Alderman MH, Madhavan S, Ooi WL, et al: Association of the renin-sodium profile with the risk of myocardial infarction in patients with hypertension. *N Engl J Med* 324:1098, 1991
5. Panthier JJ, Foote S, Chambraud B, et al: Complete amino acid sequence and maturation of the mouse submaxillary gland renin precursor. *Nature* 298:90, 1982
6. Corvol P, Panthier JJ, Foote S, et al: Structure of the mouse submaxillary gland renin precursor and a model for renin processing. *Hypertension* 5(suppl 1):13, 1983
7. Hadman JA, Mort YJ, Catanzaro DF, et al: Primary structure of human renin gene. *DNA Cell Biol* 3:457, 1984
8. Hobart PM, Fogliano M, O'Connor BA, et al: Human renin gene: structure and sequence analysis. *Proc Natl Acad Sci USA* 81:5026, 1984
9. Miyazaki H, Fukamizu A, Hirose S, et al: Structure of the human renin gene. *Proc Natl Acad Sci USA* 81:5999, 1984
10. Cohen-Haguenauer O, Soubrier F, N'Guyene VC, et al: Regional mapping of the human renin gene to 1q32 by in situ hybridization. *Ann Genet* 32:16, 1983
11. Naftilan AJ, Williams R, Burt D, et al: A lack of linkage of renin gene restriction length polymorphisms with human hypertension. *Hypertension* 14:614, 1989
12. Morris BJ, Griffiths LR: Frequency in hypertensives of alleles for a RFLP associated with the renin gene. *Biochem Biophys Res Commun* 150:219, 1988
13. Soubrier F, Jeunemaitre X, Rigat B, et al: Similar frequencies of renin gene restriction fragment length polymorphisms in hypertensive and normotensive subjects. *Hypertension* 16:712, 1990
14. Jeunemaitre X, Rigat B, Charru A, et al: Sib pair linkage analysis of renin gene haplotypes in human essential hypertension. *Hum Genet* 88:301, 1992
15. Soubrier F, Alhenc-Gelas F, Hubert C, et al: Two putative active centers in human angiotensin I converting enzyme revealed by molecular cloning. *Proc Natl Acad Sci USA* 85:9386, 1988
16. Bernstein KE, Martin BM, Edwards AS, et al: Mouse angiotensin I-converting enzyme is a protein composed of two homologous domains. *J Biol Chem* 264:11945, 1988
17. Wei L, Alhenc-Gelas F, Soubrier F, et al: Expression and characterization of recombinant human angiotensin I-converting enzyme: evidence for a C-terminal transmembrane anchor and for a proteolytic processing of the secreted recombinant and plasma enzymes. *J Biol Chem* 266:5540, 1991
18. Beldent V, Michaud A, Wei L, et al: Proteolytic release of human angiotensin-converting enzyme. *J Biol Chem* 268:26428, 1993
19. Wei L, Alhenc-Gelas F, Corvol P, et al: The two homologous domains of the human angiotensin I-converting enzyme are both catalytically active. *J Biol Chem* 266:9002, 1991
20. Wei L, Clauser E, Alhenc-Gelas F, et al: The two homologous domains of human angiotensin I-converting enzyme interact differently with competitive inhibitors. *J Biol Chem* 267:13398, 1992
21. Jaspard E, Wei L, Alhenc-Gelas F: Differences in the properties and enzymatic specificities of the two active sites of angiotensin I-converting enzyme (kininase II). *J Biol Chem* 268:9496, 1993
22. Lattion AL, Soubrier F, Allegrini J, et al: The testicular transcript of the angiotensin I-

converting enzyme encodes for the ancestral, non-duplicated form of the enzyme. *FEBS Lett* 252:99, 1989

23. Ehlers MRW, Fox EA, Strydom DJ, et al: Molecular cloning of human testicular angiotensin-converting enzyme: the testis isozyme is identical to the C-terminal half of endothelial angiotensin-converting enzyme. *Proc Natl Acad Sci USA* 86:7741, 1989
24. Kumar RS, Kusari J, Roy SN, et al: Structure of testicular angiotensin-converting enzyme: a segmental mosaic isozyme. *J Biol Chem* 264:16754, 1989
25. Hubert C, Houot AM, Corvol P, et al: Structure of the angiotensin I-converting enzyme gene: two alternate promoters correspond to evolutionary steps of a duplicated gene. *J Biol Chem* 266:15377, 1991
26. Kumar RS, Thekkumkara TJ, Sen GC: The mRNAs encoding the two angiotensin-converting isozymes are transcribed from the same gene by a tissue-specific choice of alternative transcription initiation sites. *J Biol Chem* 266:3854, 1991
27. Howard TE, Shai SY, Langford KG, et al: Transcription of testicular angiotensin-converting enzyme (ACE) is initiated within the twelfth intron of the somatic ACE gene. *Mol Cell Biol* 10:4294, 1990
28. Alhenc-Gelas F, Richard J, Courbon D, et al: Distribution of plasma angiotensin I converting enzyme levels in healthy men: relationship to environmental and hormonal parameters. *J Lab Clin Med* 117:33, 1991
29. Cambien F, Alhenc-Gelas F, Herbeth B, et al: Familial resemblance of plasma angiotensin converting enzyme levels. *Am J Hum Genet* 43:774, 1988
30. Rigat B, Hubert C, Alhenc-Gelas F, et al: An insertion/deletion polymorphism in the angiotensin I converting enzyme gene accounting for half the variance of serum enzyme levels. *J Clin Invest* 86:1343, 1990
31. Costerousse O, Allegrini J, Lopez M, et al: Angiotensin I-converting enzyme in human circulating mononuclear cells: genetic polymorphism of expression in T-lymphocytes. *Biochem J* 290:33, 1993
32. Tiret L, Rigat B, Visvikis S, et al: Evidence from combined segregation and linkage analysis that a variant of the angiotensin I-converting enzyme (ACE) gene controls plasma ACE levels. *Am J Hum Genet* 51:197, 1992
33. Hilbert P, Lindpaintner K, Beckmann JS, et al: Chromosomal mapping of two genetic loci asociated with blood-pressure regulation in hereditary hypertensive rats. *Nature* 353:521, 1991
34. Jacob HJ, Lindpaintner K, Lincoln SE, et al: Genetic mapping of a gene causing hypertension in the stroke-prone spontaneously hypertensive rat. *Cell* 67:213, 1991
35. Mattei MG, Hubert C, Alhenc-Gelas F, et al: Angiotensin I converting enzyme is on chromosome 17. Tenth International Workshop on Human Gene Mapping, New Haven, CT, June 11–17, 1989. *Cytogenet Cell Genet* 51:1041, 1989
36. Zee RYL, Lou YK, Griffiths LR, et al: Association of an insertion/deletion polymorphism of the angiotensin I-converting enzyme gene with essential hypertension. *Biochem Biophys Res Commun* 184:9, 1992
37. Jeunemaitre X, Lifton RP, Hunt SC, et al: Absence of linkage between the angiotensin-converting enzyme locus and human essential hypertension. *Nature Genet* 1:72, 1992
38. Harrap SB, Davidson HR, Connor JM, et al: The angiotensin I converting enzyme gene and predisposition to high blood pressure. *Hypertension* 21:455, 1993
39. Watt GCM, Harrap SB, Foy CJW, et al: Abnormalities of glucocorticoid metabolism and the renin angiotensin system: a four-corners approach to the identification of genetic determinants of blood pressure. *J Hypertens* 10:473, 1992
40. Higashimori K, Zhao Y, Higaki J, et al: Association of a polymorphism of the angiotensin converting enzyme gene with essential hypertension in the Japanese population. *Biochem Biophys Res Commun* 191:393, 1993
41. Schmidt S, Van Hoof IMS, Grobbee DE, et al: Polymorphism of the angiotensin I converting enzyme gene is apparently not related to high blood pressure: Dutch hypertension and offspring study. *J Hypertens* 11:345, 1993
42. Cambien F, Poirier O, Lecert L, et al: Deletion polymorphism in the gene for angiotensin-converting enzyme is a potent risk factor for myocardial infarction. *Nature* 359:641, 1992
43. Tiret L, Kee F, Poirier O, et al: Deletion polymorphism in angiotensin-converting enzyme gene associated with parental history of myocardial infarction. *Lancet* 341:991, 1993
44. Otishi M, Fujii K, Minaminot T, et al: A potent genetic risk factor for restenosis. *Nature Genet* 5:324, 1993

45. Raynolds MC, Bristow MR, Bush EW, et al: Angiotensin-converting enzyme DD genotype in patients with ischaemic or dilated cardiomyopathy. *Lancet* 342:1073, 1993

46. Marian AJ, Yu QT, Workman R, et al: Angiotensin-converting enzyme polymorphism in hypertrophic cardiomyopathy and sudden cardiac death. *Lancet* 342:1085, 1993

47. Schunkert H, Hense H-W, Holmer SR, et al: Association between a deletion polymorphism of the angiotensin-converting enzyme gene and left ventricular hypertrophy. *N Engl J Med* 330:1634, 1994

48. Cumin F, Le-Nguyen D, Castro B, et al: Comparative enzymatic studies of human renin acting on pure natural or synthetic substrates. *Biochim Biophys Acta* 913:10, 1987

49. Ménard J, El-Amrani AIK, Savoie F, et al: Angiotensinogen: an attractive and underrated participant in hypertension and inflammation. *Hypertension* 18:705, 1991

50. Gardes J, Bouhnik J, Clauser E, et al: Role of angiotensinogen in blood pressure homeostasis. *Hypertension* 4:185, 1982

51. Krakoff LR, Einsenfeld AJ: Hormonal control of plasma renin substrate (angiotensinogen). *Circ Res* 41:II-43, 1977

52. Hollenberg NK, Williams GH, Burger B, et al: Renal blood flow and its response to angiotensin II: an interaction between oral contraceptive agents, sodium intake and the renin-angiotensin system in healthy young women. *Circ Res* 38:35, 1976

53. Ueno N, Yoshida K, Hirose S, et al: Angiotensinogen-producing hepatocellular carcinoma. *Hypertension* 6:931, 1984

54. Kew MC, Leckie BJ, Greef MC: Arterial hypertension as a paraneoplastic phenomenon in hepatocellular carcinoma. *Arch Intern Med* 149:2111, 1989

55. Kageyama R, Ohkubo H, Nakanishi S: Primary structure of human preangiotensinogen deduced from the cloned DNA sequence. *Biochemistry* 23:3603, 1984

56. Tanaka T, Ohkubo H, Kakanishi S: Common structural organization of the angiotensinogen and the α–1-antitrypsin gene. *J Biol Chem* 259:8063, 1984

57. Gaillard I, Clauser E, Corvol P: Structure of human angiotensinogen gene. *DNA Cell Biol* 8:87, 1989

58. Gaillard-Sanchez I, Mattei MG, Clauser E, et al: Assignment by in situ hybridization of angiotensinogen to chromosome band 1q42: the same region as human renin gene. *Hum Genet* 84:341, 1990

59. Clouston WM, Richards RI: An allelic polymorphism of the angiotensinogen gene in mice. *Nucleic Acids Res* 17:822, 1989

60. Chirgwin JM, Schaefer IM, Diaz JA, et al: Mouse kidney renin gene is on chromosome 1. *Somat Cell Mol Genet* 10:633, 1984

61. Mori M, Ishizaki I, Yamada T, et al: Restriction fragment length polymorphisms of the angiotensinogen gene in inbred rat strains and mapping of the gene on chromosome 19q. *Cytogenet Cell Genet* 50:42, 1989

62. Pravenec M, Simonet L, Kren V: The rat renin gene assignment to chromosome 13 and linkage to the regulation of blood pressure. *Genomics* 9:466, 1991

63. Clauser E, Gaillard I, Wei L, et al: Regulation of angiotensinogen gene. *Am J Hypertens* 2:403, 1989

64. Lynch KR, Peach MJ: Molecular biology of angiotensinogen. *Hypertension* 17:263, 1991

65. Campbell DJ, Habener JF: Angiotensinogen gene is expressed and differentially regulated in multiple tissues of the rat. *J Clin Invest* 78:31, 1986

66. Ohkubo H, Nakayama K, Tanaka T, et al: Tissue distribution of rat angiotensinogen mRNA and structural analysis of its heterogeneity. *J Biol Chem* 261:319, 1986

67. Cassis LA, Lynch KR, Peach MJ: Localization of angiotensinogen messenger RNA in rat aorta. *Circ Res* 62:1259, 1988

68. Naftilan AJ, Zou WM, Ingelfinger JR, et al: Localization and differential regulation of angiotensinogen mRNA expression in the vessel wall. *J Clin Invest* 87:1300, 1991

69. Rakugi H, Jacob HZ, Krieger JE, et al: Vascular injury induces angiotensinogen gene expression in the media and neointima. *Circ Res* 87:283, 1993

70. Lindpaintner K, Jin M, Niedermaier N, et al: Cardiac angiotensinogen and its local activation in the isolated perfused beating heart. *Circ Res* 67:564, 1990

71. Schunkert H, Dzau VJ, Tang SS, et al: Increased rat cardiac angiotensin converting enzyme activity and mRNA expression in pressure overload left ventricular hypertrophy: effects on coronary resistance, contractility and relaxation. *J Clin Invest* 86:1913, 1990

72. Schunkert H, Ingelfinger J, Hirsch AT, et al: Evidence for tissue specific activation of renal angiotensinogen mRNA expression in chronic stable experimental heart failure. *J Clin Invest* 90:1523, 1992

73. Walker WG, Whelton PK, Saito H, et al: Relation between blood pressure and renin, renin substrate, angiotensin II, aldosterone and urinary sodium and potassium in 574 ambulatory subjects. *Hypertension* 1:287, 1979

74. Fasola AF, Martz BL, Helmer OM: Plasma renin activity during supine exercise in offspring of hypertensive parents. *J Appl Physiol* 25:410, 1968

75. Kotelevtsev YV, Clauser E, Corvol P, et al: Dinucleotide repeat polymorphism in the human angiotensinogen gene. *Nucleic Acids Res* 19:6978, 1991

76. Jeunemaitre X, Soubrier F, Kotelevtsev YV, et al: Molecular basis of human hypertension: role of angiotensinogen. *Cell* 71:169, 1992

77. Orita M, Iwahana H, Hayashi K, et al: Detection of polymorphisms of human DNA by gel electrophoresis as single-strand conformation polymorphisms. *Proc Natl Acad Sci USA* 86:2766, 1989

78. Jeunemaitre X, Charru A, Chatellier G, et al: M235T variant of the human angiotensinogen gene in unselected hypertensive patients. *J Hypertens* 11(suppl 5):S80, 1994

79. Caulfield M, Lavender P, Farrall M, et al: Linkage of the angiotensinogen gene to essential hypertension. *N Engl J Med* 330:1629, 1994

80. Cooper DW, Hill JA, Chesley LC: Genetic control of susceptibility to eclampsia and miscarriage. *Br J Obstet Gynaecol* 95:644, 1988

81. Liston WA, Kilpatrick DC: Is genetic susceptibility to pre-eclampsia conferred by homozygosity for the same single recessive gene in mother and fetus? *J Obstet Gynecol* 98:1079, 1991

82. Ward K, Hata PF, Jeunemaitre X, et al: A molecular variant of angiotensinogen associated with preeclampsia. *Nature Genet* 4:59, 1993

83. Arngrimsson R, Purandare S, Connor M, et al: Angiotensinogen: a candidate gene involved in preeclampsia. *Nature Genet* 4:114, 1993

Acknowledgment

This work was supported by Grants from INSERM, Collège de France, Bristol-Myers Squibb, Association Claude Bernard, and Association Naturalia et Biologia.

Figure 1 Talar Agasyan.

Figure 2 Talar Agasyan. Adapted from "Molecular Basis of Human Hypertension: Role of Angiotensinogen," by X. Jeunemaitre, F. Soubrier, Y. V. Kotelevtsev, et al., in *Cell* 71:169, 1992. Used with permission.

CHAPTER 18

Regulation of Vascular Tone

Hiroki Kurihara, M.D., Ph.D., Yoshio Yazaki, M.D., Ph.D.

Systemic blood pressure and regional blood perfusion are greatly influenced by changes in vascular resistance as well as cardiac output. This circulatory regulation is essential to maintain the appropriate blood supply to organs throughout the body. Disturbance of the circulatory regulation leads to a variety of diseases, including hypertension.

Vascular resistance is determined by the caliber of the resistance vessels (arterioles). The contractile state of vascular smooth muscle, referred to as vascular tone, modulates the caliber of arterioles. Vascular tone is regulated by several factors, such as autonomic nerves, circulating hormones, and substances produced by endothelium. In this chapter, we review the molecular mechanisms of smooth muscle contraction and their regulation as related to blood pressure control.

Molecular Mechanisms of Smooth Muscle Contraction

Contractile Apparatus

In the resistance vessels, the resting tone is in a state of partial contraction. The vascular tone can be up- or down-regulated from the resting tone to maintain an appropriate blood flow. The principal apparatus to produce contraction in smooth muscle cells is myosin and actin, as in striated muscle. Myosin consists of two intertwined heavy chains and two pairs of light chains: 20-kilodalton regulatory light chain (LC_{20}) and 17-kilodalton alkaline light chain (LC_{17}). Myosin interacts with filamentous actin to produce contraction at the expense of adenosine triphosphate (ATP). The molecular isoforms of actin and each component of myosin and their regulatory mechanism in smooth muscle differ from those in striated muscle.[1-6]

Conversion of chemical energy into mechanical contraction is mediated by actin-activated myosin ATPase. In smooth muscle cells, the activity of myosin ATPase is dependent on phosphorylation of myosin by active myosin light-chain kinase (MLCK).[6] MLCK is activated by Ca^{2+}-calmodulin complex, leading to the phosphorylation of LC_{20}. The phosphorylation of LC_{20} then activates myosin ATPase, and contraction occurs. Thus, MLCK is a key enzyme in the relation between Ca^{2+} and smooth muscle contraction. Another two actin-binding proteins, caldesmon and calponin, have been shown to inhibit the coupling of LC_{20} phosphorylation with contraction and may modulate smooth muscle contraction together with MLCK.[1,2]

Although smooth muscle contraction is triggered by phosphorylation of myosin, tonic contraction can be sustained even after myosin is dephosphorylated. This phenomenon is well explained by the latch-bridge hypothesis of Hai and Murphy.[3] It proposes that the dephosphorylated myosin crossbridge (latch bridge) remains attached to actin for some time and the latch bridge can generate force to an extent similar to that of the phosphorylated myosin crossbridge at reduced ATP consumption. The molecular mechanisms of the latch phenomenon remain unclear.

Regulation by Second Messengers

The activation of MLCK by an increase in the intracellular free Ca^{2+} concentration ($[Ca^{2+}]_i$) is considered the primary event in smooth muscle contraction. Ca^{2+} binds to calmodulin to form Ca^{2+}-calmodulin complex, which activates MLCK by removing its autoinhibition. Most contractile stimuli induce smooth muscle contraction via a $[Ca^{2+}]_i$ increase.[4,5,7-9]

Two mechanisms are postulated to be responsible for stimuli-induced increases in $[Ca^{2+}]_i$: electromechanical coupling and pharmacomechanical coupling. Electromechanical coupling is defined as the regulation of $[Ca^{2+}]_i$ associated with changes in membrane potential. For example, K^+-induced depolarization of plasma membrane results in the activation of L-type voltage-dependent Ca^{2+} channels. Increased Ca^{2+} influx through the activated Ca^{2+} channels causes an increase in $[Ca^{2+}]_i$ and contraction. The activation of L-type Ca^{2+} channels and subsequent contraction are effectively inhibited by dihydropyridine Ca^{2+} channel antagonists. The resulting $[Ca^{2+}]_i$ increase can induce subsequent release of Ca^{2+} from sarcoplasmic reticulum. This phenomenon, termed Ca^{2+}-induced Ca^{2+} release, is mediated by distinct Ca^{2+} channels in sarcoplasmic reticulum, which are sensitive to ryanodine, a plant alkaloid. In fact, vascular smooth muscle contraction can be inhibited by ryanodine, although the extent of inhibition differs among vessel types.

Another mechanism, pharmacomechanical coupling, is the regulation of $[Ca^{2+}]_i$ without membrane potential changes. Most contractile agonists that bind to G-protein–coupled receptors increase $[Ca^{2+}]_i$ through this mechanism. Agonist-receptor binding activates phospholipase C via G-protein (Gq), and phosphatidylinositol-4,5-diphosphate is hydrolyzed into inositol-1,4,5-trisphosphate and 1,2-diacylglycerol. Inositol-1,4,5-trisphosphate interacts with its receptors on sarcoplasmic reticulum and elicits Ca^{2+} release. Agonist–receptor complexes also increase Ca^{2+} influx through receptor-operated Ca^{2+} channels. In addition, agonist-induced pharmacomechanical coupling seems to involve changes in the $[Ca^{2+}]_i$ sensitivity of myosin phosphorylation, which may also contribute to the agonist-induced contraction.

Cytosolic Ca^{2+} needs to be removed to stop the contraction. After an increase in $[Ca^{2+}]_i$, several mechanisms act to remove an excess of cytosolic Ca^{2+}. Ca^{2+} uptake by sarcoplasmic reticulum is mediated by Ca^{2+}-ATPase and phospholamban. In addition, several proteins, including Na^+, K^+-ATPase, Ca^{2+} pump, Na^+-H^+ exchanger, and Na^+-Ca^{2+} exchanger in plasma membrane, can contribute to Ca^{2+} handling. The activity of these proteins is regulated by second messengers and may participate in the regulation of smooth muscle contraction [*see Figure 1*].

Ca^{2+} handling in vascular smooth muscle is also affected by the activity of K^+ channels. Smooth muscle contains several types of K^+ channels, such as Ca^{2+}-activated K^+ channels, ATP-sensitive K^+ channels, and delayed rectifier K^+ channels. Ca^{2+}-activated K^+ channels are inhibited by charybdotoxin and apamin, whereas ATP-sensitive K^+ channels are inhibited by glyburide (glibenclamide). Delayed rectifier K^+ channels are blocked by divalent cations (Ca^{2+} and Mg^{2+}), which may antagonize the membrane hyperpolarization through activation of Ca^{2+}-activated K^+ channels and implicate them as having a role in agonist-induced contraction. Activation of these channels results in hyperpolarization of plasma membrane, which leads to vasodilatation through inactivation of voltage-dependent Ca^{2+} channels and activation of Na^+-Ca^{2+} exchanger. For example, ATP-sensitive K^+ channels are reported to contribute to vasodilatation elicited by hypoxia, ischemia, or both. Recently, K^+ channel openers, which activate ATP-sensitive K^+ channels, have been considered as therapeutic drugs for cardiovascular diseases, including coronary heart disease and hypertension.

Whereas inositol-1,4,5-trisphosphate releases Ca^{2+} from its intracellular store, 1,2-diacylglycerol activates protein kinase C. The involvement of protein kinase C in smooth muscle contraction is supported by the fact that phorbol ester, which can activate protein kinase C independently of other stimuli, can induce sustained contraction and protein kinase C inhibitor can suppress agonist-induced contraction. Although several proteins, including LC_{20}, MLCK, caldesmon, calponin, and membrane proteins (L-type voltage-dependent Ca^{2+} channel, inositol-1,4,5-trisphosphate receptor, Na^+-Ca^{2+} exchanger, Ca^{2+} pump in sarcolemma, and sarcoplasmic reticulum), are phosphorylated in vitro, the physiologically important substrates have not been identified.

Cyclic adenosine monophosphate (cAMP) and cyclic guanosine monophosphate (cGMP) are also involved in the regulation of smooth muscle cell contraction. cAMP and cGMP stimulate A- or G-kinase, which, in turn, phosphorylates yet-unknown substrates that induce smooth muscle relaxation. The precise mechanism of cyclic nucleotide–induced relaxation remains little known. Possible targets of phosphorylation include phospholamban, Ca^{2+}-ATPase, and contractile proteins such as MLCK. Through phosphorylation of these proteins along with others, cAMP and cGMP are thought to cause a decrease in $[Ca^{2+}]_i$, a decrease in $[Ca^{2+}]_i$ sensitivity of myosin phosphorylation, and an uncoupling of force from myosin phosphorylation and thus lead to relaxation. In addition, cGMP and its

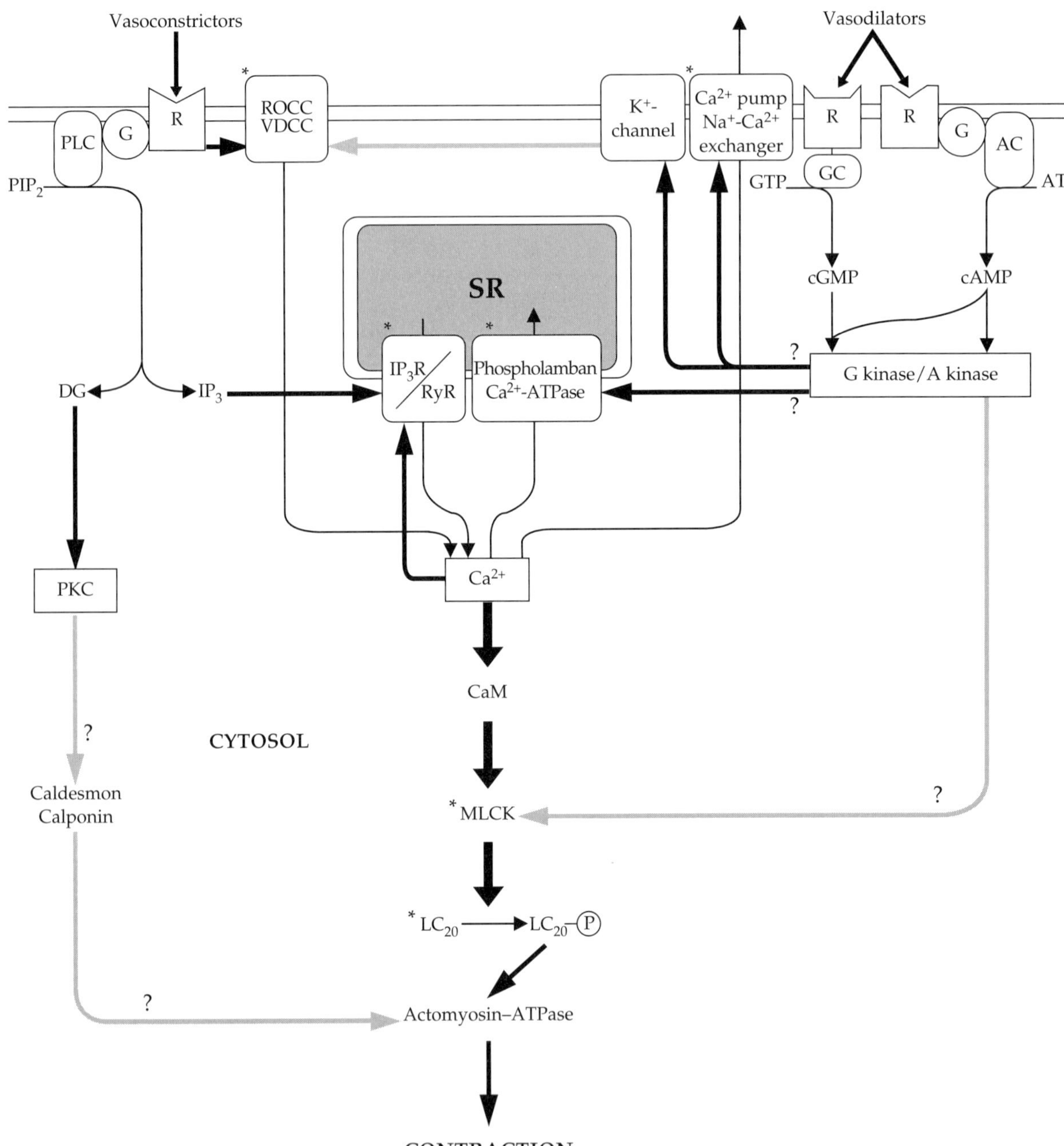

Figure 1 Intracellular signaling pathways regulating vascular smooth muscle contraction. R, receptor; G, G-protein; PLC, phospholipase C; AC, adenylate cyclase; GC, guanylate cyclase; ROCC, receptor-operated Ca^{2+} channel; VDCC, voltage-dependent Ca^{2+} channel; PIP_2, phosphatidylinositol-4,5-bisphosphate; IP_3, inositol-1,4,5-trisphosphate; DG, diacylglycerol; IP_3R, IP_3 receptor; RyR, ryanodine receptor; PKC, protein kinase C; CaM, calmodulin; MLCK, myosin light-chain kinase; LC_{20}, 20-kd myosin regulatory light chain; SR, sarcoplasmic reticulum. Thick black arrows indicate stimulation. Thick gray arrows indicate inhibition. Asterisks indicate possible targets of phosphorylation by PKC.

metabolite, 5′-GMP, are reported to activate Ca^{2+}-activated K^+ channels. The resulting hyperpolarization could cause smooth muscle relaxation through inactivation of voltage-dependent Ca^{2+} channels and activation of Na^+-Ca^{2+} exchanger.

Regulatory Mechanisms of Vascular Tone

Neural Control

Peripheral Innervation

The autonomic nervous system supplies a network of vasomotor nerve fibers, and the vasomotor center in the medulla modulates the level of vascular tone via these nerve fibers. The nerve fibers form a plexus on the adventitia of the resistance vessel wall and send extensions to form varicosities on the outer surface of the media. Neurotransmitters are released from the varicosities toward smooth muscle cells.

The nerve fibers consist of three kinds of fibers: noradrenergic, cholinergic, and nonadrenergic, noncholinergic. The distribution of fibers differs among the various types of vessels. For example, vascular beds in the skeletal muscle and mesenteric area receive a richer supply of noradrenergic fibers than in the coronary or cerebral vessels. The diversity in distribution grossly reflects the responsiveness to nervous stimulation.

The sympathetic noradrenergic fibers mediate vasoconstriction. Norepinephrine released from the nerve terminals reacts with postsynaptic alpha$_1$-adrenergic receptors. The binding of norepinephrine to alpha$_1$-adrenergic receptors elicits vasoconstriction. Norepinephrine also acts on presynaptic alpha$_2$-adrenergic receptors in the nerve terminal and suppresses the release of norepinephrine as a negative feedback. The cholinergic fibers travel with the sympathetic nerve and cause vasodilatation when stimulated.

In addition to these classic neurotransmitters, several substances exist in the nerve terminals of nonadrenergic, noncholinergic fibers in vascular beds. These include vasoconstrictors, such as ATP and neuropeptide Y, and vasodilators, such as substance P, vasoactive intestinal peptide, and calcitonin gene–related peptide (CGRP).

Recently, nitric oxide (NO) has been found to serve as a neurotransmitter in peripheral nerves. Endogenous NO was originally identified as a substance responsible for endothelium-dependent vasodilatation. However, NO is also released from nonadrenergic, noncholinergic nerve endings in cerebral arteries and causes vasodilatation. In other vessels, such as mesenteric arteries, pharmacological studies have revealed reciprocal nitroxidergic vasodilator and noradrenergic vasoconstrictor innervation in the regulation of vascular tone. Thus, these so-called nitroxidergic nerves may act as a counterpart of adrenergic vasoconstrictor nerves.[10-12]

Central Vasomotor Control

The vasomotor center, a group of neurons in the medulla oblongata, integrates information from baroreceptors and other sources. The major efferent mechanisms of the central vasomotor control include vagal discharges;

sympathetic discharges; nonadrenergic, noncholinergic discharges; and adrenorenal hormone and vasopressin release. These mechanisms participate in cardiovascular control by the baroreceptor reflex [*see Figure 2 and Figure 3*]. Although little is known about the interaction of nonadrenergic, noncholinergic innervation with other systems in the baroreceptor reflex, a role for nitroxidergic neural function in blood pressure regulation is suggested by the fact that blockade of nitroxidergic neural discharges can cause elevation of blood pressure.

Two theories are proposed on the mechanism of tonic discharge generation in vasomotor center. The pacemaker theory postulates that specific pacemaker neurons in the medulla produce tonic discharges. The other hypothesis, the oscillator theory, is that tonic discharges are generated by the network oscillator involving the neuronal feedback loop. Although the primary source of the tonic discharge is not clarified, the role of the ventrolateral medulla (VLM) in central vasomotor control has been recently emphasized.

The VLM is divided into the rostral (RVLM) and caudal (CVLM) parts. Various afferents converge on the RVLM and CVLM from peripheral and central sources, and the RVLM sends impulses to sympathetic preganglionic neurons. The vasomotor neurons in RVLM secrete L-glutamate instead of epinephrine as an excitatory neurotransmitter and provoke excitatory postsynaptic potential in sympathetic preganglionic neurons. The CVLM receives impulses from aortic baroreceptor via the nucleus tractus solitarius and transmits γ-aminobutyric acid–mediated inhibitory impulses to the RVLM. The CVLM also projects ascending axons to the hypothalamus and stimulates the secretion of vasopressin, in which the neurotransmitter is L-glutamate. The activity of RVLM and the responsiveness of RVLM to stimulatory substances are augmented in hypertensive model animals. Thus, the VLM plays a central role in the integration of neurochemical input and the modulation of vascular tone.[10-12]

Humoral Control

Various substances have been shown to have vasoconstrictor or vasodilator effects [*see Table 1*]. Angiotensin II is the most important humoral fac-

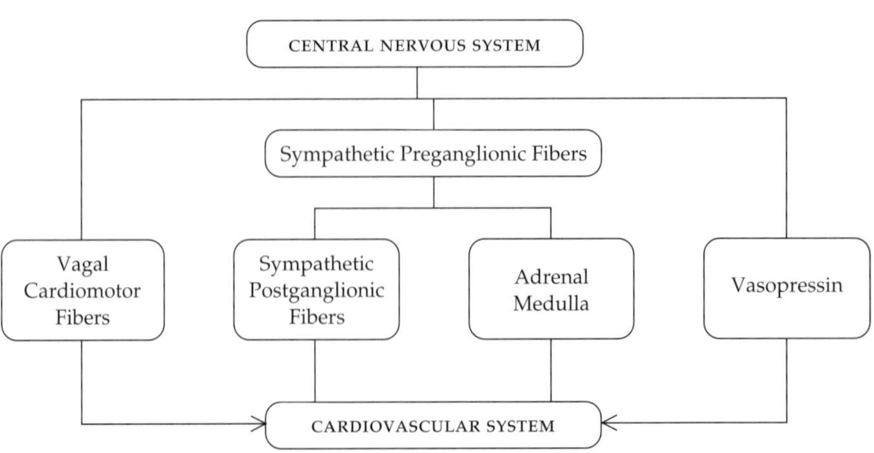

Figure 2 *Flowchart showing the mechanisms that participate in cardiovascular control by baroreceptor reflex.*

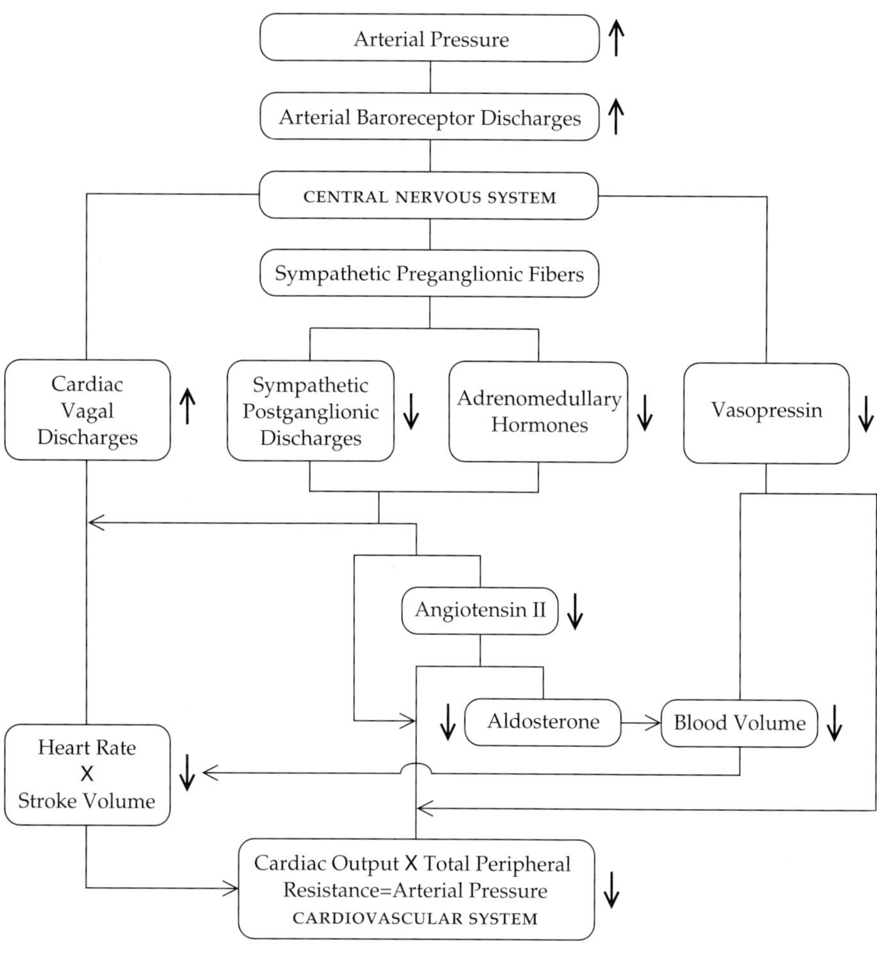

Figure 3 Flowchart showing the integration of information from baroreceptors and other sources by the central nervous system and the baroreceptor reflex control of arterial blood pressure. ↑= stimulation; ↓= inhibition.

tor in the regulation of vascular tone and is very involved in the pathophysiology of hypertension. The renin-angiotensin system is discussed in Chapter 17. Here, some of the other factors are described briefly.

Circulating Catecholamines

In circulating blood, epinephrine and norepinephrine are found in substantial amounts. Plasma epinephrine is predominantly released from the adrenal medulla and serves as a circulating hormone. In contrast, plasma norepinephrine is a result of spillover into systemic circulation from noradrenergic nerve endings. However, norepinephrine is released together with epinephrine from the adrenal medulla in large amounts in certain physiologic (e.g., vigorous exercise) or pathological (e.g., shock, hypoglycemia, and severe injury) states and acts as a hormone.

Circulating catecholamines act on alpha$_1$-adrenergic receptors on vascular smooth muscle cells and induce vasoconstriction. In certain vascular beds (e.g., skeletal muscle and liver), catecholamines can cause vasodilatation through beta$_2$-adrenergic receptors. Beta$_2$-adrenergic receptors are also found in the prejunctional terminals of sympathetic nerves and mediate the stimulation of norepinephrine release, whereas alpha$_2$-adrenergic receptors in the prejunctional terminals mediate the down-regulation of norepi-

Table 1 Neurohumoral Substances Affecting Vascular Tone

	Vasoconstrictors	*Vasodilators*
Peptides	Angiotensin II Vasopressin Endothelins Neuropeptide Y	Natriuretic peptides Kinins Substance P Calcitonin gene–related peptide Vasoactive intestinal peptide Glucagon
Nonpeptides	Catecholamine (α_1) Serotonin Thromboxane A_2 Leukotrienes Endogenous digitalislike substance	Catecholamine (β_2) Histamine Adenosine Prostacyclin Endothelium-derived relaxing factor/nitric oxide

nephrine release. The total outcome of an increase in plasma catecholamine levels is increased systemic vascular tone and blood pressure elevation. However, epinephrine tends to increase only systolic blood pressure because its affinity for beta$_2$-adrenergic receptors is higher than that of norepinephrine. Circulating catecholamines are responsible for hypertension in pheochromocytoma and, in some individuals with a genetic predisposition to hypertension, may contribute to a link between psychophysiologic stress, adrenomedullary activation, and the genesis of hypertension.[10,13]

Vasopressin

Vasopressin is a small peptide that is synthesized in the supraoptic and paraventricular nuclei in the hypothalamus and secreted from the nerve endings projecting into the posterior pituitary gland. The secretion of vasopressin is greatly stimulated by an increase in plasma osmotic pressure and a decrease in extracellular fluid volume. Angiotensin II potentiates the response of vasopressin secretion to hypovolemia.

In addition to its antidiuretic effects mediated by V_2 receptors in the distal tubules and collecting ducts of the kidney, vasopressin induces vasoconstriction through V_{1A} receptors in vascular smooth muscle cells. When vasopressin is administered in vivo, arterial blood pressure significantly increases. However, an increase in endogenous vasopressin within a physiologic range does not affect blood pressure. This is explained by the fact that vasopressin also potentiates baroreflex activities. Although vasopressin is thought to participate in plasma volume homeostasis and blood pressure control, its role in the pathophysiology of human hypertension is not yet established.[14-16]

Natriuretic Peptides

The discovery of natriuretic peptides was initially triggered by the finding that atrial cardiocytes contain secretory granules and that the content of granules is markedly decreased by volume expansion, leading to natriuresis. Now, two members of the natriuretic peptide family, atrial natriuretic peptide (ANP) and brain natriuretic peptide (BNP), are found in the heart. ANP is mainly secreted by the atria in response to myocardial stretch induced by volume expansion. BNP is predominantly produced by the ventricles. The failing heart produces more ANP and BNP than the normal heart. A third isoform, C-type natriuretic peptide (CNP), is not found in the heart but is produced by vascular endothelial cells in response to several stimuli such as cytokines. These natriuretic peptides are also broadly found in the brain and neuronal tissues and may serve as neuropeptides.

Natriuretic peptides cause natriuresis mainly through an increase in glomerular filtration rate. A decrease in sodium reabsorption in the tubules may also contribute to their natriuretic effect. In the endocrine system, natriuretic peptides inhibit renin secretion from juxtaglomerular cells and suppress aldosterone production in the adrenal gland. In the cardiovascular system, natriuretic peptides have vasodilatory effects and inhibit the vasoconstrictive effects of various substances. When natriuretic peptides are administered intravenously to mammals, they decrease arterial blood pressure. Transgenic mice overproducing ANP are reported to be hypotensive. In addition, natriuretic peptides have effects in the central nervous system to suppress angiotensin II–induced augmentation of sympathetic nerve activity and vasopressin release. Thus, the natriuretic peptide system can be regarded as a counterpart of the renin-angiotensin system and may participate in the peripheral and central regulation of vascular tone.

These activities of natriuretic peptides are mediated by two types of receptors, ANP-A and ANP-B receptors, which have cytosolic guanylate cyclase domains. Activated guanylate cyclase produces cGMP, which leads to vasodilatation. The ANP-A receptor has the highest affinity for ANP, whereas the ANP-B receptor has the highest affinity for CNP. Another type of receptor, ANP-C receptor, is regarded as a clearance receptor. The role for CNP in signal transduction remains controversial.[17-22]

Control by Endothelium

In 1980, Furchgott and Zawadzki[23] discovered that the response of vessels to various stimuli is quite different, depending on whether or not endothelium is present. Since the discovery of this fact (i.e., endothelium-dependent vasodilatation), endothelium has been recognized as a modifier of vascular tone. In addition to endothelium-derived relaxing factor (EDRF, now shown to be nitric oxide), which is a major substance mediating endothelium-dependent vasodilatation, endothelial cells produce several vasoactive substances in response to various signals [*see Figure 4*]. The balance of production of these factors by endothelial cells is thought to regulate vascular tone in a physiologic state, and the disturbance of this balance may contribute to the pathophysiology of cardiovascular diseases. Hereafter, the major endothelium-derived factors are discussed.

Endothelium-Derived Relaxing Factor

Numerous factors, such as acetylcholine, bradykinin, serotonin, histamine, ATP, shear stress, stretch, and hypoxia, can cause endothelium-dependent relaxation. EDRF, the mediator of this phenomenon, has been identified as NO and its close derivatives. NO is produced by not only endothelial cells but also smooth muscle cells, macrophages, platelets, and some neurons, and it has diverse effects including inhibition of platelet aggregation, inhibition of smooth muscle proliferation and modulation of immunologic reaction. In the central nervous system, NO is suggested to contribute to several neurologic functions, such as memory and perception.

NO is produced from L-arginine by a reduced nicotinamide adenosine dinucleotide phosphate (NADPH)-dependent dioxygenase, NO synthase (NOS). Two types of NOS are known. One is a constitutive Ca^{2+}/calmodulin-dependent NOS, which is expressed in endothelial cells and neurons, although the molecular structures are different. The constitutive NOS determines the basal release of NO and is activated by aforementioned stim-

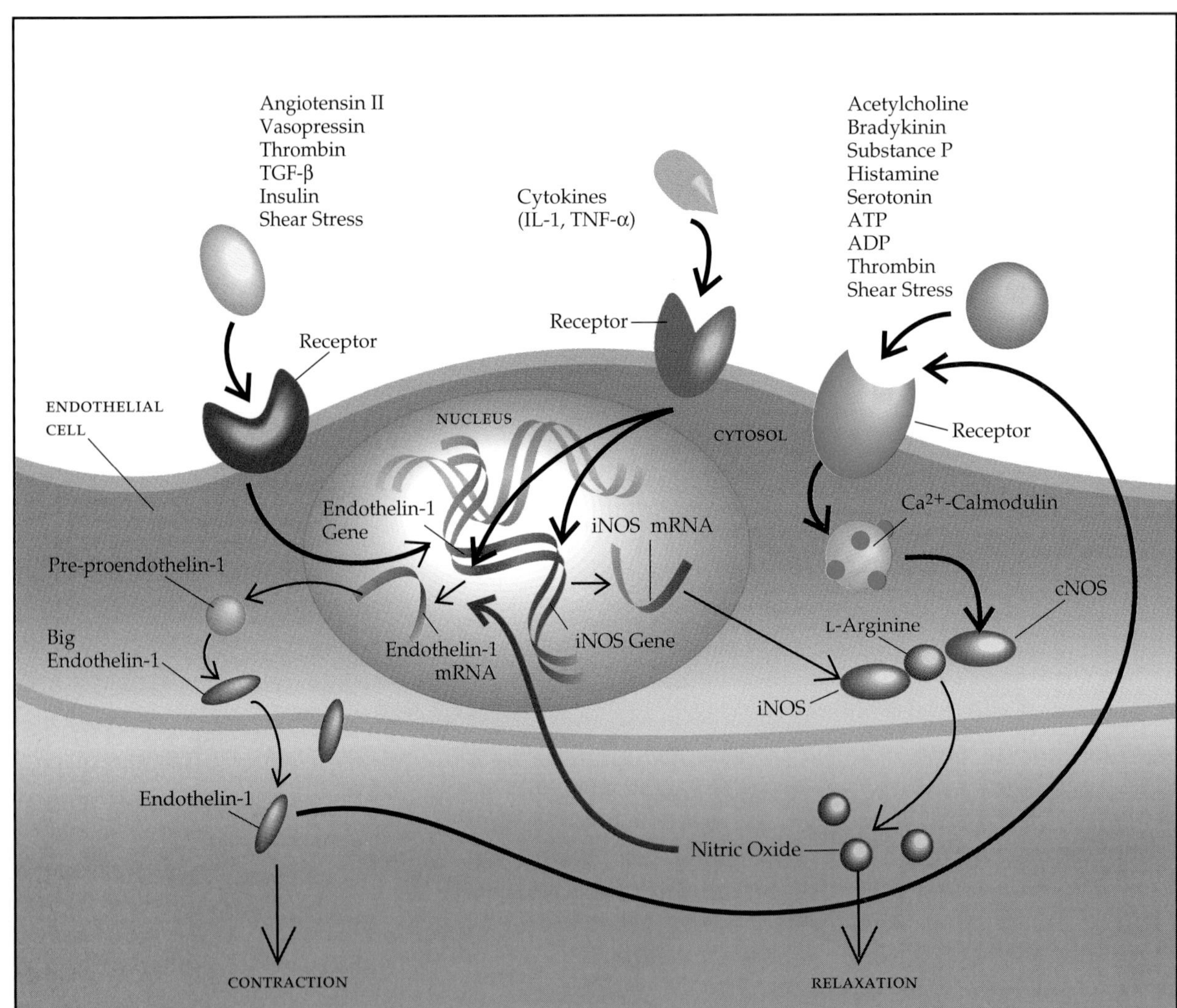

__Figure 4__ Regulatory mechanisms of nitric oxide and endothelin-1 production in vascular endothelial cells. Numerous factors can cause endothelium-dependent contraction and relaxation by stimulating endothelial cell surface receptors. The processes are mediated by endothelin-1 and by nitric oxide, which is derived both from inducible nitric oxide synthase (iNOS) and from constitutive nitric oxide synthase (cNOS). The thick black arrows indicate stimulation. The thick blue arrow indicates inhibition.

uli. The other type of NOS is an inducible, Ca^{2+}-independent NOS. Inducible NOS of the same structure is expressed in endothelial cells, smooth muscle cells, and macrophages in the presence of cytokines and lipopolysaccharides. NO production is competitively inhibited by some L-arginine analogues, such as N^G-monomethyl-L-arginine (L-NMMA).

NO activates the soluble guanylate cyclase in smooth muscle and increases cytosolic cGMP levels, leading to smooth muscle relaxation. The stimulatory effect of NO on guanylate cyclase is inhibited by hemoglobin and methylene blue.

NO is postulated to play a physiologic role in the maintenance of regional and systemic vascular tone. For example, shear stress–induced or stretch-induced release of NO is thought to be responsible for flow-induced vasodilatation. The role of NO in blood pressure control is supported by the fact that administration of L-NMMA causes an increase in blood pressure in experimental animals.

The implication of NO in the pathophysiology of hypertension is suggested by studies using L-NMMA and L-arginine. Furthermore, the preventive effects of endogenous NO on atherogenesis are suggested by the fact that treatment with L-arginine can reduce intimal thickening after vascular injury. These findings may give a feasibility to therapeutic trials targeted to NO in cardiovascular diseases.[23-27]

Endothelium-Derived Hyperpolarizing Factor

Along with the production of NO, several agonists, such as acetylcholine, bradykinin, and histamine, can cause hyperpolarization of smooth muscle cells that is not mediated by NO. This hyperpolarization is triggered by opening K^+ channels. The mediator is called endothelium-derived hyperpolarizing factor (EDHF), but no substance is identified yet. In certain vessels, EDHF seems to mediate endothelium-dependent relaxation that is not inhibited by L-NMMA.[28]

Eicosanoids

Prostacyclin and thromboxane A_2 are produced by endothelial cells from arachidonic acid via the cyclooxygenase pathway. Prostacyclin inhibits platelet aggregation and induces vasodilatation, whereas thromboxane A_2, also produced predominantly by platelets, promotes platelet aggregation and vasoconstriction. The balance of their production by endothelial cells and platelets is pivotal for local regulation of clot formation.

Prostacyclin binds to its G_s-coupled receptors in smooth muscle cells and leads to the activation of adenylate cyclase. The resulting increase in cAMP causes relaxation of smooth muscle. The thromboxane A_2–induced vasoconstriction is mediated by its receptor coupled with G-protein and phospholipase C. However, the role of these eicosanoids in endothelium-dependent relaxation or contraction is not well understood.[25,28-30]

Endothelin-1

Endothelin-1 (ET1) is a 21-amino acid polypeptide mainly produced by vascular endothelial cells. Three isopeptides, ET1, 2, and 3, form a gene family, and only ET1 is produced by endothelial cells. Endothelins have the most potent vasoconstrictor activity among known vasoactive substances. In addition, they have a diverse set of biologic activities, such as proliferative effects on various cells, stimulation of hormone release, and modulation of central nervous system activity. ET1 also acts on endothelial cells in an autocrine manner and stimulates NO and prostacyclin release.

The actions of endothelins are mediated by two types of G-protein–coupled receptors, ET1,2-selective ET-A receptor and nonselective ET-B receptor, which are distributed differently among various cell types. In vascular smooth muscle, ET-A receptor is mainly expressed, whereas ET-B receptor is dominant in endothelial cells. ET1-bound receptors activate phospholipase C and increase Ca^{2+} release from intracellular stores via inositol-1,4,5-trisphosphate. In certain vessels such as porcine coronary arteries, ET1 activates the voltage-dependent Ca^{2+} channel through G-protein. Protein kinase C activation via diacylglycerol is suggested to be involved in ET1-induced smooth muscle proliferation.

In endothelial cells, ET1 is produced through a constitutive pathway, and its production is mainly regulated at the level of gene expression. ET1 gene expression is induced by various factors. Several factors stimulate both NO and ET1 production by endothelial cells, and NO can inhibit the stimulated ET1 production. ET1 gene expression is also induced in vascular smooth muscle cells by certain endothelial cell–derived substances, including platelet-derived growth factor. Thus, the production of NO and ET1 is interrelated and regulated in a complicated manner through autocrine and paracrine mechanisms.

When ET1 is administered intravenously to experimental animals, it causes an initial transient decrease in arterial blood pressure, followed by a long-lasting blood pressure elevation. The initial decrease in blood pressure is thought to be the result of ET-B receptor–mediated stimulation of NO release, and the following blood pressure increase is the result of its direct constrictive effect on vascular smooth muscle cells predominantly mediated by ET-A receptor.

The involvement of ET1 in hypertension is suggested by studies of plasma ET1 levels, which increase in hypertensive patients and model animals. In animal models, such as sodium-depleted squirrel monkeys, blood pressure is decreased by endothelin antagonists. However, this decrease does not always occur in all populations of hypertensive patients or all model animals. Furthermore, mice in which ET1 production is decreased by gene targeting have higher blood pressure than normal mice, indicating that ET1 may act predominantly as a depressor rather than as a pressor. Accordingly, the net effect of local production of ET1 in vessels may not be simply vasoconstrictive under physiologic conditions. Thus, further investigation is needed to clarify the role of ET1 in physiologic blood pressure regulation and the pathophysiology of hypertension.[25,31-37]

Summary

The systemic and regional vascular tone is determined by the vascular smooth muscle contractile state. Actin and myosin join to form actomyosin, the principal contractile apparatus in smooth muscle. Actomyosin is functionally regulated by second messengers via regulatory proteins such as myosin light-chain kinase. Neural, humoral, and endothelial control mechanisms affect the regulation of vascular tone. It is difficult to rank the large number of regulatory factors according to their relative importance in systemic and regional regulation. Rather, these factors are thought to provide a feedback system in the regulation of vascular tone. The disturbance of these regulatory mechanisms may be involved in the pathophysiology of cardiovascular diseases, including hypertension.

References

1. Sobue K, Kanda K, Tanaka T, et al: Caldesmon: a common actin-linked regulatory protein in the smooth muscle and nonmuscle contractile system. *J Cell Biochem* 37:317, 1988
2. Takahashi K, Hiwada K, Kokubu T: Vascular smooth muscle calponin: a novel troponin T-like protein. *Hypertension* 11:620, 1988
3. Hai C-M, Murphy RA: Ca^{2+} crossbridge phosphorylation and contraction. *Annu Rev Physiol* 51:285, 1988
4. Hathaway DR, March KL, Lash JA, et al: Vascular smooth muscle: a review of the molecular basis of contractility. *Circulation* 83:382, 1991
5. Rembold CM: Regulation of contraction and relaxation in arterial smooth muscle. *Hypertension* 20:129, 1992
6. Hartshorne DJ, Matsushima S, Ito M, et al: Myosin light chain kinase: structure-function relationships. *Jpn J Pharmacol* 5817P, 1992
7. Rasmussen H, Takuwa Y, Park S: Protein kinase C in the regulation of smooth muscle contraction. *FASEB J* 1:177, 1987
8. Means AR, VanBerkum MFA, Bagchi I, et al: Regulatory functions of calmodulin. *Pharmacol Ther* 50:255, 1991
9. Andrea JE, Walsh MP: Protein kinase C of smooth muscle. *Hypertension* 20:585, 1992
10. Loewy AD, Spyer KM, Eds. *Central Regulation of Autonomic Functions*. Oxford University Press, New York, 1990
11. Kumada M, Terui N, Kuwaki T: Arterial baroreceptor reflex: its central and peripheral neural mechanisms. *Prog Neurobiol* 35:331, 1990
12. Toda N, Kitamura Y, Okamura T: Neural mechanism of hypertension by nitric oxide synthase inhibitor in dogs. *Hypertension* 21:3, 1993
13. Floras JS: Epinephrine and the genesis of hypertension. *Hypertension* 19:1, 1992
14. Jard S, Barberis C, Audiger S, et al: Neurohypophyseal hormone receptor systems in brain and periphery. *Prog Brain Res* 72:173, 1987
15. Share L: Role of vasopressin in cardiovascular regulation. *Physiol Rev* 68:1248, 1988
16. Berecek KH, Swords BH: Central role for vasopressin in cardiovascular regulation and the pathogenesis of hypertension. *Hypertension* 16:213, 1990
17. de Bold AJ: Atrial natriuretic factor: a hormone produced by the heart. *Science* 230:767, 1985
18. Sudoh T, Kangawa K, Minamino N, et al: A new natriuretic peptide in porcine brain. *Nature* 332:78, 1988
19. Ruskoaho H: Atrial natriuretic peptide: synthesis, release, and metabolism. *Pharmacol Rev* 44: 479, 1992
20. Koller KJ, Goeddel DV: Molecular biology of the natriuretic peptides and their receptors. *Circulation* 86:1081, 1992
21. Atlas S, Maack T: Atrial natriuretic factor. *Handbook of Physiology: Renal Physiology*. Windhager EE, Ed. Oxford University Press, New York, 1992, pp 157
22. Koh GY, Klug MG, Field LJ: Atrial natriuretic factor and transgenic mice. *Hypertension* 22:634, 1993
23. Furchgott RF, Zawadzki JV: The obligatory role of endothelial cells in the relaxation of arterial smooth muscle by acetylcholine. *Nature* 288:373, 1980
24. Palmer RMJ, Ashton DS, Moncada S: Vascular endothelial cells synthesize nitric oxide from L-arginine. *Nature* 333:664, 1988

25. Vane JR, Änggard EE, Botting RM: Regulatory functions of the vascular endothelium. *N Engl J Med* 323:27, 1990
26. Snyder SH, Bredt DS: Biological roles of nitric oxide. *Sci Am* 266: 68, 1992.
27. Moncada S, Higgs A: The L-arginine-nitric oxide pathway. *N Engl J Med* 329:2002, 1993
28. Vanhoutte PM: Other endothelium-derived factors. *Circulation* 87: V9, 1993
29. Moncada S, Gryglewski R, Bunting S, et al: An enzyme isolated from arteries transforms prostaglandin endoperoxidase to an unstable substance that inhibits platelet aggregation. *Nature* 263:663, 1976
30. Dusting GJ, MacDonald PS: Prostacyclin and vascular function: implications for hypertension and atherosclerosis. *Pharmacol Ther* 48:323, 1990
31. Yanagisawa M, Kurihara H, Kimura S, et al: A novel potent vasoconstrictor produced by vascular endothelial cells. *Nature* 332:411, 1988
32. Arai H, Hori S, Aramori I, et al: Cloning and expression of a cDNA encoding an endothelin receptor. *Nature* 348:730, 1990
33. Sakurai T, Yanagisawa M, Takuwa Y, et al: Cloning of a cDNA encoding a non-isopeptide-selective subtype of the endothelin receptor. *Nature* 348:732, 1990
34. Masaki T, Kimura S, Yanagisawa M, et al: Molecular and cellular mechanism of endothelin regulation: Implications for vascular function. *Circulation* 84:1457, 1991
35. Lüscher T, Boulanger CM, Dohi Y, et al: Endothelium-derived contracting factors. *Hypertension* 19:117, 1992
36. Clozel M, Breu V, Burri K, et al: Pathophysiological role of endothelin revealed by the first orally active endothelin receptor antagonist. *Nature* 365:759, 1993
37. Kurihara Y, Kurihara H, Suzuki H, et al: Elevated blood pressure and craniofacial abnormalities in mice deficient in endothelin-1. *Nature* 368:703, 1994

Acknowledgments

Figures 1, 2, 3 Talar Agasyan.

Figure 4 Dana Burns-Pizer.

CHAPTER 19

Immunobiology of Transplantation

Peter Parham, Ph.D.

Thymus-derived lymphocytes (T cells) are the principal controllers of immune reactions,[1] particularly those directed against allografts.[2,3] Their antigen receptors respond only to peptide antigens and only then when the peptide is bound to either a class I or a class II human leukocyte antigen (HLA) molecule.[4] The defining characteristic of HLA proteins is high genetic polymorphism, which causes HLA proteins to create the strongest antigenic stimulus in transplantion. Immune responses to tissue of a different HLA type (allogeneic tissue) are called alloresponses and the responding lymphocytes, alloreactive B and T cells. The unique combination of antigen-presenting function and extraordinary polymorphism has led the chromosomal region containing the HLA genes to be termed the major histocompatibility complex (MHC).

Transplant Rejection

Transplant rejection may occur in different ways.[3,5] Preformed antibodies in the recipient's circulation, which are the result of an earlier alloresponse caused by such events as blood transfusion, a previous transplant, or pregnancy, induce hyperacute rejection. Although the antibodies mediating hyperacute rejection are made by B cells, T cells provide essential help in their production. Acute rejection is the direct result of T cell–mediated immune responses, provoked during and after the time of transplantation and probably involving both cytotoxic T cells and other effector cells, such as macrophages and polymorphonuclear cells, which are recruited by the cytokines released by activated T cell reactions. In bone marrow transplantation,[6] in which alloreactive T cells are components of the allograft, acute rejection manifests as graft-versus-host disease.[7]

"Approximately 70% of heart transplant patients will have one or two (T) cell–mediated rejection episodes in the first 3 months post transplant."[8] Rejection is characterized by infiltrating T cells and myocyte necrosis, which are monitored by histologic examination of endomyocardial biopsy specimens.[9] Six operational grades of acute rejection are currently defined [*see Table 1*]. Unlike acute rejection, chronic rejection occurs over a period of years after transplantation, and its underlying mechanisms are poorly understood.

Hyperacute rejection has been greatly reduced by the use of the cross-match test, which consists of comparing cells in the patients' sera against the cells of potential donors to test for preformed antibodies.[10,11] Donors are then matched to recipients who have the least reactivity. Acute and chronic rejection can be reduced by matching for HLA type, as the survival curves for patients who received kidney or bone marrow transplants from an HLA-identical family member convincingly demonstrate.[6,12,13] HLA matching also aids in donor selection from HLA-disparate family members and from unrelated donors.[14,15] However, for most patients who need transplants, and obviously for those who require heart transplants, donation from an HLA-identical family member is not possible. Limited organ supplies further reduce the possibilities for HLA matching, and in practice, many transplantations are performed between donors and recipients with considerable HLA differences.[8] In these circumstances, nonspecific suppression of the immune response has been the practical and routine remedy for rejection.

Combinations of immunosuppressive drugs, such as steroids, purine analogues, cyclosporine, FK506, and rapamycin, are given to inhibit the recipient's immune system before transplantation and to prevent rejection afterward.[16,17] T cell–specific antibodies are used for similar reasons.[18] Depleting the T cells in the bone marrow before transplantation reduces the severity

Table 1 Morphological Grading of Acute Rejection*

Old Grading	*New ISHT† Grading*	*Characteristics*
Focal mild rejection	Grade IA	Focal aggregates of perivascular-activated lymphocytes; rarely interstitial foci
Diffuse mild rejection	Grade IB	Diffuse but sparse interstitial foci; activated lymphocytes
Focal moderate rejection	Grade II	One focus of perimyocytic-activated lymphocytes with myocyte damage
Moderate rejection	Grade IIIA	Multifocal areas of myocyte damage caused by activated lymphocytes and eosinophils
Diffuse moderate rejection	Grade IIIB	Borderline severe rejection
Severe acute rejection	Grade IV	Diffuse mixed (eosinophils, often neutrophils) infiltrate with vasculitis, hemorrhage, and myocyte necrosis

*Graded on a minimum of four good pieces of myocardium obtained by endomyocardial biopsy.
†International Society for Heart Transplantation.

of graft-versus-host disease[19] but in so doing increases both the frequency of graft rejection and the recurrence of the leukemia for which the bone marrow recipient is being treated.[20] Under all these regimens, transplantation patients remain perpetually immunosuppressed, prone to opportunistic infections and malignancies.[21,22]

Since the first successful kidney grafts were performed in the 1950s, the survival times for transplanted organs have increased, as have the range of organs transplanted.[23] More important, the quality of life after transplantation for the kidney and heart transplantation patient is much improved.[24] Rejection remains a formidable problem, as do the side effects of the drugs used for its prevention. The goal of transplantation immunology research is to gain an understanding of the workings of human T cells and the specificity of their response to transplanted tissues. Investigators hope that such an understanding will lead to the development of therapies that ensure acceptance of a specified foreign tissue while preserving immunocompetence against other antigens.

Class I and II Human Leukocyte Antigen Genes

The HLA region is contained in the MHC of humans. The term human leukocyte antigen reflects the discovery of class I molecules as cell-surface antigens of peripheral blood leukocytes. The HLA region is located on the short arm of chromosome 6 [*see Figure 1*] and encompasses approximately 4 million base pairs of DNA: in *Escherichia coli* , an equivalent amount codes for the entire organism. Because of its role in transplantation, the HLA region has become the best-characterized segment of the human genome: it constitutes about 20 percent of chromosome 6 and 0.1 percent of the entire genome. At least 200 genes have been identified so far, and the work is far from finished.[25] The number of genes and their proximity have been something of a surprise: molecular biologists expected to find much more DNA that was not organized into genes (open reading frames).

The HLA region can be divided into three subregions: a telomeric class I region, which contains the class I heavy chain genes; a centromeric class II region, which contains genes for the α and β chains of class II molecules; and an intervening class III region, which contains a mixture of genes, including those for tumor necrosis factor and the complement components C2, C4, and factor B. (A telomere is an end of a chromosome; a centromere is the central point at which the chromosome attaches to the spindle during mitosis.) Until the 1980s, only genes for known proteins could be mapped. With subsequent advances in recombinant DNA technology, those genes served as embarkation points for the mapping of many newly discovered genes that encoded proteins of unknown function. These genes, some of which are associated with defense and immunity, are spread throughout the HLA region.[25]

Every human possesses two chromosomes 6, one inherited from each parent. In the HLA region of each chromosome, a large number of loci may differ in DNA sequence among individuals. Hereditable differences at each locus are called alleles. The combination of all the alleles within the HLA region of an individual chromosome is known as a haplotype.

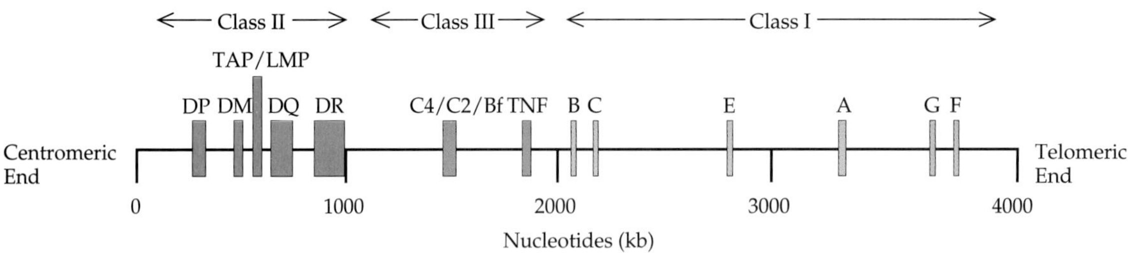

Figure 1 *Physical map of genes in the human leukocyte antigen (HLA) region on the short arm of chromosome 6. The approximate locations of selected genes and clusters of genes are shown. In the class II region, DP, DQ, and DR indicate the locations of genes encoding the* α *and* β *chains of the DP, DQ, and DR class II molecules that present peptide antigens to CD4 T cells; DM is the location of genes encoding the* α *and* β *chains of the DM molecule, an intracellular class II–like molecule that plays a critical but as yet unspecified role in loading other class II molecules with peptide; TAP/LMP is the site of genes encoding the transporter of antigen processing that pumps class I molecule–binding peptides into the endoplasmic reticulum and the site of genes (LMP, for low-molecular-weight proteins) encoding two subunits of the proteasome. In the class III region, the site of genes encoding the complement proteins C4, C2, Bf, and tumor necrosis factor (TNF) are shown. In the class I region, A, B, and C show the location of the HLA-A, HLA-B, and HLA-C genes, respectively. These encode the classic class I molecules, which present peptides to CD8 T cells. The heavy chains encoded by the HLA-E, -F, and -G genes form nonclassic class I molecules whose functions are unknown.*

Genetic recombination within the HLA region is sufficiently infrequent that the matching of siblings for HLA type usually requires only discrimination of the four possible haplotype pairs obtained from one maternal and one paternal haplotype. Thus, if the mother has HLA haplotypes a and b and the father, haplotypes c and d, each child will have the a+c, a+d, b+c, or b+d haplotype combination, and the probability that any two children are HLA identical is one in four. In contrast, HLA matching within the unrelated population necessitates discrimination of many thousands of haplotype combinations and thus much higher resolution in HLA typing methods.

The success of a transplant is improved with the degree of HLA match. However, in the practice of heart and kidney transplantation, the limiting supply of donor organs, the importance of their rapid use, and the relative ease with which immunosuppression can be employed to overcome rejection allow transplantation to be frequently performed despite considerable HLA mismatches.

Transplantation of bone marrow is far more sensitive to HLA differences than are heart and kidney transplantations—single amino acid differences can be critical[26]—and in allogeneic bone marrow transplantation, the problems of HLA diversity must be addressed. Approximately 1.5 million potential donors are listed among bone marrow registries world wide. For patients with common caucasoid HLA types, searching these registries yields many well-matched individuals; however, this is not the case for patients with rare combinations of HLA alleles, many of whom are from minority populations.

Typing for the class I antigens HLA-A, -B, and -C has changed little in the past 30 years. Panels of alloantibodies, selected by screening of sera from multiparous women, and some monoclonal antibodies are used in a microcytotoxicity assay. The class I molecules consist of a polymorphic heavy chain that is noncovalently associated with β_2-microglobulin, a smaller monomorphic polypeptide encoded by a gene on chromosome 15 [*see Figure 2*]. Separate genes within the HLA region code for the HLA-A, -B, and -C heavy chains [*see Figure 1*], and each of these genes has many alleles. The three genes are expressed codominantly, so that cells of a heterozygous person express two HLA-A, two HLA-B, and two HLA-C molecules. HLA-A, -B, and -C proteins present antigens to cytotoxic CD8 T cells[27] and inhibit the functions of natural killer cells.[28] (Many lymphocyte cell surface proteins are named as part of the CD series. They were defined by the capacity of specific monoclonal antibodies to bind to the lymphocyte surface. At a workshop held in 1982 in Paris, France, these monoclonal antibodies were grouped into clusters of differentiation, each defining different molecular species on the lymphocyte surface.) Mechanisms that viruses and tumors use to evade cytotoxic T cell responses interfere with the surface expression of class I HLA molecules on virus-infected and tumor cells. Such cells, which lack class I HLA molecules, are then susceptible to attack by natural killer cells. Thus, the positive regulation of cytotoxic T cells and negative regulation of natural killer by class I molecules create complementary arms of the immune response.

In addition to HLA-A, -B, and -C, the class I region encodes other class I heavy chains (HLA-E, -F, and -G) that associate with β_2-microglobulin and have unknown function. Found only on the trophoblast, HLA-G has been speculated to contribute to maternal-fetal tolerance. In contrast with the highly polymorphic HLA-A, HLA-B, and HLA-C genes, HLA-E, HLA-F, and HLA-G exhibit much less variability. Trophoblast cells are noted for their

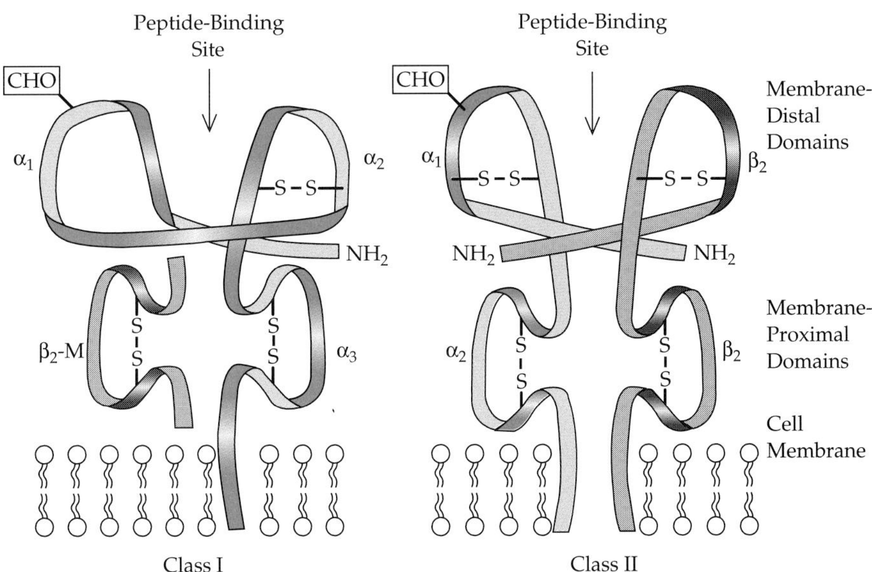

Figure 2 *Structures of the class I and class II HLA molecules. The ribbons represent the polypeptide chains, with -S-S- showing the positions of intrachain disulfide bonds and CHO, the positions of covalently attached carbohydrate structures. In the class I molecule, β_2-microglobulin (β_2-M) and the α_3 domain of the class I heavy chain are immunoglobulin-like domains proximal to all cell surfaces; the α_1 and α_2 domains of the heavy chain are distal to the cell surface and form the peptide-binding site. In class II molecules, the α_2 domain of the α chain and the β_2 domain of the β chain are immunoglobulin-like domains proximal to the cell surface. The peptide-binding site is formed by the α_1 domain of the α chain and the β_1 domain of the β chain, which are distal to the cell surface.*

absence of HLA-A, -B, and -C molecules, a characteristic that provides a type of barrier that prevents maternal cytoxic T cells from responding to the foreign paternal HLA-A, -B, and -C of the fetus. HLA-G may act to inhibit the activities of maternal natural killer cells.

The class II HLA molecules, HLA-DP, -DQ, and -DR, were first defined using the mixed lymphocyte culture and other in vitro assays of the alloresponse.[28] They present antigens to CD4 T cells, the cells that initiate most, if not all, effector mechanisms in immunity through production of secreted lymphokines. Unsatisfactory attempts to define class II molecules serologically stimulated a systematic characterization of class II genes and the development of typing for polymorphism based on the DNA sequences.[29] Panels of sequence-specific oligonucleotides are now used for routine class II typing in many transplantation centers, and analogous systems for class I typing are currently being developed. DNA typing will likely replace serologic class I typing in the very near future.

DNA-based methods have revealed that HLA polymorphism is much greater than has been detected by routine serologic tissue typing: the class I HLA-B27 serotype, for example, represents at least seven different alleles.[30] The imprecision of HLA typing conducted in the past tended to overestimate the degree of match between unrelated individuals. Projects that rely on DNA matching to type pairs of unrelated donors and recipients retrospectively are under way and will enable reassessment of the correlations between HLA match and transplantation outcome.

Class II molecules are composed of heterodimers of α and β chains [*see Figure 2*]. The genes encoding complementary α and β chains are closely juxtaposed and coordinately regulated.[31] The HLA-DR α chain is monomorphic, and the HLA-DR β chain, polymorphic. For HLA-DP and -DQ molecules, both α and β chains are polymorphic. Five HLA-DR β chain genes exist, and certain haplotypes express multiple HLA-DR molecules in which different β chains are associated with the same α chain.

Class I molecules are constitutively expressed on most cell types, but at differing levels,[32] whereas class II molecule expression is restricted to specialized antigen-presenting cells (dendritic cells, macrophages, B cells, thymic epithelium) and also activated T cells. Expression of both class I and II molecules is increased by interferon gamma, a product of activated CD4 T cells that also induces expression of class II molecules on various cell types of epithelial or mesenchymal origin, including vascular endothelium.[31,33] Antigen presentation is thereby increased in inflammatory sites. Before transplantation, class I molecules cannot be detected on the myocardium of the donor heart, and class II molecules cannot be detected on the vascular endothelium; however, after transplantation, strong expression of class I molecules by the myocardium, and of class II molecules by the endothelium, is induced.[8] This environment allows a strong alloreactive T cell response to be triggered.

Class I and II Human Leukocyte Antigen Proteins

Similarities in the amino acid sequences of class I and II HLA proteins suggest they share a common three-dimensional structure, and crystallographic structures of three human class I molecules[34-36] and one human class II molecule[37] have proved this hypothesis correct. Sites of antigen binding and of interaction with the T cell receptor complex are formed by four extracellular protein domains [*see Figure 2*]. Two immunoglobulin-like domains [*see membrane proximal, Figure 2*] combine to provide a support for the two domains that form the peptide-binding site [*see membrane distal, Figure 2*]. The extracellular domains are held to the membrane by short hydrophobic sequences that extend into the cytoplasm as hydrophilic tails. Although the amino acid sequences and three-dimensional structures of the class I and class II molecules are similar, the polypeptide chains of class I and II molecules connect differently [*see Figure 2*]. β_2-Microglobulin supplies one immunoglobulin-like domain to the class I molecule, and the heavy chain supplies the remaining three extracellular domains (α_1, α_2, and α_3), the transmembrane anchor, and the cytoplasmic tail. In class II molecules, the α and β chains each provide one domain of the peptide-binding site, an immunoglobulin-like domain, a transmembrane anchor, and a cytoplasmic tail.

Peptide antigens bind to HLA proteins in an extended conformation, lying within a deep groove flanked by two α helices atop a floor of β pleated sheet. The size of the peptides bound by class I molecules is restricted, usually to nine amino acids, because the two ends must bind within proscribed subsites (pockets) of the groove. Peptides longer than nine residues are forced to bulge in the middle [*see Figure 3*]. In contrast, peptides bound by class II molecules can extend beyond the binding groove; they are longer than those bound by class I molecules (12 to 25 residues) and often do not have precisely defined ends.[38] Thus, structural analysis of bound peptides to isolated class II molecules often reveals families of sequences with the same central class II–binding epitope but different numbers of flanking residues.

Sequences for 47 HLA-A, 88 HLA-B, and 29 HLA-C alleles have been determined. For the class II loci, 93 HLA-DRB1, four HLA-DRB3, two HLA-DRB4, five HLA-DRB5, 11 HLA-DQA1, 21 HLA-DQB1, seven HLA-DPA1,

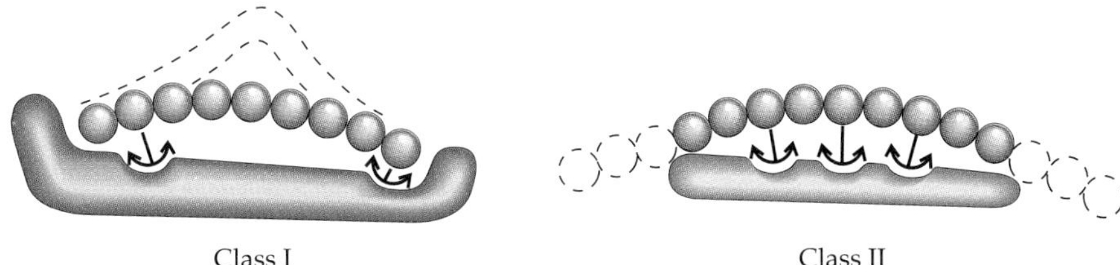

Figure 3 *The peptide-binding sites of class I and class II HLA molecules showing how peptides of different length are accommodated within the groove. Class I molecules bind peptides of restricted length, generally eight or nine amino acid residues. Hydrogen bonds made to conserve residues of class I heavy chains position the N- and C-terminals of the peptide within the binding site. Allele-specific binding is due to selection of sequences with specific "anchor" residues at particular positions. Anchors at positions 2 and 9, as shown, are common. Class II molecules bind longer peptides, averaging 15 amino acids but varying in their length and extending beyond the limits of the groove. Often found are nested sets of peptides sharing the same core sequence but possessing ragged ends. Hydrogen bonds made with conserved features of the central part of the peptide form the basis for high-affinity binding.*

and 52 HLA-DPB1 sequences have been identified.[39] Pairs of alleles differ by one to 50 amino acid substitutions, depending on the locus. Within any set of alleles, the pattern of substitution is far from random; substitutions that change amino acid residues within the peptide-binding groove are the likeliest to occur. Each locus has its nuances, but the inescapable conclusion is that HLA polymorphism results from natural selection for peptide-binding sites of different specificity.[40]

The peptides isolated from purified class I and II molecules are extraordinarily heterogeneous, and fractionation reveals thousands of separate species. Thus, the site determined by a single allele can bind peptides with many different amino acid sequences. However, the binding properties are not random. Class I–binding peptides usually have two anchor positions. The amino acids at these anchor positions are highly restricted because of the requirements for fitting into a particular pocket of the binding groove. These pockets have been designated by capital letters A through F.[36] For example, peptides binding to B*2705 have arginine at position 2, whereas those binding to B*4001 and B*0702 have glutamic acid and proline, respectively. (B*2705, B*4001, and B*0702 are examples of the official World Health Organization nomenclature now used to designate HLA alleles. Each corresponds to a unique sequence. The letter indicates the locus, in this case HLA-B; the first two digits indicate the allelic family; and the last two digits the various subtypes within a family. A fifth digit is used to distinguish alleles that differ only at one or more silent nucleotide substitutions—that is, substitutions that do not result in amino acid replacement.) These differences correlate with polymorphism in the HLA-B heavy chain that changes the B pocket of the peptide-binding groove. Such data provide a direct demonstration that natural HLA polymorphisms create sites of different peptide-binding specificity. For class II molecules, the peptide-binding motifs are less clear-cut, and certain peptides are not selective in their binding. Nevertheless, the HLA class II alleles have distinctive peptide-binding specificities.[38]

The major benefit of HLA polymorphism appears to be that of heterozygote advantage.[41] Heterozygotes, which most humans are, have two distinct peptide-binding specificities per locus and are likely to present more peptides and have a stronger immune response to any pathogen than are homozygotes. Thus, someone who is heterozygous at all HLA loci will express six class I and six class II molecules, compared to three class I and three class II for a homozygote. Resistance to a disease caused by a particular pathogenic organism can be associated with expression of a particular HLA allele. The reason for resistance is probably the favorable presentation to T cell receptors of peptides derived from the pathogen by the associated HLA molecule. Resistance to severe malaria in West Africans has been associated with the presence of HLA-B53, an antigen-presenting molecule that is frequently present in West African populations and recently derived populations, such as African Americans, and is rare elsewhere.[42]

The HLA alleles present in different populations, and their frequency, vary greatly. In the past, these differences were underestimated because of the imprecisions of serologic and cellular typing. In the search for HLA-matched organs for transplantation, the benefit of screening donors whose ethnic origins are similar to those of patients cannot be overestimated.[43]

Pathways of Antigen Processing and Presentation

The distinctive properties of the peptide-binding grooves of class I and class II MHC molecules reflect specializations that facilitate the binding of peptides in different cellular compartments [*see Figure 4*].[44] Class I and class II polypeptides are formed on membrane-associated ribosomes and are translocated into the endoplasmic reticulum. At this site, their pathways of peptide acquisition diverge: class I molecules bind peptides in the endoplasmic reticulum, whereas class II molecules are assembled and transported out of the endoplasmic reticulum in the absence of peptide [*see Figure 4*].

Proteins made on membrane-associated ribosomes and destined for secretion into the extracellular space or for insertion into membranes are synthesized with an amino terminal hydrophobic sequence, or signal peptide, that is cleaved off during translocation of the protein into the endoplasmic reticulum. Some peptides bound by class I molecules, such as cleaved signal peptides, are made in the endoplasmic reticulum; others are derived from cytoplasmic or nuclear proteins and are pumped into the endoplasmic reticulum by a peptide transporter. Genes in the class II HLA region, *TAP1* (transporter of antigen processing) and *TAP2*, encode the subunits of the transporter, which is a member of the family of adenosine triphosphate—dependent transporters.[45] Another pair of genes in the class II region, *LMP2* (low-molecular-weight protein) and *LMP7*, encode subunits of the proteasome, which is a large intracellular protease involved in the production of peptides for presentation.[46] Like class I and class II genes, expression of the *TAP* and *LMP* genes is increased by interferon gamma, which probably facilitates the supply of peptides to the elevated numbers of class I molecules. In the endoplasmic reticulum, the transporter interacts with newly synthesized class I molecules,[47] providing for targeted delivery of peptides.

The association of class I heavy chains with β_2-microglobulin and the binding of peptide are concomitant processes that are facilitated by calnexin and perhaps other molecular chaperones.[48] In the absence of either β_2-microglobulin or appropriate peptides, class I heavy chains fold poorly and fail to reach the cell surface. Polymorphism also affects the rate of class I assembly, possibly because of intrinsic folding properties of the different heavy chains or because of the availability of suitable binding peptides.

In the endoplasmic reticulum, class II α and β chains form a complex with a third polypeptide that is also interferon regulated and has no genetic polymorphism. This invariant chain forms a trimer in which each invariant chain binds an $\alpha\beta$ heterodimer.[49] The invariant chain serves three purposes: (1) it chaperones assembly of the α and β chains, (2) it prevents peptide binding of class II molecules to the $\alpha\beta$ heterodimers, and (3) it targets them to organelles—endosomes and lysosomes—of the endocytic pathway.[44] Once in the endocytic pathway, the lower pH of the endocytic organelles and their resident proteases act to degrade the invariant chain away from the class II molecules, thereby exposing the peptide-binding site and allowing peptides to bind.[48] A class II–like molecule called HLA-DM, which is encoded in the class II region of the HLA region, is found in intracellular compartments and is important for the loading of class II molecules with peptides.[50] Its function is not yet known. One theory is that HLA-DM competes

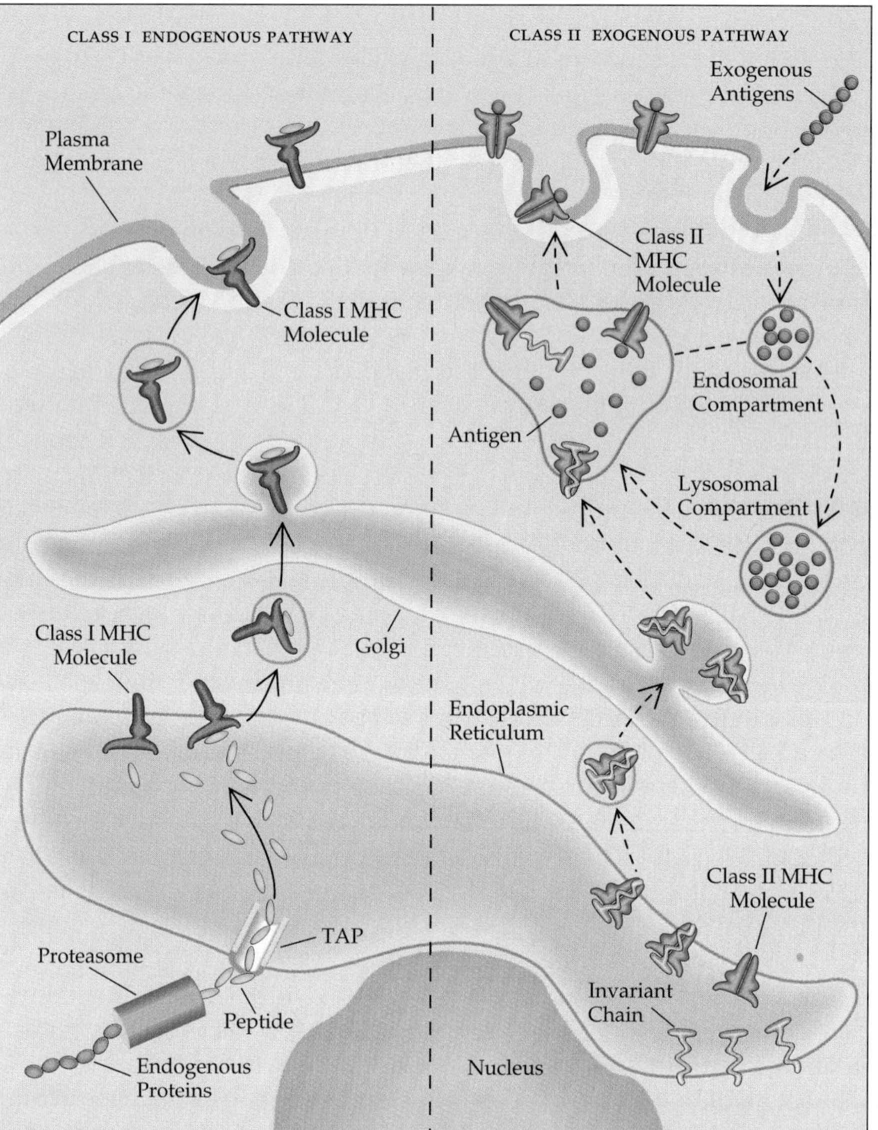

Figure 4 *Cellular processing and presentation of antigens. Endogenous proteins are degraded into peptides by the proteasomes and transported into the endoplasmic reticulum by the transporter of antigen processing, or TAP, protein. In the endosplasmic reticulum, peptides are bound by class I MHC molecules and then transported through the Golgi apparatus to the plasma membrane. Exogenous antigens enter the cell by endocytosis and are degraded to endosomal and lysosomal compartments. Peptides encounter class II MHC molecules in a poorly defined cellular compartment before transport to the plasma membrane. The invariant chain transiently associates with class II MHC molecules during exocytosis.*

for binding of invariant chain fragments, thereby freeing up the binding sites of HLA-DP, -DQ, and -DR molecules for antigenic peptides to bind.

The endocytic pathway is full of proteins taken up from the cell's environment that are in various states of degradation. Most of the proteins that have undergone endocytosis were synthesized by other cells and tissues or by microorganisms that have penetrated the tissues. Such proteins are called exogenous. Peptides bound by class II HLA molecules are primarily derived from exogenous proteins; secondary sources are the endogenous membrane proteins that enter the endocytic pathway, including class I molecules.[26] Peptides derived from the invariant chain are frequently found associated with class II molecules and may represent the segment of the invariant chain that blocks the peptide-binding site en route from the endoplasmic reticulum.

Having bound peptide, a class II molecule then travels to the plasma membrane. Subsequent recycling of class II molecules between the plasma membrane and the endosomes may permit an exchange of peptides, so that a single class II molecule can present a succession of different peptides. In contrast, class I molecules present a single, tightly bound peptide in their lifetime.

This difference can be explained in terms of the functions of the two HLA classes. Class I molecules carry peptides derived from endogenously synthesized proteins. The class I molecule–peptide complex interacts with cytotoxic CD8 T cells, which, if stimulated, kill the antigen-presenting cell. In this manner, virus-infected cells are destroyed, preventing viral replication and spread of infection. It makes sense from a functional perspective that class I molecules would bind peptides tightly; otherwise, viral peptides would dissociate from the class I molecules of an infected cell and rebind to those of a healthy cell, signaling for its destruction by cytotoxic T cells.

In contrast, class II molecules bind to peptides derived from the fragmentation of exogenous proteins. For this reason, class II molecules need not be expressed on all cell types, but only on professional antigen-presenting cells posted at intervals throughout the tissues. These cells, which include dendritic cells, macrophages, B cells, and thymic epithelial cells, are specialized in the initiation of primary immune responses; they have high levels of adhesion and costimulatory molecules that provide strong activation signals to T cells. In the presence of foreign proteins, class II molecule–foreign peptide complexes trigger cytokine secretion from CD4 T cells, which stimulate B cells to make antibody[51] and/or other effector cells, including macrophages[52] and polymorphonuclear leukocytes, which remove cellular and bacterial debris.[1] It is the exceptional CD4 T cell that kills its antigen-presenting cell, and it is perhaps of little consequence if peptides presented by one cell dissociate and are bound to another.

Through their different pathways of assembly and intracellular traffic, class I and class II molecules display a selection of endogenous and exogenous peptides at the plasma membrane [*see Figure 4*]. This display of cell-surface peptides in association with class I and class II molecules reflects what is going on inside and outside the antigen-presenting cell, respectively. The displayed molecules are bound by circulating T cells through their receptors.

T Cell Receptors and Their Selection for Binding to HLA Proteins

T cells descend from stem cells that migrate from the bone marrow to the thymus, where they undergo a program of differentiation and selection in which variable antigen receptors are assembled and tested for their usefulness.[53] T and B cells are derived from a common stem cell precursor, and the T cell receptor (TCR) has many similarities to the immunoglobulins that form the antigen receptors of B cells: they both consist of two chains that have variable and constant regions, which are the products of somatically rearranged genes.[54] Much of the machinery of gene rearrangement is shared by B and T cells, and in both lineages, the end product is a cell that expresses a single type of receptor. TCRs can be made either from α and β chains or from γ and δ chains, producing T cells with very different properties. The $\alpha\beta$

T cells have the capacity to interact with class I and class II HLA molecules, whereas that does not seem to be the case for γδ T cells. Although much of a descriptive nature is known about the γδ T cells, their functional importance in the human immune response is unclear.

Within the thymus, the TCR genes rearrange, first the β and then the α. The α and β chains assemble in the endoplasmic reticulum, forming a variable binding site. The three-dimensional structure of this binding site is not known, but not surprisingly, it is speculated to be similar to that of an immunoglobulin. In the endoplasmic reticulum, the αβ chain heterodimer associates noncovalently with five invariant polypeptides, known collectively as the CD3 complex. (The OKT3 antibody used to prevent acute rejection of transplanted organs is directed against an epitope of this complex.) The CD3 polypeptides form part of the TCR complex; they are essential for cell-surface expression of the αβ heterodimer and provide a part of the signal-transducing machinery that converts antigen recognition into a cellular response.[54,55]

Along with the TCR–CD3 complex, thymocytes begin to express the CD4 and CD8 molecules on their cell surface. CD4 and CD8 bind to sites in the immunoglobulin-like domains of class II and class I HLA molecules, respectively.[55,56]

Rearrangement of α and β genes creates a random collection of TCR-binding sites, possibly as many as 10^{16}.[54] From this collection, the thymus selects T cells that might be effective in providing protective immunity against foreign antigens. Such T cells have receptors that recognize peptides bound to one of the class I or class II HLA molecules. The interaction takes place on an extended surface consisting of the upper faces of the HLA helices and the bound peptide. T cells are selected through the interactions of their TCRs with the class I and II molecules of thymic epithelial cells. When a TCR and a particular HLA molecule are compatible, a positive signal transmitted to the thymocyte initiates further differentiation.

Historically, a T cell was said to be "restricted" by the HLA molecule on which it was positively selected. If the TCR is being positively selected by a class I molecule, CD8 will form part of the receptor complex through its interactions with class I. In contrast, when a TCR is positively selected by a class II molecule, CD4 forms part of the receptor complex through its interactions with class II. CD4 and CD8 are therefore known as T cell coreceptors. Immature T cells express both CD4 and CD8 and are said to be double positive.

Two models have been postulated to explain how class I–restricted T cells lose expression of CD4, whereas class II–restricted T cells lose expression of CD8. In the *instructive model*, positive selection occurs on double-positive cells, and selection of a TCR by a class I molecule, with consequent engagement of CD8, maintains CD8 expression while CD4 is turned off.[53] Alternatively, if the TCR is being positively selected by a class II molecule, expression of the CD4 coreceptor will be maintained and CD8 turned off.

In the *stochastic model*, double-positive cells randomly lose expression of either CD4 or CD8, giving rise to populations of immature T cells that are single positive. Positive selection is postulated to occur on populations of these single-positive cells, and for each cell, the expression of either CD4 or CD8 predetermines whether positive selection occurs on class I or class II molecules. At present, the evidence favors the stochastic model, but both mechanisms may contribute to the commitment of a T cell to either a CD4 or a CD8 phenotype.

Thymocytes also undergo a negative selection. Cells bearing receptors that interact too strongly with an HLA molecule, or a particular HLA–peptide complex, receive a signal that leads to programmed cell death (apoptosis). Negative selection is thought to take place before positive selection and may involve a different set of antigen-presenting cells (bone marrow–derived dendritic cells) within the thymus. The effect of negative selection is to eliminate potentially autoreactive cells before they enter the circulation.

Thymocytes with TCRs that interact poorly with the HLA molecules encountered in the thymus die because they do not receive the signal to proceed to the next stage of differentiation. In reality, most (>95 percent) thymocytes die, and only a small fraction of the cells enter the circulation as mature T cells. Until they encounter specific antigens, they are called naive T cells, and many remain that way because their TCRs are directed against antigens to which the individual is never exposed.

During negative selection in the thymus, an immature T cell is not exposed to the diversity of HLA–peptide complexes that will be encountered subsequently during circulation through the tissues. Thus, some T cells emerge from the thymus with specificity for peptides derived from self proteins—in particular, tissue-specific proteins. These T cells, however, are prevented from responding to their target by mechanisms of peripheral tolerance.[57] To respond aggressively to an antigen, the T cell needs to receive two signals: first, an antigen-specific signal through the TCR complex on engagement of an appropriate HLA–peptide ligand, and second, a signal that is generated when costimulatory molecules of the T cell engage their ligands on an antigen-presenting cell. Ligands for the costimulators are expressed by a restricted set of professional antigen-presenting cells. If a T cell receives only the antigen-specific signal without the costimulatory signal, it enters an inactive state, called anergy, that is resilient to subsequent reception of either signal.[58] In this manner, T cells directed to tissue-specific peptides may be rendered anergic on their first encounter with the target antigen.

T Cell Activation

In the course of its lifetime, a functioning CD4 T cell will have encountered its class II restricting molecule in four distinctive situations: positive and negative selection in the thymus, and primary and secondary stimulation by a specific antigen. Each of these encounters triggers a different response in the CD4 T cell. The consequences of interactions between different types of antigen-presenting cells may differ because the antigen-presenting cells may vary in their repertoires of costimulators and adhesion molecules.[59] CD28 and CTLA-4 are related molecules that are expressed on T cells and are their costimulators. They both bind to the B7-1 and B7-2 ligands, which are constitutively expressed on dendritic cells and on activated B cells and monocytes. Other sets of interacting adhesion molecules that affect the response of the T cells are lymphocyte function antigen–1, intercellular adhesion molecules–1 and –2, very late antigen–4, vascular cell adhesion molecule–1, and CD2–lymphocyte function antigen–3.

The quality of the costimulatory signal appears to vary with the type of antigen-presenting cell, as does the range of lymphokines produced by the CD4 T cell in response. In the laboratory, two extreme phenotypes of activated CD4 T cells have been characterized: TH_1 cells secrete interferon gamma and interleukin-2 (IL-2), which promote phagocyte-mediated defense mechanisms. TH_2 cells secrete interleukin-4 and interleukin-10, which cause resting B cells to produce antibodies.[60] TH_1 cells are likelier to arise from antigen presentation by macrophages, TH_2 cells, from antigen presentation by B cells. Once a CD4 T cell response starts to be either TH_1-like or TH_2-like, it tends to remain that way as a result of positive reinforcement from the lymphokines produced.

The professional antigen-presenting cells are thymic epithelial cells, dendritic cells, macrophages, and B cells. Thymic epithelial cells are instrumental in thymic selection, and dendritic cells are the most potent stimulators of naive cells. Dendritic cells are present as minor subpopulations in all tissues and include Langerhans and Kupffer cells.[61-63] They express high levels of class II HLA molecules and, over extended periods of time, present antigens that have previously entered the cell through endocytosis at a site of injury or infection.

Under the influence of inflammatory cytokines, dendritic cells migrate via the afferent lymph to the draining lymph node, where they home to the T cell areas. There they encounter naive T cells, which have entered the lymph node from the blood by passage across high endothelial venules. Particulate antigen that reaches the lymph node is phagocytosed and presented by macrophages, as well as by B cells through antigen-specific, receptor-mediated endocytosis using the immunoglobulin receptors. Antigen-presenting cells express thousands of different peptide–class II complexes at varying levels of abundance. Just a few hundred identical class II–peptide complexes are sufficient to stimulate a T cell that expresses the complementary TCR.

Receptor engagement results in a clustering of TCRs and their associated coreceptors, costimulators, and transducing molecules into the region of contact with the antigen-presenting cells. Tyrosine kinases and phosphatases are the instruments of signal transduction [*see Figure 5*]. The CD3 ζ chain is phosphorylated rapidly on activation, possibly by the lymphocyte-specific kinase $p56^{lck}$, which binds to the cytoplasmic tail of the CD4 and CD8 coreceptors. This action may in turn induce the activation of the $p59^{fyn}$ and ZAP-70 kinases, which associate with the ζ chain tail. An intracellular phosphatase, CD45, regulates the kinases. Through the use of different exons of the CD45 gene, T cells at different stages of activation change the extracellular recognition domains of CD45 while retaining the same intracellular catalytic domain.[55,64] The $p59^{fyn}$ kinase phosphorylates and activates phosphoinositol-specific phospholipase C, which hydrolyzes phosphatidylinositol bisphosphate to inositol trisphosphate. This product causes elevation in the intracellular stores of Ca^{2+}.[65-67]

Elevated intracellular calcium levels activate calcineurin, a protein phosphatase believed to control expression of the *IL-2* gene. It is the secreted product IL-2 that drives the expansion and differentiation of T cells. The transcription factor NFAT (nuclear factor for activating T cells), which is essential for turning on IL-2 transcription, is prevented from moving from its site of synthesis, the cytoplasm, to its site of action, the nucleus, by phosphorylation. Calcineurin removes the phosphate and permits nuclear localization. By this sequence, events at the T cell surface lead to a change in gene expression.[68,69]

Cyclosporine, the immunosuppressive drug widely used in clinical transplantation, inhibits activation of CD4 T cells by interfering with induction of IL-2. Cyclosporine penetrates cell membranes and binds to cyclophilin A, a cytoplasmic protein. This complex inhibits calcineurin activity. Another immunosuppressive drug, FK506, also acts to inhibit calcineurin, by binding to an intracellular cyclophilin protein different from the protein bound by cyclosporine.[68] Unfortunately, not only T cells are dependent on calcineurin, and these drugs have toxic effects in other tissues, notably the kidney.[22]

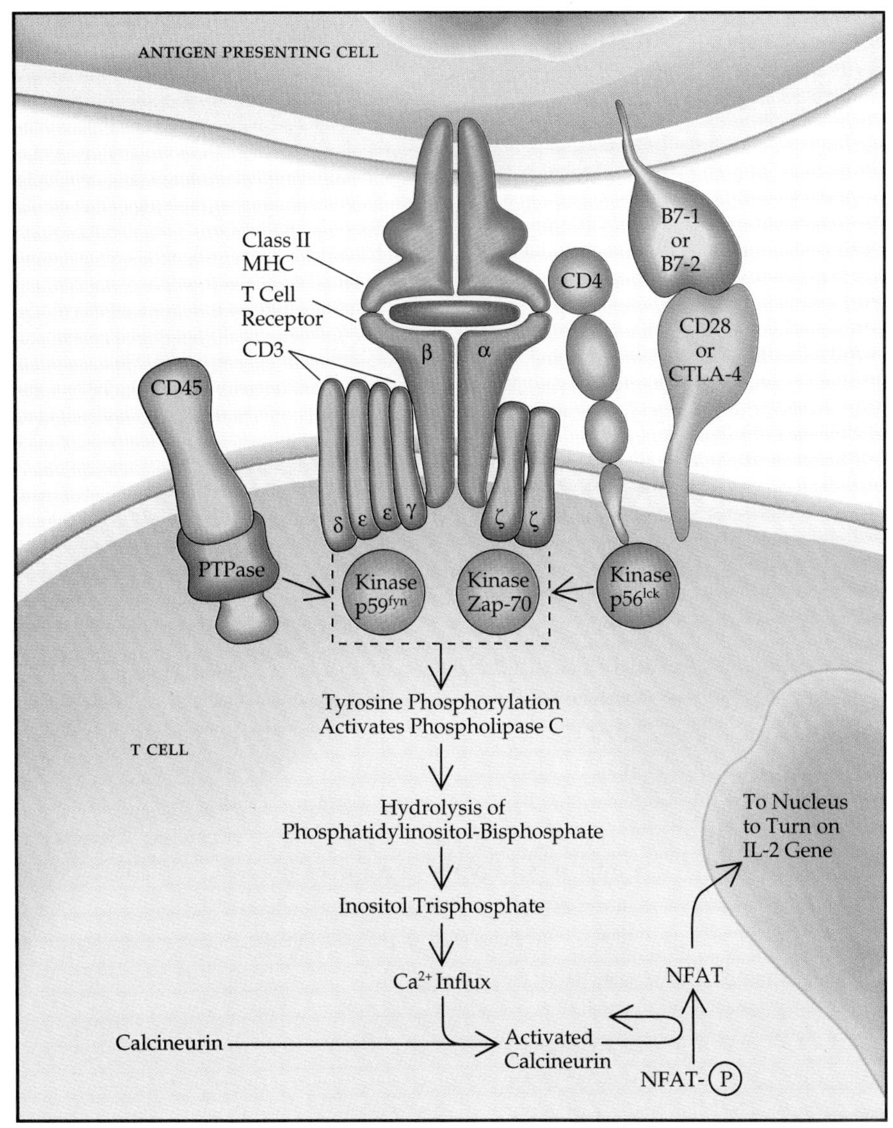

Figure 5 *Activation of a CD4 T cell by an antigen-presenting cell that shows components of the T cell receptor complex and elements involved in signal transduction. NFAT— nuclear factor for activating T cells; PTPase—phosphotyrosine phosphatase.*

The second signal given through the T cell costimulators CD28 and CTLA-4 also involves tyrosine phosphorylation by the $p56^{lck}$ and c-$p59^{fyn}$ kinases. It acts to increase the production and stability of IL-2 mRNA, thus increasing the output of IL-2 protein. Unlike that of the TCR-mediated signal, the effect of the second signal on IL-2 production is not affected by the administration of cyclosporine.[59]

In addition to IL-2 production, antigen activation of CD4 T cells is accompanied by induction of the IL-2 receptor, transferrin receptor, class II HLA antigens, initiation of the cell cycle, and thus cell division. Proliferation produces short-lived effector cells that remain in the lymph node. All these events persist only in the presence of antigen. Other, longer-lived changes that characterize the memory phenotype are decreased cell surface levels of a lymph node–homing receptor, lymphocyte endothelium cell adhesion molecule–1,[70] and expression of the RO form of the CD45 phosphatase rather than the RA form. RA and RO correspond to two of the alternatively spliced forms of CD45, which were originally distinguished on the basis of differential binding by monoclonal antibodies. Increased levels of adhesion and costimulatory molecules are also the property of memory T cells.[71]

Memory T cells leave the lymph node for the peripheral circulation and move to the sites of tissue damage that stimulate their activation. Memory T cells express adhesion molecules for endothelial cells that facilitate their entry into inflamed tissue from the blood. Interferon gamma produced by inflammatory cells induces class II expression on vascular endothelial cells, which also have costimulatory activity.[33,72] Thus, in sites of inflammation, such as a newly transplanted heart, the endothelium in addition to tissue macrophages and dendritic cells presents antigen. Stimulation of memory CD4 T cells produces lymphokine release that activates macrophages and other effector cells. In sites of viral infection, tumor growth, or transplanted allogeneic tissue, CD8 T cells are stimulated by IL-2 and by the viral, tumor, or allogeneic peptides presented by class I molecules.

Strength and Specificity in the Alloreactive T Cell Response

Historically, there has been much discussion as to which T cells mediate transplant rejection, CD4 or CD8.[2,73] Now there seems to be consensus that cytotoxic CD8 cells are the effector cells that ultimately mediate graft destruction but that their activation depends on CD4 T cells [*see Figure 6*]. For heart transplants, the presence of cells expressing perforin and granzyme A, which are markers of activated cytotoxic CD8 T cells, in the lymphocyte infiltrate appears to be a reliable indicator of rejection.[74] Investigators are uncertain whether the role of the CD4 T cells in transplant rejection is simply to provide IL-2 or whether other cytokines and interactions with CD8 T cells contribute, possibly through engagement with the same antigen-presenting cell.[75]

A full-blown alloreactive response against both class I and class II differences leads to activation of about one to 10 percent of peripheral T cells, compared with 0.01 percent of T cells activated by challenge with a normal

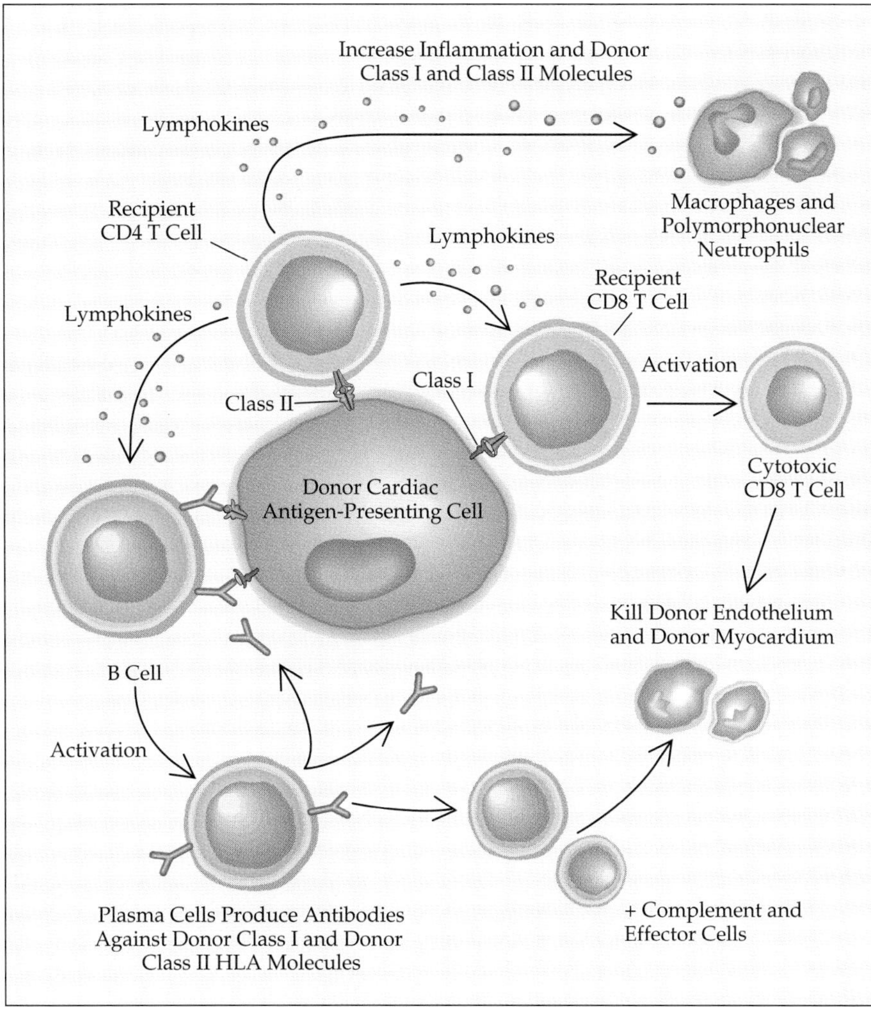

Figure 6 *Shown are possible immune responses to a transplanted allogeneic heart. Recipient CD4 T cells are activated by peptide-bound class II HLA molecules on the surface of the donor cardiac antigen-presenting cell. Recipient CD4 T cells secrete various lymphokines that, in conjunction with peptide-bound class I HLA molecules, activate recipient CD8 T cells to become cytotoxic. Lymphokines secreted by recipient CD4 T cells also activate macrophages and polymorphonuclear neutrophils that in turn increase inflammation and expression of donor class I and class II HLA molecules. B cells, which are activated by class I and class II HLA molecules from the donor cardiac antigen-presenting cells and by lymphokines from recipient CD4 T cells, become antibody-secreting plasma cells, producing antibodies against donor class I and class II HLA molecules. The antibodies, along with complement and effector cells, act with the CD8 T cells in the destruction of donor endothelium and myocardium.*

protein antigen. This quantitative difference in the T cell response is the nub of the transplantation problem.[76]

In transplantation, the recipient's T cells engage the HLA–peptide complexes expressed at the surface of donor antigen-presenting cells. The donor's HLA molecules have different peptide-binding specificities than those of the recipient and therefore display a different set of peptides on the surface of donor antigen-presenting cells than those of the recipient, even though most proteins from which the peptides are derived are identical in both the donor and the recipient. In a case of complete HLA mismatch, the six class I and six class II molecules might present over 20,000 different peptides not presented by the recipient's HLA molecules.

The recipient's TCR repertoire will have been neither negatively selected nor made peripherally tolerant to the HLA–peptide ligands presented by the donor's antigen-presenting cells. However, these HLA–peptide complexes represent ligands with which TCRs of the recipient's T cells can potentially engage, and because donor and recipient are from the same species, all the adhesion molecules, coreceptors, and costimulators are compatible.

In the course of conventional immunization, T cells respond to peptides presented by antigen-presenting cells of the same HLA type (syngeneic) and are blind to most presented peptides, which are derived from self proteins and to which the T cells have been made tolerant. In contrast, after organ transplantation, the recipient's T cells are tolerant to few of the peptides presented by the allogeneic cell. Thus, the allogeneic antigen-presenting cell displays a large array of different HLA–peptide ligands, each potentially capable of stimulating a different alloreactive T cell. Furthermore, many of these HLA–peptide ligands will be at higher abundance (perhaps up to 10,000 copies per cell) than is normal in a syngeneic system (commonly a few hundred copies per cell). For responses against such high-abundance ligands, there may not be as great a need for costimulators and coreceptors because of the increased numbers of specific TCR-peptide-HLA interactions. This may explain why unusual CD4 T cells that are cytotoxic and CD8 cells with helper function can be found in alloreactive populations.

From the perspective of this analysis of the difference between conventional immunization and allogeneic transplantation, the problem is not just the HLA difference but the total compatibility between donor and recipient in the rest of the machinery involved in the T cell response. That compatibility turns the recognition event between TCR and HLA–peptide into a large, aggressive, fundamentally normal immune response.

Xenotransplantation

A way to avoid the ferocity of the allogeneic cytotoxic T cell response is to transplant organs between different species (xenotransplantation). This possible benefit and the increasing discrepancy between the number of patients who need a transplant and the number of available organs have led to renewed enthusiasm for xenotransplantation.[77,78]

As the evolutionary distance between two species increases, the fundamental nature of the immune response to a xenotransplant changes. In addition, the capacity of the T cells from one species to productively engage with the antigen-presenting cells of the other species is reduced. For example, the response of mouse cytotoxic CD8 T cells to human antigen-presenting cells is poor; however, responses that involve processing of donor antigens by the recipient's antigen-presenting cells become stronger because the sequence differences between the proteins of two species increase as the evolutionary distance between them increases. All such differences are a source of potential epitopes against which either CD4 T cells or B cells can respond. Thus, with increased evolutionary distance, the alloreactive antibody responses and CD4 T cell–mediated inflammation tend to increase.

The pig is currently being presented as a candidate source of organs for transplantation. Organs are of similar size and capacity to those of humans, and the animals are cheap and easy to raise. Pigs are judged to be sufficiently distant from humans to attenuate the $CD8^+$ T cell response, yet close enough so that the antibody and CD4 responses can be managed. A genetic approach to managing rejection is envisaged through engineering human genes in and pig genes out of the porcine genome. The possibilities are many: animals made transgenic for the appropriate human genes could be rendered tolerant to dominant human antigens to prevent graft-versus-host effects; expression of porcine MHC genes can be eliminated, either completely or in a tissue-specific form, by gene knockout technology; and resistance of xenogeneic cells to human antibodies might be induced by the introduction of transgenes for decay-accelerating factor, a cell surface molecule that inhibits complement action.

Components of the immune system frequently differ between species in ways that complicate extrapolation of the transplantation experience from one species to another, as is readily appreciated from a comparison of transplantation models in rats and mice. Xenotransplantation is full of unknowns and must be approached with a knowledge of the differences between the immune system of the pig, or any other species being considered (kangaroos apparently have a lobby[79]), and that of humans.

Immunosuppressive Monoclonal Antibodies and Recombinant Proteins

Natural mechanisms that induce tolerance turn off T cells in ways that are antigen specific and long lasting: the goal of transplantation immunologists is to do the same. The signals received by a T cell during an encounter with antigens depend on arrays of interacting proteins on the surface of both the T cell and the antigen-presenting cell. Almost all these cell surface molecules were defined using monoclonal antibodies, and those same antibodies have been tested for their capacity in vitro to inhibit T cell function and in vivo to prevent transplant rejection. Antibodies against the coreceptors and costimulators have proved particularly effective in inhibiting T cell function. If either the coreceptor or the costimulator is disengaged from the TCR, a signal to tolerate rather than to activate is delivered.

In rodent models, administration of single doses of antibodies against the coreceptors CD4 and CD8 can enable a subsequent transplant to be accepted with no further therapy, and with time, immunocompetence is recovered.[80] Disruption of coreceptor function provides a time window in which T cells are made tolerant to introduced antigens. An active T cell–mediated suppressor mechanism appears to be in effect because tolerance can be transmitted to a naive animal by transfer of T cells. Furthermore, this transferred tolerance prevented rejection of a cardiac allograft.[81]

Increased understanding of the mechanism of costimulation allows other targeted strategies to be applied. Disruption of the costimulatory interaction of CTLA-4 and the B7-1 and B7-2 ligands by use of a soluble recombinant protein (consisting of the extracellular domain of CTLA-4 fused to the Fc domain of human immunoglobulin [IgG_1]) permits acceptance of an allogeneic heart transplant in rats.[82] The very complexity of antigen presentation in the natural setting may be an advantage in the development of novel immunosuppressive therapies.

References

1. Abbas AK, Williams ME, Burstein HJ, et al: Activation and functions of CD4+ T-cell subsets. *Immunol Rev* 123:5,1991
2. Hall BM: Cells mediating allograft rejection. *Transplantation* 51:1141, 1991
3. Mandel TE: Basic immunology of transplantation. *Med J Aust* 157:126, 1992
4. Lanzavecchia A: Identifying strategies for immune intervention. *Science* 260:937, 1993
5. Ettenger R, Ferstenberg LB: Basic immunology of transplantation. *Perspect Pediatr Pathol* 14:9, 1991
6. Storb R: Marrow transplantation. *Curr Top Microbiol Immunol* 177:169, 1992
7. Korngold R: Biology of graft-vs.-host disease. *Am J Pediatr Hematol Oncol* 15:18, 1993
8. Rose ML, Yacoub M: Heart transplantation: cellular and humoral immunity. *Springer Semin Immunopathol* 11:423, 1989
9. Hunt S, Billingham M: Long-term results of cardiac transplantation. *Annu Rev Med* 42:437, 1991
10. Patel R, Terasaki PI: Significance of the positive crossmatch test in kidney transplantation. *N Engl J Med* 280:735, 1969
11. Anonymous: Antibodies as a barrier to kidney transplantation. *Lancet* 1:357, 1989
12. Frei U, Brunkhorst R, Schindler R, et al: Present status of kidney transplantation. *Clin Nephrol* 38:S46, 1992
13. Morris PJ: Histocompatibility antigens and transplantation: reflections over 20 years. *Immunol Lett* 21:25, 1989
14. Thorogood J, Persijn GG, Schreuder GMT, et al: The effect of HLA matching on kidney graft survival in separate post transplantation intervals. *Transplantation* 50:146, 1990
15. Thorogood J, van Houwelingen JC, Persijn GG, et al: Prognostic indices to predict survival of first and second renal allografts. *Transplantation* 52:831, 1991
16. Russ GR: Immunosuppression in transplantation. *Med J Aust* 157:198, 1992
17. Salomon DR: The use of immunosuppressive drugs in kidney transplantation. *Pharmacotherapy* 11:153S, 1991
18. Sablinski T, Hancock WW, Tilney NL, et al: CD4 monoclonal antibodies in organ transplantation: a review of progress. *Transplantation* 52:579, 1991
19. Marmont AM, Gale RP, Butturini A, et al: T-cell depletion in allogeneic bone marrow transplantation: progress and problems. *Haematologica* 74:235, 1989
20. Hows JM: Mechanisms of graft failure after human marrow transplantation: a review. *Immunol Lett* 29:77, 1991
21. Disney APS: Complications of immunosuppressive therapy in transplantation: neoplasia and infection. *Med J Aust* 157:262, 1992
22. Russ GR: Complications of immunosuppressive therapy in transplantation: specific immunosuppressive agents. *Med J Aust* 157:264, 1992
23. Murray JE: Human organ transplantation: background and consequences. *Science* 256:1411, 1992
24. Molzahn AE: Quality of life after organ transplantation. *J Adv Nurs* 16: 1042, 1991
25. Campbell DR, Trowsdale J: Map of the human MHC. *Immunol Today* 14:349, 1993
26. Fleischhauer K, Kernan NA, O'Reilly RJ, et al: Bone marrow–allograft rejection by T lymphocytes recognizing a single amino acid difference in HLA-B44. *N Engl J Med* 323:1818, 1990
27. Townsend A, Bodmer H: Antigen recognition by class I–restricted T lymphocytes. *Annu Rev Immunol* 7:601, 1989
28. Storkus WJ, Dawson JR: Target structures involved in natural killing (NK): characteristics, distribution, and candidate molecules. *Crit Rev Immunol* 10:393, 1991
29. Dyer P, Middleton D, Eds. *Histocompatibility Testing: A Practical Approach*. Oxford University Press, Oxford, 1993
30. Benjamin RJ, Parham P: Guilt by association: HLA-B27 and ankylosing spondylitis. *Immunol Today* 11:137, 1990
31. Glimcher LH, Kara CJ: Sequences and factors: a guide to MHC class-II transcription. *Annu Rev Immunol* 10:13, 1992
32. Daar AS, Fuggle SV, Fabre JW, et al: The detailed distribution of HLA-A, B, C antigens in normal human organs. *Transplantation* 38:287, 1984
33. Pober JS, Cotran RS: Immunologic interactions of T lymphocytes with vascular endothelium. *Adv Immunol* 50:261, 1991
34. Bjorkman PJ, Saper MA, Samraoui B, et al: Structure of the human class I histocompatibility antigen, HLA-A2. *Nature* 329:506, 1987

35. Bjorkman PJ, Saper MA, Samraoui B, et al: The foreign antigen binding site and T cell recognition regions of class I histocompatibility antigens. *Nature* 329:512, 1987
36. Madden DR, Gorga JC, Strominger JL, et al: The three-dimensional structure of HLA-B27 at 2.1Å resolution suggests a general mechanism for tight peptide binding to MHC. *Cell* 70:1035, 1992
37. Brown JH, Jardetsky TS, Gorga JC, et al: Three-dimensional structure of the human class II histocompatibility antigen HLA-DR1. *Nature* 364:33, 1993
38. Barber LD, Parham P: Peptide binding to major histocompatibility complex molecules. *Annu Rev Cell Biol* 9:163, 1993
39. The WHO Nomenclature Committee for Factors of the HLA System: Nomenclature for factors of the HLA system, 1990. *Immunogenetics* 33:301, 1991
40. Lawlor DA, Zemmour J, Ennis PD, et al: Evolution of class I MHC genes and proteins: from natural selection to thymic selection. *Annu Rev Immunol* 8:23, 1990
41. Hughes AL, Nei M: Pattern of nucleotide substitution at major histocompatibility complex class I loci reveals overdominant selection. *Nature* 335:167, 1988
42. Hill AVS, Allsopp CEM, Kwiatkowski D, et al: Common West African HLA antigens are associated with protection from severe malaria. *Nature* 352:595, 1991
43. Parham P: HLA, anthropology and transplantation. *Transplant Proc* 25:159, 1993
44. Brodsky FM, Guagliardi LE: The cell biology of antigen processing and presentation. *Annu Rev Immunol* 9:707, 1991
45. Monaco JJ: Genes in the MHC that may affect antigen processing. *Curr Opin Immunol* 4:70, 1992
46. Goldberg AL, Rock KL: Proteolysis: proteasomes and antigen presentation. *Nature* 357:375, 1992
47. Ortmann B, Androlewicz MJ, Cresswell P: MHC class I/β_2-microglobulin complexes associate with TAP transporters before peptide binding. *Nature* 368:864, 1994
48. Bijlmakers MJ, Ploegh HL: Putting together an MHC class I molecule. *Curr Opin Immunol* 5:21, 1993
49. Cresswell P: Chemistry and functional role of the invariant chain. *Curr Opin Immunol* 4:87, 1992
50. Kelly AP, Monaco JJ, Cho S, et al: A new human HLA class II-related locus, DM. *Nature* 353:571, 1991
51. Parker DC: T cell-dependent B cell activation. *Annu Rev Immunol* 11:331, 1993
52. Paulnock DM: Macrophage activation by T cells. *Curr Opin Immunol* 4:344, 1992
53. Pardoll D, Carrera A: Thymic selection. *Curr Opin Immunol* 4:162, 1992
54. Moss PAH, Rosenberg WMC, Bell JI: The human T cell receptor in health and disease. *Annu Rev Immunol* 10:71, 1992
55. Janeway CA Jr: The T cell receptor as a multicomponent signaling machine: CD4/CD8 coreceptors and CD45 in T cell activation. *Annu Rev Immunol* 10:645, 1992
56. Miceli MC, Parnes JR: The roles of CD4 and CD8 in T cell activation. *Semin Immunol* 3:133, 1991
57. Miller JFAP, Morahan G: Peripheral T cell tolerance. *Annu Rev Immunol* 10:51, 1992
58. Schwartz RH: T cell anergy. *Sci Am* 269:62, 1993
59. Jenkins MK, Johnson JG: Molecules involved in T-cell costimulation. *Curr Opin Immunol* 5:361, 1993
60. Scott P: Selective differentiation of $CD4^+$ T helper cell subsets. *Curr Opin Immunol* 5:391, 1993
61. Steinman RM: The dendritic cell system and its role in immunogenicity. *Annu Rev Immunol* 9:271, 1991
62. Austyn JM, Larsen CP: Migration patterns of dendritic leukocytes: implications for transplantation. *Transplantation* 49:1, 1990
63. Romani N, Schuler G: The immunologic properties of epidermal Langerhans cells as a part of the dendritic cell system. *Springer Semin Immunopathol* 13:265, 1992
64. Koretszky GA: Role of the CD45 tyrosine phosphatase in signal transduction in the immune system. *FASEB J* 7:420, 1993
65. Klausner RD, Samelson LE: T cell antigen receptor activation pathways: the tyrosine kinase connection. *Cell* 64:875, 1991
66. Cambier JC: Signal transduction by T- and B-cell antigen receptors: converging structures and concepts. *Curr Opin Immunol* 4:257, 1992
67. DeFranco AL: Signaling pathways activated by protein tyrosine phosphorylation in lymphocytes. *Curr Opin Immunol* 6:364, 1994

68. Siekierka JS, Sigal NH: FK-506 and cyclosporin A: immunosuppressive mechanism of action and beyond. *Curr Opin Immunol* 4:548, 1992
69. Jain J, McCaffrey PG, Miner Z, et al: The T-cell transcription factor $NFAT_p$ is a substrate for calcineurin and interacts with Fos and Jun. *Nature* 365:352, 1993
70. Picker LJ: Physiological and molecular mechanisms of lymphocyte homing. *Annu Rev Immunol* 10:561, 1992
71. Mackay CR: Homing of naive, memory and effector lymphocytes. *Curr Opin Immunol* 5:423, 1993
72. Shimizu Y, Newman W, Tanaka Y, et al: Lymphocyte interactions with endothelial cells. *Immunol Today* 13:106, 1992
73. Steinmuller D: Which T cells mediate allograft rejection? *Transplantation* 40:229, 1985
74. Griffiths GM, Namikawa R, Mueller C, et al: Granzyme A and perforin as markers for rejection in cardiac transplantation. *Eur J Immunol* 21:687, 1991
75. Gill RG: T-cell–T-cell collaboration in allograft responses. *Curr Opin Immunol* 5:782, 1993
76. Sherman LA, Chattopadhyay S: The molecular basis of allorecognition. *Annu Rev Immunol* 11:385, 1993
77. White DJG: Transplantation of organs between species. *Int Arch Allergy Immunol* 98:1, 1992
78. Auchincloss H: Xenogeneic transplantation: a review. *Transplantation* 46:1, 1988
79. Mandel TE: Future directions in transplantation. *Med J Aust* 158:269, 1993
80. Qin S, Cobbold SP, Pope H, et al: "Infectious" transplantation tolerance. *Science* 259:974, 1993
81. Waldmann H, Cobbold S: Monoclonal antibodies for the induction of transplantation tolerance. *Curr Opin Immunol* 5:753, 1993
82. Lenschow DJ, Bluestone JA: T cell co-stimulation and in vivo tolerance. *Curr Opin Immunol* 5:747, 1993

Acknowledgments

Table 1 Data from "Long-Term Results of Cardiac Transplantation," by S. Hunt, M. Billingham, in *Annual Review of Medicine* 42:437, 1991.

Figure 1 Talar Agasyan. Adapted from "Map of the Human MHC," by D.R. Campbell, J. Trowsdale, in *Immunology Today* 14:349, 1993.

Figure 2 Talar Agasyan.

Figures 3, 4, 5, 6 Dimitry Schidlovsky.

CHAPTER 20

Arteriosclerosis of Cardiac Transplantation

Peter Libby, M.D., Frederick J. Schoen, M.D., Ph.D., Jordan S. Pober, M.D., Ph.D.

Since the introduction of cardiac transplantation some 25 years ago, many advances have led to the widespread use of this modality for the treatment of end-stage heart disease. Notably, the addition of cyclosporine A to the immunosuppressive armamentarium has permitted excellent one-year survival of heart transplant recipients. Surveillance biopsies and current immunosuppressive regimens limit morbidity and mortality resulting from acute myocardial rejection. Cardiac transplantation teams have also gained greater experience with the diagnosis and management of opportunistic infections. Now that these limiting factors have come under control, cardiac allografts routinely survive several years.

The very success of clinical cardiac transplantation has led to the emergence of transplantation-associated arteriosclerosis as the limiting factor in the survival of cardiac allografts.[1-4] Transplantation-associated arteriosclerosis affects the arteries of all types of solid organ allografts, although the manifestations in the coronary arteries are particularly prevalent and dramatic. When a kidney allograft fails, the patient can be treated with dialysis. However, retransplantation remains the only definitive solution for transplantation-associated arteriosclerosis that affects the coronary arteries. In addition to its clinical importance, transplantation-associated arteriosclerosis provides an unusual opportunity for analysis of a special type of arteriosclerosis in which immunologic factors may play a decisive role. Because immune and inflammatory phenomena contribute to typical atherosclerosis as well,[5] the study of transplantation-associated arteriosclerosis may help elucidate the pathogenesis of typical atherosclerosis.

Pathology of Coronary Arteriosclerosis in Transplanted Hearts

As recognized by the early students of this disease,[1] transplantation-associated arteriosclerosis often involves the artery concentrically rather than in the eccentric fashion typically encountered in atherosclerosis [*see Figure 1*]. Moreover, graft coronary disease typically affects not just the epicardial conduit coronary arteries but the smaller intramyocardial branches as well. This distribution presents a particular therapeutic challenge. Modalities such as bypass surgery and angioplasty, which are well suited for the treatment of segmental atherosclerosis, prove less apt to treat arteriosclerosis of transplanted coronary arteries because of the diffuse nature of this disease and its involvement of the small vessels.

Although it is usually manifested by diffuse concentric intimal thickening, transplantation-associated arteriosclerosis occasionally occurs superimposed on a preexisting atherosclerotic lesion in the donor coronary vessel.[2] Such composite lesions may be eccentric and may exhibit a histologic appearance distinct from the transplant disease that occurs in previously normal coronary arteries [*see Figure 2*]. Clinically, these superimposed lesions may appear more segmental and thus more amenable to angioplasty or bypass grafting than those usually caused by transplantation-associated arteriosclerosis. The superimposed lesions may represent a distinct clinical and pathologic subgroup of coronary artery disease in transplanted hearts.

The plaque of typical atherosclerosis contains a necrotic core of hypocellular debris rich in lipid, macrophage foam cells, and even extracellular crystals of cholesterol. In contrast, lesions of graft coronary disease contain much less obvious accumulations of extracellular lipid [*see Figure 1*]. When

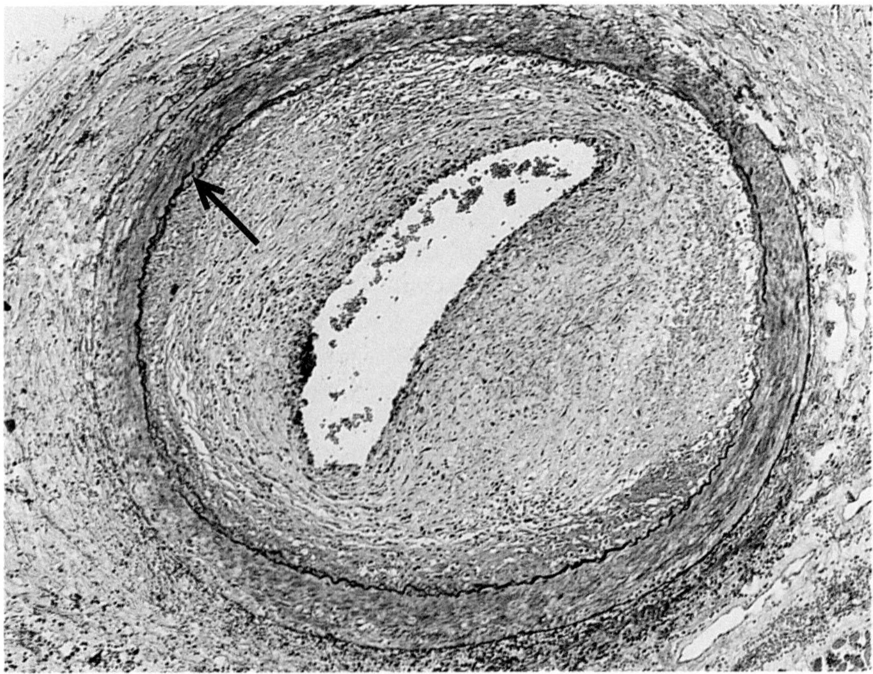

Figure 1 *Histologic appearance of graft arteriosclerosis. Low-power photomicrograph of vessel cross-section demonstrating severe, near-complete, concentric occlusion by intimal proliferation. The intimal elastic lamina (arrow) is virtually completely intact. Verhoeff–von Giessen stain (elastin black), ×22.*

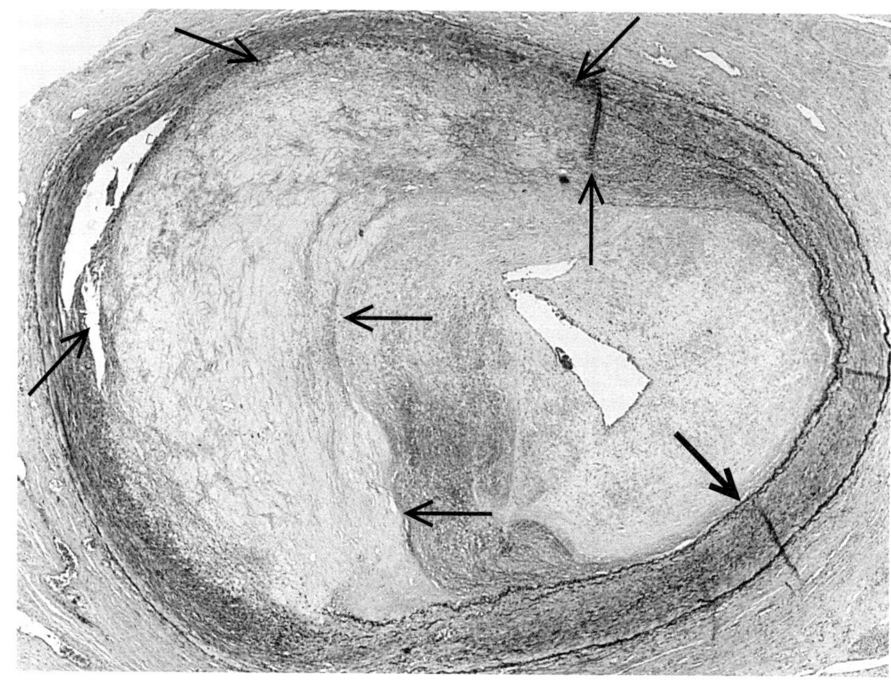

Figure 2 *Graft arteriosclerosis superimposed on typical atherosclerosis originating from a donor. The original atherosclerotic lesion is outlined by the arrowheads. The elastic lamina is intact (bold arrow) beneath the graft arteriosclerosis, but not below the preexisting atherosclerotic lesion. Verhoeff–von Giessen stain (elastin black), ×22.*

found in graft arteriosclerosis, lipid deposits occur in a concentric distribution more commonly in the base of the intimal lesion than just beneath a fibrous cap, as is the case with typical atherosclerosis. Although histologically evident lipid accumulation appears less common in graft coronary disease than in usual atherosclerosis, some investigators find correlations with hyperlipidemia or high levels of extractable lipid in transplantation-associated arteriosclerotic lesions.[6] Nevertheless, lipid deposition does not appear to be essential to the pathogenesis of graft arteriosclerosis. Because the intimal lesions that develop in transplanted coronary arteries contain inconstant amounts of lipid and lack the typical necrotic core, we prefer to use the more general term *arteriosclerosis* (hardening of the arteries) rather than *atherosclerosis* (gruel-like) to underscore the distinct structure of these transplantation-associated lesions.[7]

Engrafted coronary arteries typically develop intimal disease more quickly than do arteries affected by usual atherosclerosis. Although highly variable, graft arterial disease commonly develops over months to a few years of engraftment.[3] Arteriography provides a notoriously inaccurate method for the assessment of graft coronary artery disease because of the concentric and diffuse nature of this process. However, even this relatively insensitive tool reveals that approximately 40 percent of transplant recipients will develop angiographic signs of graft arterial disease within three years postimplantation. Recently, the use of intravascular ultrasound to assess the coronary arteries has yielded preliminary data indicating that the angiographic studies have indeed underestimated the incidence of this process.[3,8]

Functional assessments of grafted coronary arteries also suggest a high prevalence of early graft arterial disease as manifested by abnormal vasomotor responses. Coronary arteries affected by allograft arteriosclerosis have attenuated vasodilator responses to the endothelium-independent agent nitroglycerin.[9] This result suggests a defect in smooth muscle cell function or altered dilatory capacity resulting from a structural change, such as matrix accumulation, in affected arteries. Normal coronary arteries dilate in response to the endothelium-dependent vasodilator acetylcholine, whereas atherosclerotic vessels typically constrict when challenged with this pharmacological probe. Transplant recipients exhibit paradoxical vasoconstriction in epicardial vessels and microvessels in response to acetylcholine within a year of transplantation.[10-12] This apparent defect in endothelium-dependent vasodilatation can actually precede intimal thickening, as detected by intravascular ultrasound.[13] Thus, data from numerous independent investigations indicate that the development of graft arterial disease in transplanted hearts occurs over months to a few years rather than over decades. For this reason, graft coronary disease constitutes an accelerated form of arteriosclerosis.

Recent studies have characterized the nature of the intimal thickening of engrafted coronary arteries. These lesions contain the same cell types found in usual atherosclerotic plaques, including smooth muscle cells, macrophages, and T cells.[14,15] We have found approximately equal numbers of T cells bearing the CD4 marker (helper/inducer phenotype) and those bearing the CD8 marker (typically cytotoxic T cells).[15] Hruban et al. have encountered a higher number of CD8-bearing cells in their series.[14] Members of this research group also have recently studied the expression of perforin, a molecule that plays an important role in the increase in permeability of the membrane of target cells attacked by cytolytic T cells.[16] They found that a small number of T cells (approximately five percent) within most transplantation-associated arteriosclerosis lesions stained for this marker for killer T cells.

Although the lesions of transplantation-associated arteriosclerosis contain the same types of cells as in ordinary atherosclerotic plaques, their distribution appears quite distinct. These lesions typically lack necrotic cores rich in macrophages. Rather, variable numbers of macrophages localize throughout the expanded intima. In typical atherosclerosis, T cells reside prominently on the lateral borders of the necrotic core.[17] In contrast, the T cells in the lesions of graft arteriosclerosis localize in an annular pattern encircling and immediately subjacent to the luminal endothelial cells, which typically remain intact in these lesions[14,15] [*see Figure 3*]. As in the case of usual atherosclerosis, in addition to the cells, the expanded intima contains abundant extracellular matrix. The constituents of this matrix and the types of collagens, glycosaminoglycans, elastin, and other matrix constituents in relation to ordinary atherosclerosis remain unexplored.

Pathogenesis of Transplantation-Associated Accelerated Arteriosclerosis

As in usual atherosclerosis, understanding of the pathogenesis of the transplantation-associated disease is incomplete. Any model for the development of this disease must explain the involvement of the engrafted arteries and the sparing of the host's own vessels. This observation indicates that nonspecific effects of the medications that recipients receive and of

a

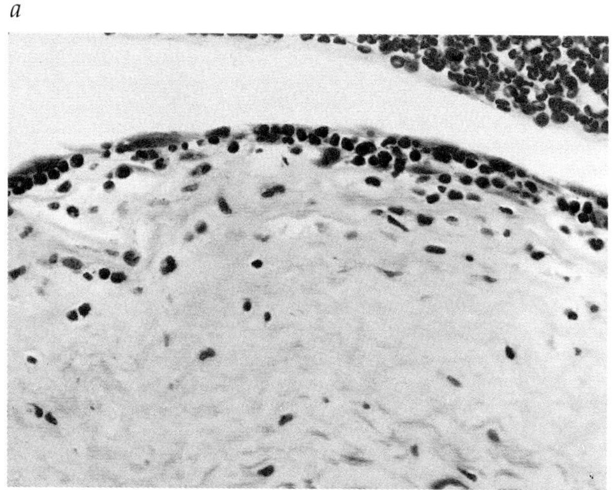

b

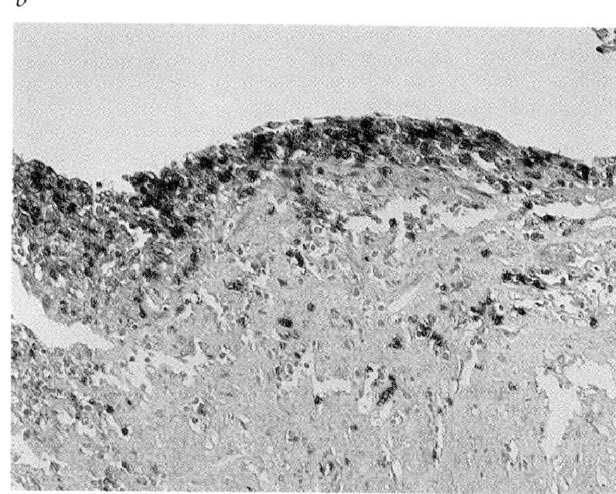

Figure 3 *Subendothelial lymphocytes in graft arteriosclerosis. (a) High-power photomicrograph of luminal surface of coronary artery from cardiac transplant recipient late postoperatively that demonstrates subendothelial mononuclear infiltrate, with morphologic characteristics of lymphocytes (round, darkly stained nuclei in cells with scant cytoplasm). Hematoxylin-eosin, ×315. (b) Immunohistochemical verification that abundant T cells are distributed in the subendothelial cellular band (the cells stained brown). Immunoperoxidase staining (×150) with an antibody that recognizes T cells through the Leu 4 antigen.*

the transplanted state itself do not underlie the pathogenesis of this process. Some studies have implicated cytomegalovirus infection as a common concomitant of transplantation arteriosclerosis[18-21]; however, the association between these two common complications of transplantation may be fortuitous. Also, a systemic infection would be expected to affect host as well as donor arteries, a pattern not observed in graft-associated arterioclerosis. Ischemic injury to the coronary arteries in the time between harvesting and reestablishing of coronary flow could explain selective involvement of the donor arteries. However, scant evidence supports this possibility. In rat aortic interposition grafts using inbred strains, isografts (from immunologically identical donors) do not develop intimal lesions, whereas those transplanted across major histocompatibility barriers do.[22] These results point to an immunologic basis for the development of graft arteriosclerosis.

In this context, the ability of engrafted coronary artery endothelial cells to express major histocompatibility antigens likely holds a key to our understanding of the immunopathogenesis of this type of coronary artery disease. The endothelial cells overlying transplantation-associated arteriosclerotic lesions uniformly express major histocompatibility complex (MHC) class II antigens.[14,15] Recognition of cells as foreign by host helper T cells ($CD4^+$) requires the surface expression of such histocompatibility antigens. Although most human arteries appear not to express MHC class II antigen constitutively, coronary arteries may be an exception.[23] Regardless of whether the MHC class II expression is constitutive or induced, the presence of these markers on the surface of graft endothelial cells indicates an inciting stimulus for the host's allogeneic immune response.

We have formulated a model of the pathogenesis of transplantation-associated arteriosclerosis based on an allogeneic immune response.[7] We hy-

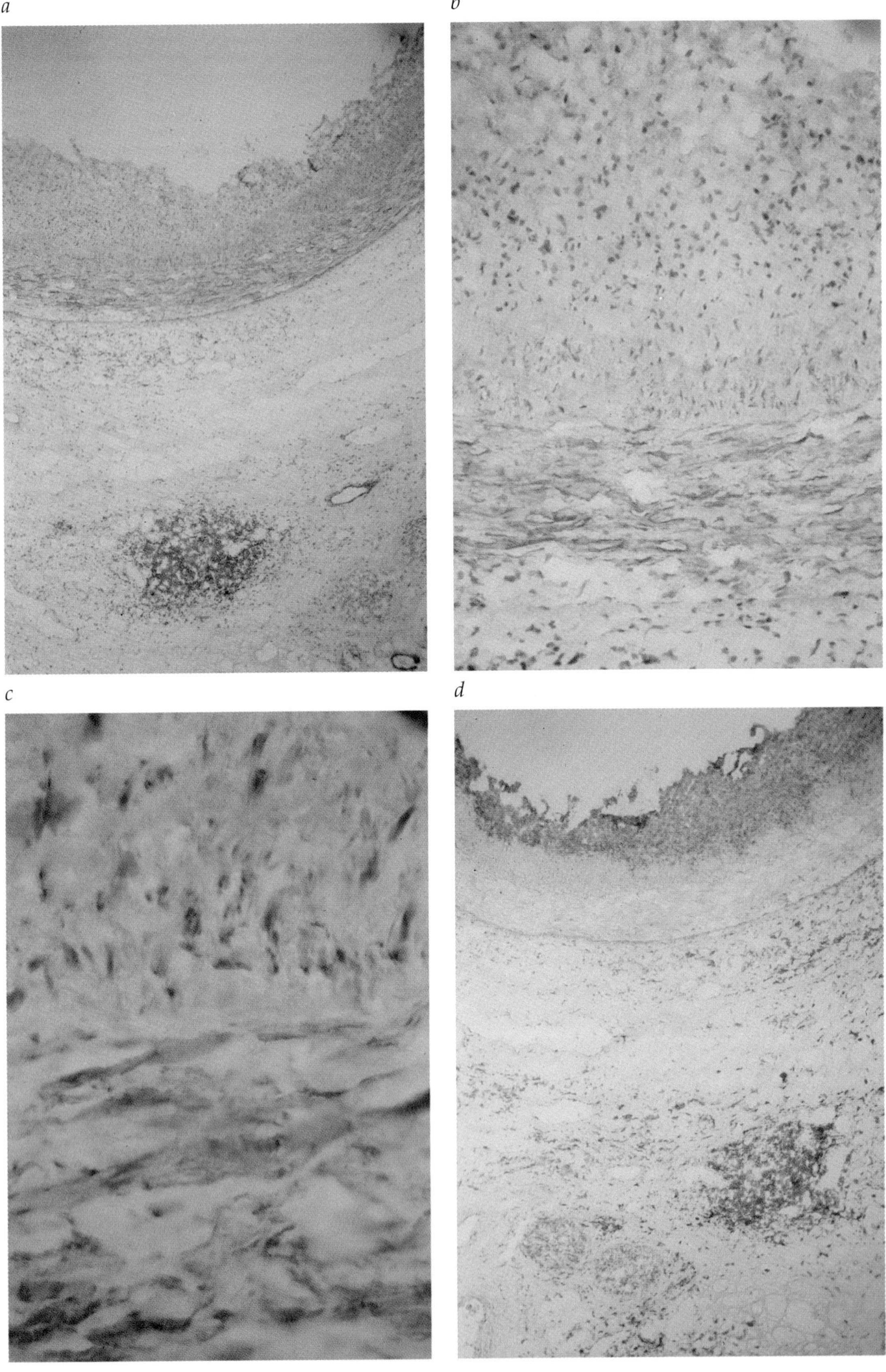
a
b
c
d

pothesize that the helper T cells of the recipient engage the foreign class II antigens on the surface of the engrafted endothelial cells. Having encountered an activating stimulus, these T cells in turn augment their expression of high-affinity receptors for the autocrine growth stimulus interleukin-2 (IL-2). In addition, activated helper T cells secrete IL-2, which leads to proliferation of the alloreactive clone of T cells via this autocrine growth loop.

In addition to IL-2–induced expansion of alloreactive helper T cells, the activated T cell secretes another cytokine, interferon gamma, also known as immune interferon. This cytokine increases the expression of MHC class II antigens on vascular wall cells, thereby promoting the continued presence of this stimulus for alloreactive T-cell activation. Furthermore, interferon gamma activates macrophages to produce other cytokines, some of which may promote the proliferation of, and matrix synthesis by, vascular smooth muscle cells. The morphology of the human transplantation-associated arteriosclerotric lesion suggests that some of the intimal smooth muscle cells migrate from the media [*see Figures 4a through 4c*]. This cell type likely produces the abundant extracellular matrix found in these lesions. Stimulators of growth or matrix production secreted by activated macrophages include transforming growth factors (TGFs) α and β; interleukin-1 (IL-1); tumor necrosis factor (TNF); and heparin-binding growth factors, including acidic and basic fibroblast growth factors and a novel heparin-binding epidermal growth factor–like molecule. In addition to IL-2 and interferon gamma, the activated T cell can elaborate cytokines that target mesenchymal cells, such as TNF-α or lymphotoxin, also known as TNF-β.

How might leukocytes such as T cells and mononuclear phagocytes, cells not present in substantial numbers in normal vessels, accumulate in transplanted arteries? Recruitment of leukocytes involves several steps, including initial adherence to the endothelium and subsequent migration through the endothelial monolayer and into the arterial wall. Increasingly well-characterized cell surface molecules mediate the adhesion of leukocytes to endothelial cells [*see Chapter 4*]. Several of these recognized endothelium-leukocyte adhesion molecules may participate in the recruitment of T cells and mononuclear phagocytes in transplanted coronary arteries. Notably, vascular cell adhesion molecule–1 (VCAM-1) and intercellular adhesion molecule–1 (ICAM-1) can mediate the adhesion of these classes of leukocytes to endothelial cells. Coronary artery endothelial cells express relatively low levels of ICAM-1 in the basal state in humans and in other species studied. Under normal conditions, coronary arteries express VCAM-1 slightly or not at all.[23]

Some investigators have disclosed increased levels of expression of ICAM-1 and VCAM-1 in coronary arteries from transplanted human hearts, although specimens suitable for such analysis seldom become available.[24-27]

Figure 4 *Serial sections of a human coronary artery affected by arteriosclerosis after transplantation. (a through c) Smooth muscle cells stained red by immunoperoxidase staining for muscle α-actin (antibody HHF-35) photographed at low (a), medium (b), and high (c) power. Note the intense staining of medial smooth muscle cells (b) and of cells oriented perpendicular to the medial cells in the base of the expanding intima (c). The less intensely stained cells in the more luminal portions of the intima probably represent modulated smooth muscle cells with reduced α-actin expression. (d) Low-power view stained for macrophages (stained brown) that reveals substantial accumulation of these phagocytes in the luminal portion of the expanded intima.*

Animal studies permit more systematic evaluation of such endothelial functions as the expression of adhesion molecules. VCAM-1 and ICAM-1 expression on the surface of endothelial cells occurs as early as 24 hours after transplantation of arteries in rabbits. Administration of antibodies that neutralize very late antigen–4 (VLA-4), the cognate ligand for VCAM-1 on leukocytes, reduces arterial leukocyte recruitment in transplanted rabbit hearts.[28] Cytokines expressed by activated T cells (e.g., lymphotoxin, TNF, and interferon gamma), macrophages, or even the intrinsic vascular wall cells (e.g., IL-1 or TNF) can enhance the expression of VCAM-1 and ICAM-1 on endothelial cells. Thus, cytokine-induced increases in leukocyte adhesion molecules likely contribute to the first step in leukocyte recruitment in the early phases of transplantation-associated arteriosclerosis, a scenario thought also to pertain to typical atherosclerosis.

Engagement of the cognate ligand on the leukocyte surface may promote leukocyte transmigration through the endothelial monolayer. Directed migration of leukocytes may also result from local production of chemoattractant molecules, such as the chemokine monocyte chemoattractant protein–1 (MCP-1), also known as monocyte chemoattractant and activating factor–1 and, in the mouse, JE.[29] Human transplantation-associated arteriosclerotic lesions contain substantial amounts of MCP-1 protein and messenger RNA, which indicates that this molecule may indeed participate in monocyte recruitment in this context.[30] Surface-bound forms of the chemokines may also function as adhesion molecules by binding their receptors on target cells,[31] further promoting recruitment and contact between the cells involved in signaling pathways.

The initial allogeneic stimulation of T cells and the subsequent recruitment and activation of mononuclear phagocytes and intrinsic vascular wall cells (as indicated by increased expression of adhesion molecules) lead to the chronic fibroproliferative stage of lesion development. No formal measurements of cellular proliferation have established this mechanism for the accumulation of smooth muscle cells in human transplantation-associated arteriosclerosis. However, we have documented replication of smooth muscle cells within the coronary arteries of transplanted rabbit hearts. The mode of stimulation of smooth muscle cell proliferation may include paracrine mediators released by activated neighboring cells, as well as autocrine mediators (e.g., TNF-α). Many of the same factors that stimulate smooth muscle cell mitogenesis also induce their migration, and migration of smooth muscle cells may also contribute to intimal thickening in transplantation-associated arteriosclerosis.

Increased synthesis of extracellular matrix constituents by smooth muscle cells likely contributes to the accumulation of matrix materials, such as interstitial collagen, within the developing arteriosclerotic lesion in transplanted arteries. Some of the cytokines and growth factors that stimulate smooth muscle cell proliferation (e.g., IL-1 and TNF) can also enhance interstitial collagen gene expression in human smooth muscle cells. However, the effects of such mediators on matrix metabolism are complex. For example, TGF-β probably inhibits smooth muscle proliferation under most circumstances, yet TGF-β potently stimulates interstitial collagen gene expression by the cells. Conversely, interferon gamma can retard smooth muscle cell proliferation and can inhibit interstitial collagen gene expression.[32]

The model that we proposed in 1989 for the pathogenesis of transplantation-associated arteriosclerosis represents a special case of a delayed-type hypersensitivity reaction.[7] This classic immunopathological mechanism involves an antigen-specific cellular immune response initiated by T cells. The T cells recognize antigen that consists of a peptide associated with an MHC class II molecule on the surface of an antigen-presenting cell. In the classic delayed-type hypersensitivity reaction, the antigenic peptide would be derived from a microorganism, and the presenting cell would be a macrophage. In the case of transplantation-associated arteriosclerosis, we have hypothesized that foreign class II antigens on the donor endothelium provide the initial antigenic stimulus for this delayed-type hypersensitivity reaction. Thus, in this special case, the endothelial cell assumes the role of the macrophage, and the donor MHC class II molecule, that of the invading pathogen. In the familiar example of delayed hypersensitivity reaction, the cutaneous response to injected antigens, such as *Candida*, mumps, or purified protein derivative of the tubercle bacillus, the reaction subsides within a matter of days as the antigens are cleared. However, in the case of transplantation-associated arteriosclerosis, viable endothelial cells expressing class II antigens persist. This ongoing antigenic stimulation prolongs the delayed-type hypersensitivity response. In both the classic and the transplantation-associated delayed hypersensitivities, a cytokine network mediates intercellular communication and orchestrates the behavior of the cell types that participate.

This schema, although almost certainly oversimplified, fits the data currently available and provides a useful intellectual construct for further testing. In addition, it permits distinctions between transplantation-associated arteriosclerosis and other types of vascular diseases that may complicate heart transplantation. These other processes may involve fundamentally different mechanisms. Therefore, it is important to emphasize the differences because amalgamation of the various types of pathology occurring in transplanted arteries may impede progress in understanding their pathogenesis and devising therapeutic strategies. Distinct pathogenic mechanisms likely underlie the development of these various processes, including

Table 1 Potential Mediators of Certain Immunologic Complications of Transplantation

Complication	*Mediator*
Acute rejection	$CD8^+$ T cells
Hyperacute rejection	Ab + C′, PMN
Vascular rejection	Ab + C′
Chronic rejection	$CD4^+$ T cells
Endotheliitis	$CD8^+$ T cells
Vasculitis	PMN, elastase

Ab—antibody; C′—complement; PMN—polymorphonuclear leukocytes.

hyperacute rejection, acute myocardial rejection, vascular rejection, and chronic rejection [*see Table 1*].

Hyperacute rejection refers to a reaction that occurs within minutes of the establishment of blood perfusion in an allografted organ, such as a heart. Hyperacute rejection probably results from natural antibodies against foreign histocompatibility antigens in the case of xenotransplantation, or other circulating antibodies to alloantigens in the case of intraspecies transplants. This process probably involves complement-mediated injury and may also result in disruption of the heparin sulfate–like molecules on the endothelial surface.[33,34] This inhibition of a natural anticoagulant mechanism can lead to intravascular thrombosis during hyperacute rejection. The humoral mechanism involving preformed antibody differs fundamentally from the chronic cell-mediated response that probably occurs during transplantation-associated arteriosclerosis.

Acute myocardial rejection doubtless involves many of the same effector mechanisms that occur in transplantation-associated arteriosclerosis. For example, microvessels perfusing the myocardium express increased levels of leukocyte adhesion molecules during acute rejection. These adhesion molecules probably function in the recruitment of T cells. Cytokines are very likely to participate in the recruitment and activation of these T cells. However, the effector mechanisms of acute myocardial rejection differ in important ways from the pathway we propose for the development of transplantation-associated arteriosclerosis. Myocardial cytolysis remains the hallmark of acute myocardial rejection.[35] Histologically, disrupted cardiac myocytes co-localize with T cells. T cells of the cytolytic, CD8-bearing type probably play a key role in the pathogenesis of acute rejection.[36] In contrast, cytolytic damage is not apparent in transplantation-associated arteriosclerosis. Although the arteriosclerotic lesions contain both $CD4^+$ and $CD8^+$ T cells, we postulate a primary role for helper T cells rather than cytolytic T cells in the genesis of the arteriosclerotic lesion. Although probably oversimplified, the dichotomy between $CD8^+$, lymphocyte-mediated cytolysis and CD4-mediated chronic fibrotic responses points to a major difference between these two pathological processes that can occur in transplanted hearts. Although the number of episodes of acute rejection does not consistently correlate with the development of transplantation-associated arteriosclerosis, repeated episodes of myocardial cytokine release might ultimately influence the development of arteriosclerotic changes, particularly in the smaller intramyocardial arteries.

In the context of cardiac transplantation, *vascular rejection* refers to subacute accumulations of immunoglobulin and complement within the walls of the coronary arteries.[37] Hammond et al. have proposed that this process represents a precursor to the chronic fibrotic stage of transplantation arteriosclerosis.[38] The extent to which deposition of immune complexes and local intramural complement fixation occur in this context remains uncertain. Many of the patients whose endomyocardial biopsies show arterial mural IgG and complement have received mouse monoclonal antibodies directed against T cells (OKT3). These patients may be predisposed to form human antimouse antibodies. It is also important to distinguish from an active immune complex–type vasculitis mere inspissation of immunoglobulin and complement permeating through endothelium damaged by ischemia or other trauma during transplantation. In this regard, it would be important to demonstrate the presence of activated membrane attack complex of the terminal cytolytic phase of complement activation. Such data would help to establish a pathogenic effect of local deposition of complement and antibody in transplanted arteries.

In the context of cardiac allografts, the term *chronic rejection* is confusing. Some transplantation pathologists use this term to refer to the chronic intimal thickening that we refer to as *transplantation-associated accelerated arteriosclerosis* or *graft arterial disease.* We avoid using this term to refer to this chronic vascular disease because the term may be confused with *acute rejection,* which is commonly used to refer to a myocardial rather than a vascular process. Because of this potential ambiguity, we advocate avoiding the term chronic rejection altogether. We prefer to use *persistent myocardial rejection* to describe the smoldering or indolent process seen at endomyocardial biopsy.

Conclusions

Although the pathogenic schema that we have proposed for the development of transplantation-associated arteriosclerosis fits with most of the current data, it remains to be fully validated experimentally. Certain questions remain, such as Why are transplanted veins less affected by this process than arteries, even though veins are also presumably lined with allogeneic endothelium?[39] Perhaps the hemodynamic differences between the arterial and the venous trees fosters the development of the sclerosis.

Our pathogenic model has therapeutic implications. If an allogeneic reaction leads to a chronic, delayed-type hypersensitivity response, increased or more selective or effective immunosuppression should interrupt the development of graft arteriosclerosis. The advent of new immunosuppressive agents, including the macrolides, deoxyspergualin, and mycophenolate mofetil, which have molecular mechanisms of action distinct from those of cyclosporine, may provide tools for such selective therapeutic intervention. In vitro data support the concept that these agents differ in their ability to impede allogeneic responses to endothelial cells. Perhaps a combination of agents with distinct but complementary mechanisms of action may yield more effective immunosuppression with less net toxicity. Treatment of rats with experimental heart transplantation with rapamycin may retard the development of graft arterial disease.[40] This is a fertile area for further research based on sound knowledge of the pathogenesis of the disease and of the mechanisms of action of the newly available immunosuppressive agents.

We hypothesize that an allogeneic response to foreign histocompatibility antigens from members of the same species provides the inciting stimulus for the development of graft arterial disease. Considerable interest currently focuses on the use of xenografts instead of allografts. Xenografting could obviate the shortage of human donor hearts, which currently limits broader application of this heart transplantation. Hyperacute rejection currently renders xenografting clinically impractical in humans. Basic research in complement regulatory proteins associated with cell surfaces suggests avenues for modulating the complement-mediated hyperacute rejection. However, even if hyperacute rejection could be limited, xenogeneic tissues may not evade some of the cellular immune responses, including myocardial rejection and allograft vascular disease, elicited by allogeneic MHC class II antigens.

Ultimately, basic research may provide insights into the prevention and treatment of cardiovascular diseases that may render cardiac transplantation obsolete. At present, however, this modality presents the only option in selected patients with end-stage cardiac or cardiopulmonary disease. Unfortunately, heart transplantation exemplifies a clinical solution based on inadequate technology rather than on a fundamental understanding of the pathophysiology of the underlying diseases. When we achieve true understanding of cardiovascular diseases, more satisfying, enduring, and perhaps less expensive approaches may replace transplantation.

References

1. Billingham ME: Cardiac transplant atherosclerosis. *Transplant Proc* 19:19, 1987
2. Schoen FJ, Libby P: Cardiac transplant graft arteriosclerosis. *Trends Cardiovasc Med* 1:216, 1991
3. Schroeder JS, Gao SZ, Hunt SA, et al: Accelerated graft coronary artery disease: diagnosis and prevention. *J Heart Lung Transplant* 11:S258, 1992
4. Hosenpud JD, Shipley GD, Wagner CR: Cardiac allograft vasculopathy: current concepts, recent developments, and future directions. *J Heart Lung Transplant* 11:9, 1992
5. Libby P, Hansson GK: Involvement of the immune system in human atherogenesis: current knowledge and unanswered questions. *Lab Invest* 64:5, 1991
6. Winters GL, Kendall TJ, Radio SJ, et al: Posttransplant obesity and hyperlipidemia: major predictors of severity of coronary arteriopathy in failed human heart allografts. *J Heart Lung Transplant* 9:364, 1990
7. Libby P, Salomon RN, Payne DD, et al: Functions of vascular wall cells related to the development of transplantation-associated coronary arteriosclerosis. *Transplant Proc* 21:3677, 1989
8. Ventura HO, Ramee SR, Jain A, et al: Coronary artery imaging with intravascular ultrasound in patients following cardiac transplantation. *Transplantation* 53:216, 1992
9. Pinto FJ, St. Goar FG, Fischell TA, et al: Nitroglycerin-induced coronary vasodilation in cardiac transplant recipients: evaluation with in vivo intracoronary ultrasound. *Circulation* 85:69, 1992
10. Fish RD, Nabel EG, Selwyn AP, et al: Responses of coronary arteries of cardiac transplant patients to acetylcholine. *J Clin Invest* 81:21, 1988
11. Treasure CB, Vita JA, Ganz P, et al: Loss of the coronary microvascular response to acetylcholine in cardiac transplant patients. *Circulation* 86:1156, 1992
12. Mills RM Jr, Billett JM, Nichols WW: Endothelial dysfunction early after heart transplantation: assessment with intravascular ultrasound and Doppler. *Circulation* 86:1171, 1992
13. Anderson TJ, Meredith IT, Uehata A, et al: Functional significance of intimal thickening as detected by intravascular ultrasound early and late after cardiac transplantation. *Circulation* 88:1093, 1993
14. Hruban RH, Beschorner WE, Baumgartner WA, et al: Accelerated arteriosclerosis in heart transplant recipients is associated with a T-lymphocyte-mediated endothelialitis. *Am J Pathol* 137:871, 1990
15. Salomon RN, Hughes CCW, Schoen FJ, et al: Human coronary transplantation-associated arteriosclerosis: evidence for a chronic immune reaction to activated graft endothelial cells. *Am J Pathol* 138:791, 1991
16. Fox WM III, Hameed A, Hutchins GM, et al: Perforin expression localizing cytotoxic lymphocytes in the intimas of coronary arteries with transplant-related accelerated arteriosclerosis. *Hum Pathol* 24:477, 1993

17. Jonasson L, Holm J, Skalli O, et al: Regional accumulations of T cells, macrophages, and smooth muscle cells in the human atherosclerotic plaque. *Arteriosclerosis* 6:131, 1986
18. Grattan MT, Moreno-Cabral CE, Starnes VA, et al: Cytomegalovirus infection is associated with cardiac allograft rejection and atherosclerosis. *JAMA* 261:3561, 1989
19. Loebe M, Schuler S, Zais O, et al: Role of cytomegalovirus infection in the development of coronary artery disease in the transplanted heart. *J Heart Lung Transplant* 9:707, 1990
20. Everett JP, Hershberger RE, Norman DJ, et al: Prolonged cytomegalovirus infection with viremia is associated with development of cardiac allograft vasculopathy. *J Heart Lung Transplant* 11:S133, 1992
21. Lemstrom K, Persoons M, Bruggeman C, et al: Cytomegalovirus infection enhances allograft arteriosclerosis in the rat. *Transplant Proc* 25:1406, 1993
22. Mennander A, Tiisala S, Halttunen J, et al: Chronic rejection in rat aortic allografts: an experimental model for transplant arteriosclerosis. *Arterioscler Thromb* 11:671, 1991
23. Page C, Rose M, Yacoub M, et al: Antigenic heterogeneity of vascular endothelium. *Am J Pathol* 141:673, 1992
24. Briscoe DM, Schoen FJ, Rice GE, et al: Induced expression of endothelial-leukocyte adhesion molecules in human cardiac allografts. *Transplantation* 51:537, 1991
25. Carlos TM, Schwartz BR, Kovach NL, et al: Vascular cell adhesion molecule-1 mediates lymphocyte adherence to cytokine-activated cultured human endothelial cells [published erratum appears in *Blood* 76:2420, 1990]. *Blood* 76:965, 1990
26. Taylor PM, Rose ML, Yacoub MH, et al: Induction of vascular adhesion molecules during rejection of human cardiac allografts. *Transplantation* 54:451, 1992
27. Qiao JH, Ruan XM, Trento A, et al: Expression of cell adhesion molecules in human cardiac allograft rejection. *J Heart Lung Transplant* 11:920, 1992
28. Sadahiro M, McDonald TO, Allen MD: Reduction in cellular and vascular rejection by blocking leukocyte adhesion molecule receptors. *Am J Pathol* 142:675, 1993
29. Rollins BJ: *JE/MCP-1*: an early-response gene encodes a monocyte-specific cytokine. *Cancer Cells* 3:517, 1991
30. Nelken N, Coughlin S, Gordon D, et al: Monocyte chemoattractant protein-1 in human atheromatous plaques. *J Clin Invest* 88:1121, 1991
31. Tanaka Y, Adams DH, Hubscher S, et al: T-cell adhesion induced by proteoglycan-immobilized cytokine MIP-1 beta. *Nature* 361:79, 1993
32. Amento EP, Ehsani N, Palmer H, et al: Cytokines positively and negatively regulate interstitial collagen gene expression in human vascular smooth muscle cells. *Arteriosclerosis* 11:1223, 1991
33. Dalmasso AP, Vercellotti GM, Fischel RJ, et al: Mechanism of complement activation in the hyperacute rejection of porcine organs transplanted into primate recipients. *Am J Pathol* 140:1157, 1992
34. Geller RL, Bach FH, Vercellotti GM, et al: Activation of endothelial cells in hyperacute xenograft rejection. *Transplant Proc* 24:592, 1992
35. Billingham ME, Cary NR, Hammond ME, et al: A working formulation for the standardization of nomenclature in the diagnosis of heart and lung rejection: Heart Rejection Study Group. The International Society for Heart Transplantation. *J Heart Lung Transplant* 9:587, 1990
36. Mason DW, Morris PJ: Effector mechanisms in allograft rejection. *Annu Rev Immunol* 4:119, 1986
37. Hammond EH, Yowell RL, Nunoda S, et al: Vascular (humoral) rejection in heart transplantation: pathologic observations and clinical implications. *J Heart Lung Transplant* 8:430, 1989
38. Hammond EH, Yowell RL, Price GD, et al: Vascular rejection and its relationship to allograft coronary artery disease. *J Heart Lung Transplant* 11:S111, 1992
39. Oni AA, Ray J, Hosenpud JD: Coronary venous intimal thickening in explanted cardiac allografts: evidence demonstrating that transplant coronary artery disease is a manifestation of a diffuse allograft vasculopathy. *Transplantation* 53:1247, 1992
40. Meiser BM, Billingham ME, Morris RE: Effects of cyclosporin, FK506, and rapamycin on graft-vessel disease. *Lancet* 338:1297, 1991

Acknowledgments

This work was supported by grant HL-43364 to Peter Libby, Jordan S. Pober, and Frederick J. Schoen from NHLBI.

Figures 1 through 3 reprinted from "Cardiac Transplant Graft Arteriosclerosis," by F. J. Schoen and P. Libby, in *Trends in Cardiovascular Medicine* 1:216, 1991. Used by permission.

Figure 4 micrographs were prepared by Dr. Robert N. Salomon when he was a fellow of the American Heart Association Massachusetts Affiliate in the laboratory of Dr. Peter Libby.

Index

A

B

D

G

H

I

J

K

L

M

N

O

P

R

U

V

W

X

Z